Osteotomy Essentials - From Basic Techniques to Advanced Practices

Edited by Alessandro Rozim Zorzi

Published in London, United Kingdom

Osteotomy Essentials - From Basic Techniques to Advanced Practices
http://dx.doi.org/10.5772/intechopen.110962
Edited by Alessandro Rozim Zorzi

Contributors
Aleksandar Stanković, Alexis Fernández, Amr Gibaly, André Carvalho, Arda Buyuksungur, Diego Delgado, Dragan Gabrić, Dragiša Stamenković, Filipa Goncalves Pereira, Harry John Visser, Ibrahim H. Garoushi, Ivan Marjanović, Jaime Oraa, Jin Young Choi, Ji Youn Maeng, Jorge Guadilla, Jung-Pin Hung, Kyle Williams, Kyun-Ho Shin, Leonor López de Dicastillo, Levent Ciğerim, Li-Chan Chou, Masataka Deie, Mehmet Eray Kolsuz, Mehmet Faruk Çatma, Mikel Sánchez, Mohammed Atef, Munehiro Ogawa, Nadan Mikić, Nicolás Fiz, Ramy R. Elbeialy, Ricardo Sousa, Seung-Beom Han, Seyide Tugce Gokdeniz, Shaw-Ruey Lyu, Tihomir Kuna, Tomislav Katanec, Vesna Ranković, Vladimir Gordić, Xabier Sánchez, Yasuhito Tanaka, Yuki Yamanashi, Zehra Irem Ozturk Barut, Zeynep Dilan Orhan

First published in London, United Kingdom, 2025 by IntechOpen
IntechOpen is the global imprint of INTECHOPEN LIMITED, registered in England and Wales, registration number: 11086078, 167-169 Great Portland Street, London, W1W 5PF, United Kingdom

For EU product safety concerns: IN TECH d.o.o., Prolaz Marije Krucifikse Kozulić 3, 51000 Rijeka, Croatia, info@intechopen.com or visit our website at intechopen.com.

British Library Cataloguing-in-Publication Data
A catalogue record for this book is available from the British Library

Osteotomy Essentials - From Basic Techniques to Advanced Practices
Edited by Alessandro Rozim Zorzi
p. cm.
Print ISBN 978-0-85466-038-4
Online ISBN 978-0-85466-037-7
eBook (PDF) ISBN 978-0-85466-039-1

Meet the editor

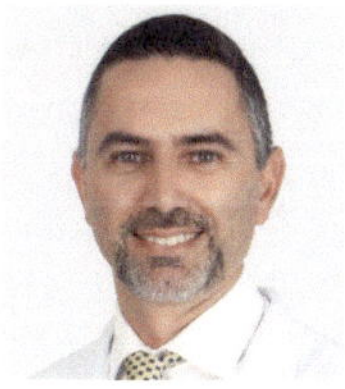

Dr. Alessandro Zorzi is a Medical and Postgraduate Sciences Professor at Faculdade São Leopoldo Mandic and a researcher in knee surgery, osteoarthritis and cartilage cell therapy. He is a member of the Knee Surgery Medical Assistance Group at Hospital Israelita Albert Einstein and the Regenerative Medicine Committee of the Brazilian Society of Orthopedics and Traumatology (SBOT). He is also an orthopedic surgeon at the University Hospital of Universidade Estadual de Campinas (UNICAMP). Dr. Zorzi earned his medical degree from the Faculty of Medicine of Ribeirão Preto at USP in 1999. He completed his Master's and Ph.D. in Surgical Sciences at UNICAMP. He further specialized in clinical research at Harvard Medical School and in research ethics involving human subjects through UNESCO.

Contents

Preface **IX**

Section 1
Osteotomies around the Knee **1**

Chapter 1 **3**
Osteotomies around the Knee: Indications, Planning, and Surgery
by Filipa Goncalves Pereira, André Carvalho and Ricardo Sousa

Chapter 2 **23**
High Tibial Osteotomy within the Knee Health Promotion Option for Knee Osteoarthritis
by Jung-Pin Hung, Li-Chan Chou and Shaw-Ruey Lyu

Chapter 3 **39**
Concomitant High Tibial Osteotomy with Medial Meniscus Posterior Root Repair in Medial Knee Joint Osteoarthritis
by Kyun-Ho Shin and Seung-Beom Han

Chapter 4 **53**
Optimal Corrective Angle in Recent High Tibial Osteotomies
by Masataka Deie and Yuki Yamanashi

Chapter 5 **65**
Design and 3D Printing of Customized Osteosynthesis Instruments for Osteotomies
by Mikel Sánchez, Alexis Fernández, Leonor López de Dicastillo, Jaime Oraa, Xabier Sánchez, Jorge Guadilla, Nicolás Fiz and Diego Delgado

Chapter 6 **81**
Infection Control
by Munehiro Ogawa and Yasuhito Tanaka

Section 2
Osteotomies in the Hip and Foot **103**

Chapter 7 **105**
Osteotomy Techniques in Total Hip Arthroplasty for Severe Dysplasia
by Mehmet Faruk Çatma

Chapter 8 117
Surgical Correction of the Cavovarus Foot Deformity with Utilization of Osteotomy and Arthrodesis Technique
by Harry John Visser and Kyle Williams

Chapter 9 133
Proximal and Distal Osteotomies in Treatment of Hallux Valugs
by Nadan Mikić, Ivan Marjanović, Aleksandar Stanković, Dragiša Stamenković, Vesna Ranković and Vladimir Gordić

Section 3
Osteotomies of the Facial Bones 163

Chapter 10 165
Technological Advances in Maxillofacial Surgery: Function and Esthetics
by Ji Youn Maeng and Jin Young Choi

Chapter 11 177
Osteotomy Challenges for Implant Placement in Posterior Mandible
by Ibrahim H. Garoushi, Ramy R. Elbeialy, Amr Gibaly and Mohammed Atef

Chapter 12 191
Temporomandibular Disorders: Current Diagnosis and Treatment Methods
by Seyide Tugce Gokdeniz, Zehra Irem Ozturk Barut, Arda Buyuksungur and Mehmet Eray Kolsuz

Chapter 13 215
Use of Statins after Bone Osteotomy and Augmentation and their Antibacterial Effect: Narrative Review of Literature
by Tomislav Katanec, Tihomir Kuna and Dragan Gabrić

Chapter 14 227
The Effect of Different Osteotomy Techniques on Implant Stability in Implant Socket Design
by Levent Ciğerim and Zeynep Dilan Orhan

Preface

Osteotomies have played a crucial role in orthopedic and maxillofacial surgery, effectively correcting deformities, restoring joint alignment, and improving function in various anatomical regions. This edited volume, Osteotomy Essentials – From Basic Techniques to Advanced Practices, aims to provide a comprehensive overview of the latest advancements, techniques, and clinical insights in this field.

The book is divided into three sections, each dedicated to a specific anatomical region where osteotomies are commonly performed. The first section, "Osteotomies around the Knee", covers the most extensive range of procedures, reflecting the widespread application of osteotomies for knee realignment and joint preservation. It begins with *Osteotomies around the Knee: Indications, Planning, and Surgery*, which provides an essential foundation for understanding patient selection and surgical planning. Subsequent chapters delve into high tibial and distal femoral osteotomies, addressing their role in treating knee osteoarthritis, ligament insufficiency, and mechanical axis correction. Other topics include the integration of meniscus repair with high tibial osteotomy and the role of 3D printing in customizing osteosynthesis instruments for osteotomies.

The second section, "Osteotomies in the Hip and Foot", extends the discussion to other key weight-bearing joints. It explores osteotomy techniques in total hip arthroplasty for severe dysplasia, the surgical correction of cavovarus foot deformities, and the application of proximal and distal osteotomies in hallux valgus treatment. These chapters highlight the importance of osteotomies in managing congenital and acquired deformities in the lower limb beyond the knee.

Finally, the third section, "Osteotomies of the Facial Bones", focuses on craniofacial surgery. It includes discussions on technological advances in maxillofacial surgery, osteotomy techniques for implant placement in the posterior mandible, and treatment approaches for temporomandibular disorders. Additionally, the section explores the use of statins in bone healing after osteotomies and the effects of different osteotomy techniques on implant stability, offering valuable insights into maxillofacial and dental applications.

This book results from the collaborative efforts of leading orthopedic and maxillofacial surgeons, researchers, and engineers worldwide. We hope that it serves as a valuable resource for both seasoned professionals and trainees seeking to enhance their knowledge of osteotomies.

I want to express my sincere gratitude to all the contributing authors for their dedication and expertise. I also extend my appreciation to Mr. Josip Knapic, Publishing Process Manager, for his invaluable support throughout the editorial process.

Alessandro Zorzi
Department of Orthopedics,
Faculdade São Leopoldo Mandic,
Campinas, Brazil

Section 1

Osteotomies around the Knee

Chapter 1

Osteotomies around the Knee: Indications, Planning, and Surgery

Filipa Goncalves Pereira, André Carvalho and Ricardo Sousa

Abstract

Indications of knee osteotomy: coronal, sagittal or axial malalignment, knee ligament instability, association with intraarticular procedures, unicompartmental pain in association of meniscal deficit or osteonecrosis, unicompartmental osteoarthrosis and mal union after trauma. Explaining the role of the X rays, CTscan and MRI when planning an osteotomy. Short description of basic principles of limb alignment surgery including important angle calculation which are needed to understand the planning procedure of a knee osteotomy. Description of several planning methods and the role of patient specific cutting guides and implants. Surgical tips to perform a knee osteotomy and avoid complications.

Keywords: knee osteotomy, limb alignment, proximal high tibial osteotomy, distal femoral osteotomy, double level osteotomy

1. Introduction

Knee osteotomies have been used since the nineteenth century to treat knee pain caused by cartilage wear [1] and developmental disorders [2]. Since the development of unicompartmental and total knee arthroplasty, the use of osteotomies has declined due to their technical complexity, the need for closer follow-up, and the more demanding recovery process for patients. Recently, however, there has been a growing interest in osteotomies, as they are no longer solely viewed as a treatment for osteoarthrosis and coronal malalignments. They are now recognized as coadjuvant therapies for treating many other pathologies, such as chondral, meniscal, and ligament injuries.

Osteotomies are a powerful tool to correct coronal and sagittal malalignments as well as torsional malalignments, which can lead to patellar maltracking. In this chapter, we will not address derotational osteotomies or tibial tuberosity osteotomies, as these are better discussed in the context of patellar instability. Instead, we will focus on tibial, femoral, double, and biplanar osteotomies.

There are several types of knee osteotomies, including opening- and closing-wedge osteotomies, each of which has its own advantages and disadvantages, which we will explore in this chapter. Historically, a proximal tibial osteotomy was performed to correct a varus knee, while distal femur osteotomy was used to correct a valgus knee. However, with the evolution of surgical techniques and the comprehension of limb alignment, we can address deformities more precisely.

This chapter discusses osteotomy indications, limb alignment concepts, planning methods, surgical techniques, and tips to avoid complications during the procedure.

2. Osteotomy indications and contraindications

In the presence of a coronal malalignment there are several indications for osteotomies, including unicompartmental knee osteoarthritis, avascular osteonecrosis, unicompartmental pain with meniscus deficiency or insufficiency without osteoarthrosis, concomitant preservation procedures (e.g., meniscal repair or transplant, cartilage repair), malunion, ligament insufficiency, or ligament revision surgery.

Regarding unicompartmental knee arthritis, there is conflicting data. Some studies suggest that high-grade osteoarthritis (Kellgren-Lawrence grade IV) in the affected compartment is a contraindication for knee osteotomy [3], while other studies do not consider this a contraindication [4].

When preforming articular preservation procedures, such as meniscal repair, meniscal root repair, meniscal transplant, cartilage repair, autologous or allograft osteochondral transplant, or treating osteochondritis dissecans, the affected knee compartment should be unloaded. Failure to correct the malalignment is the most significant factor responsible for clinical failure [5]. Most studies advise corrections for deviations greater than 5° from neutral or when the mechanical axis deviates beyond the tip of the tibial spine of the affected knee compartment. In these cases, the osteotomy should aim to neutralize the mechanical axis so that the weight-bearing line passes through 50% of the tibial plateau.

In cases of anterior cruciate ligament (ACL) revision surgery, both coronal and sagittal alignment of the knee should be evaluated. It has been proven that varus alignment increases stress on the ACL, and an osteotomy should be considered where there is ACL reconstruction failure accompanied by a varus malalignment of 5° or greater [6–8]. The tibial slope should also be measured and corrected, particularly in cases of ACL revision with a tibial slope greater than 12° or in primary ACL reconstructions where the slope exceeds 16° [9, 10].

An osteotomy should also be considered in cases of varus malalignment and lateral knee instability, especially due to posterolateral corner (PLC) injury, where the ability to control varus caused by the dynamic adduction moments of the knee is diminished. Both acute and chronic PCL injuries may be eligible for an osteotomy. In acute cases, an osteotomy can be considered when varus malalignment exceeds 3-6° or when the mechanical axis hits the tip of the medial spine, as this has been shown to increase the risk of PLC reconstruction failure [11].

Biplanar osteotomies are indicated when there is a coronal and sagittal malalignment. The most frequent indication is a varus knee with a high tibial slope that requires a valgus-producing, slope-decreasing osteotomy [12]. Other less frequent indications include valgus knee with recurvatum needing a varus-producing, slope-decreasing osteotomy, and a varus knee with PCL insufficiency requiring a valgus-producing, slope-increasing osteotomy.

In cases where the deformity arises from intra-articular defects, such as tibial plateau malunions, a tibial condylar osteotomy may be required to reestablish joint congruence and stability. This type of procedure is an intra-articular osteotomy that must be patient specific [13, 14].

Several contraindications to knee osteotomy have been identified in the literature, including patient age older than 60, tricompartmental arthritis, inflammatory arthritis, and limited range of motion.

Most studies consider the presence of tricompartmental and patellofemoral osteoarthritis as contraindications to knee osteotomy [3], but some studies argue that an osteotomy can still be performed in the presence of cartilage lesions of the patellofemoral joint [15].

While most studies recommend osteotomy for patients younger than 60 years, others prioritize physiological status over chronological age when determining candidacy. Inflammatory arthritis should be evaluated on an individual basis, as recent advances in treatment have improved disease control, potentially making younger patients candidates for knee osteotomy.

Regarding range of motion, a flexion contracture of 10° with a total range of motion less than 100° is predictive of early osteotomy failure [16]. In addition, high body mass index (BMI) is considered a relative contraindication for this procedure, as this condition may increase complications such as nonunion due to increased micromotion at the osteotomy site [17]. Smoking significantly increases the risk of nonunion, with some studies indicating a 2.2-fold increase [18]. Patients should be strongly advised to stop smoking at least 3 weeks before the surgery.

In conclusion, the ideal candidate for a knee osteotomy is an active, nonsmoking patient younger than 60 years with a normal BMI, normal range of motion, and unicompartmental knee pain without severe osteoarthrosis.

3. Deformity evaluation

To understand lower extremity alignment, it is essential to evaluate three planes: coronal, sagittal, and axial, while recognizing that there are two types of axes: anatomic and mechanical.

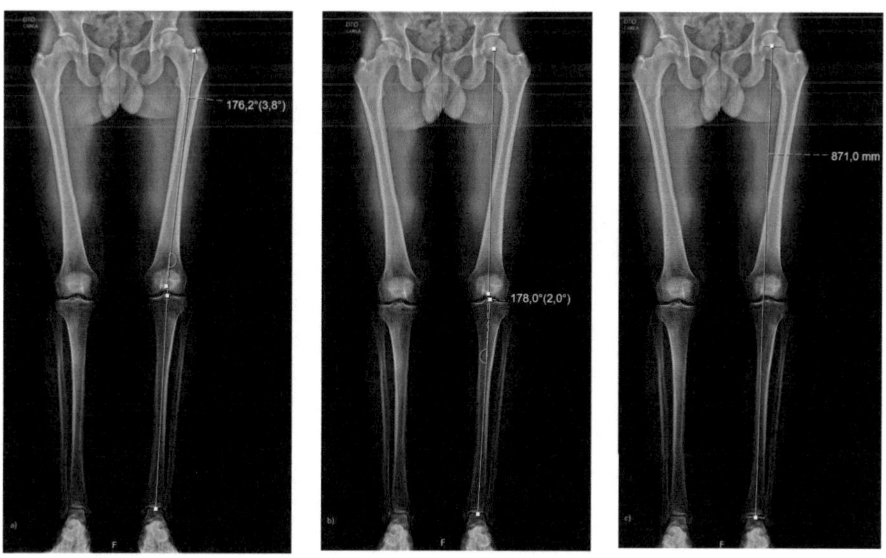

(a) (b) (c)

Figure 1.
(a) anatomic axis; (b) mechanical axis; (c) weight-bearing line.

The anatomical axis is defined by a line drawn in the medullary canal of the tibial and femoral diaphysis, and the anatomical tibiofemoral angle is calculated using those two lines (**Figure 1**).

The mechanical axis of the femur is defined by a line from the center of the femoral head to the center of the knee, which can be defined as the center of the condylar notch or the center of the tibial spines. The tibial mechanical axis is a line from the center of the tibial spines to the center of the ankle, which can be represented by the center or the talus. The mechanical tibiofemoral angle is defined as the angle between those two lines (**Figure 1**).

The Mikulicz line, also known as the weight-bearing line (WBL) or the mechanical axis of the lower limb, is defined as a line extending from the center of the femoral head to the center of the ankle (**Figure 1**).

Evaluating these angles and axes is important for determining limb alignment and classifying the limb as neutrally aligned, varus, or valgus (**Figure 2**). To properly evaluate the axes and calculate the relevant angles, which we will discuss later, it is crucial to obtain the correct radiologic images.

A complete radiologic evaluation includes an anteroposterior weight-bearing knee X-ray, Rosenberg view (weight bearing with the knees at 45° of flexion), a sagittal knee view, a Merchant view (axial patellofemoral image with the knee in 30° flexion), a sagittal leg view, and a full-length leg X-ray to ensure accurate planning and to avoid under or overcorrections in knee osteotomy. Several factors can affect the hip–knee ankle angle (HKA), such as leg rotation, foot position, knee flexion, and weight bearing. Multiple methods to obtain accurate and reproducible X-rays have been described, with the most commonly used method developed by Paley and Herzenberg [19]. This method relies on the position of the patella in the femoral condyles to achieve proper rotation.

With this information, it is possible to classify osteoarthrosis and coronal alignment as normally aligned (with the mechanical axis in the central part of the medial

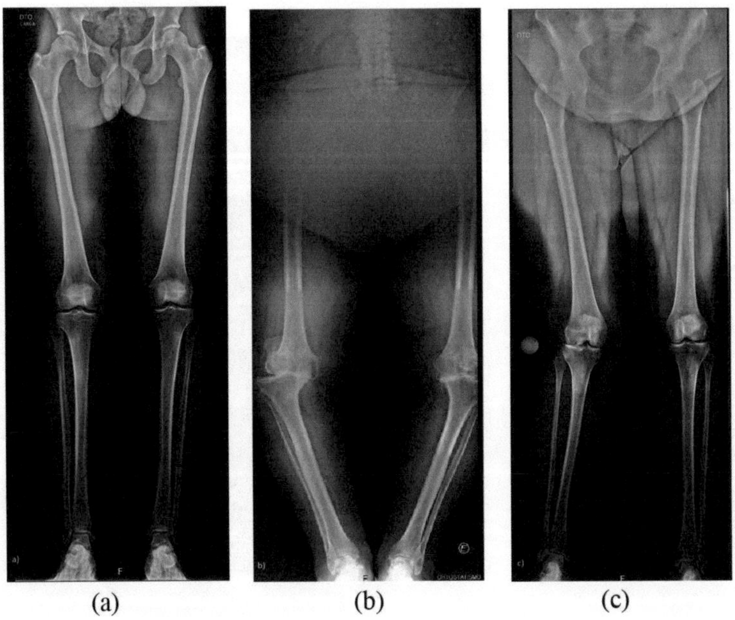

Figure 2.
(a) neutrally aligned knee; (b) varus knee; (c) valgus knee.

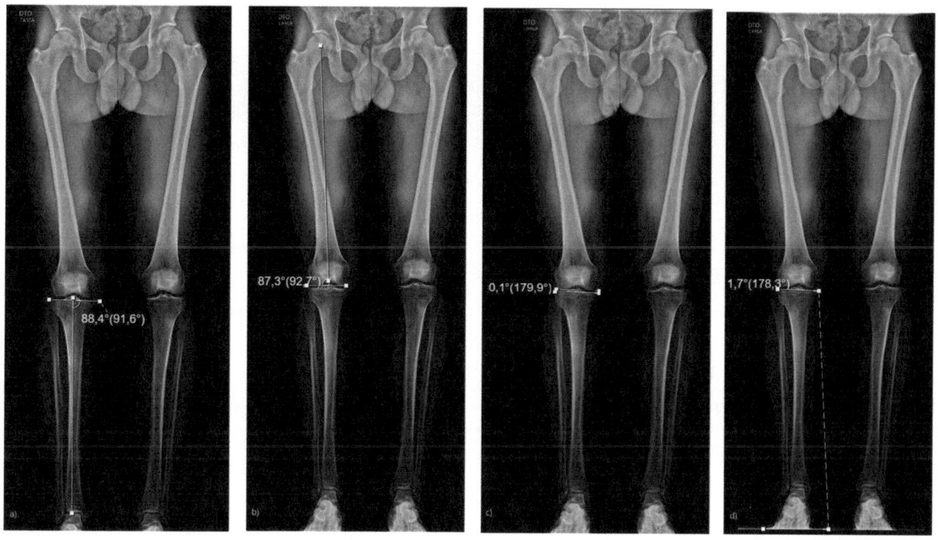

(a) (b) (c) (d)

Figure 3.
(a) medial proximal tibial angle (MPTA); (b) lateral distal femur angle (LDFA); (c) joint line convergence angle (JLCA); (d) joint line obliquity (JLO).

compartment and a mechanical angle of 0-3° of valgus), valgus (with an external shift of the axis), or varus (with a medial shift of the axis).

It is then important to determine if the coronal deformity lies in the femur, tibia, or both by calculating the distal femoral and proximal tibial angles. The mechanical medial proximal tibial angle (mMPTA) is defined as the medial angle formed by a tangential line to the tibial plateau and the mechanical axis of the tibia, with a normal value of 87° and a range from 85° to 90°. The mechanical lateral distal femur angle (mLDFA) is defined as the lateral angle formed by a tangential line to the distal femur condyles and the mechanical axis of the femur, with a normal value of 87° and a range from 85° to 90° (**Figure 3**).

By evaluating these angles, it is possible to identify the location of the bone deformity in the coronal plane. In this same plane, two additional important angles are measured: the joint line convergence angle (JLCA) and joint line obliquity (JLO). JLCA is measured using a tangential line to the tibial plateau and a tangential line to the distal femoral condyles, reflecting the intra-articular deformity of the knee, which is an important consideration when planning osteotomy. JLO can be measured using different reference lines at the joint level, with the most common method using a tangential line to the tibial plateau and a tangential line to the ground (**Figure 3**). In the sagittal plane, using a proper lateral knee and leg X-ray, it is possible to measure the tibial posterior slope. This angle is formed by a tangential line to the tibial plateau and a line perpendicular to the longitudinal axis of the tibia. The slope can also be divided into medial or lateral tibial slope depending on where the tangential line is drawn.

4. Osteotomy planning

The purpose of an osteotomy is to correct an extra-articular deformity while simultaneously unloading a knee compartment or adjusting the tibial slope to reduce stress on intra-articular ligaments.

In the coronal plane, unloading one compartment of the knee requires shifting the weight-bearing line (WBL), also known as the Mikulicz line, to the contralateral compartment. This reduces contact forces in the unloaded compartment. [20–22]

Historically, a high tibial osteotomy was performed to shift the WBL in a varus knee, while a distal femur osteotomy was performed for a valgus knee [23, 24]. Nowadays, modern osteotomy planning involves studying the origin of the deformity by measuring the axes and angles previously mentioned. This means that a valgus deformity is not always attributed to the femur, nor is a varus deformity always attributed to the tibia. These deformities may originate in one or both bones, and the correction, whether varus or valgus, must be performed at the site of the deformity, which could involve the tibia, femur, both, or even the intra-articular structures.

To correct coronal alignment, osteotomies are classified as valgus or varus producing (**Table 1**). Choosing the degree of correction is an important step in planning an osteotomy. To better understand the position of the WBL in the knee joint, it is often described as a percentage of the articular surface of the proximal tibia, with 0% corresponding to most medial part and 100% to the most lateral part of the tibial plateau.

The ideal positioning of the WBL involves minimal overcorrection, sufficient to unload the affected compartment without overloading the contralateral compartment. This position varies depending on factors such as the degree of osteoarthritis, the alignment of the contralateral limb, and ligament insufficiency. Historically, all valgus-producing osteotomies were planned to place the WBL at the Fujisawa point (62.5%) based on retrospective studies showing higher survival rates and cartilage regeneration with overcorrected valgus knees [25]. More recent studies have found that correcting the WBL to 55% of the tibial width creates an optimal distribution of contact stress between the medial and lateral compartments [26]. An easily reproducible landmark for achieving 55% correction is the lateral tibial spine [27].

In varus osteotomies, overcorrection is typically avoided. Usually, the WBL is positioned to pass through 45–50% of the tibial plateau [28]. Even a varus deformity greater than 2° increases the probability of developing knee osteoarthritis [29].

After deciding where the WBL should pass, it is time to calculate the degree of correction. Several methods can be used for this calculation: the Hernigou table for the tibia, the Dugdale method to calculate the alpha angle, and the Miniaci method.

The Hernigou table involves measuring the length of the osteotomy and the desired correction, then consulting the table for the osteotomy height in millimeters to achieve the desired correction (**Figure 4**).

The Dugdale method marks the desired WBL position on the tibial plateau and calculates the alpha angle between two lines: one from the new WBL point to the center of the femoral head and another from the same point to the center of the talus (**Figure 5**).

	Valgus-producing osteotomy	**Varus-producing osteotomy**
Tibia	Medial opening-wedge high tibia osteotomy	Medial closing-wedge high tibial osteotomy
	Lateral closing-wedge high tibia osteotomy	Lateral opening-wedge high tibial osteotomy
Femur	Lateral closing-wedge distal femur osteotomy	Lateral opening-wedge distal femur osteotomy
	Medial opening-wedge distal femur osteotomy	Medial closing-wedge distal femur osteotomy

Table 1.
Types of osteotomies.

β	4	5	6	7	8	9	10	11	12	13	14	15	16*	17	18	19
M																
50	3	4	5	6	7	8	9	10	10	11	12	13	14	15	16	16
55	4	5	6	7	8	9	10	10	11	12	13	14	15	16	17	18
60	4	5	6	7	8	9	10	11	12	14	15	16	17	18	19	20
65*	5	6	7	8	9	10	11	12	14	15	16	17	18*	19	20	21
70	5	6	7	8	10	11	12	13	15	16	17	18	20	21	22	23
75	5	6	8	9	10	12	13	14	16	17	18	20	21	22	24	25
80	6	7	8	10	11	13	14	15	17	18	19	21	22	24	25	26

Figure 4.
Hernigou table (HT).

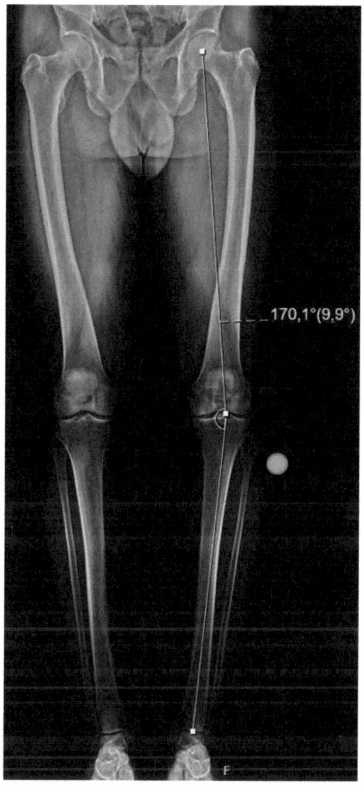

Figure 5.
Dugdale method - alpha angle.

The Miniaci method is commonly used in English-speaking countries to plan an open wedge tibial osteotomy. In this method, the Mikulicz line is drawn from the center of the femoral head to the desired point on the tibial plateau (line A), ensuring that it has the same length as the original Mikulicz line. The hinge point is marked (in this case on the proximal lateral tibial cortex), ideally more than 1 cm distal to the articular surface. The correction angle is the one formed between a line drawn to the center of the talus and the hinge point and a line drawn from the hinge point to the end of line A (line C) (**Figure 6**) [30].

The Miniaci method can also be used in a reverse fashion, known as the inverted-Miniaci method, to calculate the correction in distal femur osteotomies [28]. In this method, the original Mikulicz line and the new Mikulicz line passing the knee at the desired point (line A) should be drawn. The hinge point should be marked just above the femur epicondyle (medial or lateral whether there is an opening or closing wedge osteotomy). The lines are drawn from the hinge to the center of the femur head (line

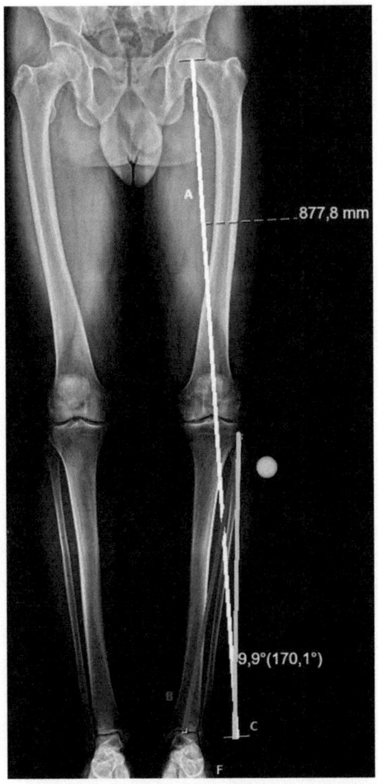

Figure 6.
Miniaci method.

B) and the hinge point to end of line A (the new center of femoral head) (line C). The angle formed between lines B and C is the correction angle (**Figure 7**).

Regardless of the method used, the angle of correction should be converted to millimeters to allow precise surgical control. Using a calibrated X-ray, the calculated angle is projected onto the bone (distal femur or proximal tibia), starting at the hinge point and ending on the opposite cortex. The height between the lines at the cortex level corresponds to the wedge size that should be resected or created. When planning an opening-wedge osteotomy, the thickness of the sawblade should be added to the calculated height.

Evaluation of the joint line obliquity angle (JLCA) is of great importance after defining the degree of the bone correction.

It has been shown that the JLCA decreases after a high tibial osteotomy [31, 32]; the greater the change between preoperative and postoperative JLCA the greater the risk of overcorrection. Risk factors to predict a JLCA change of more than 2° include a preoperative JLCA >3° and a significant difference between standing and supine JLCA measurements (>1.7°). This is particularly important in osteoarthritic varus knee because the deformity is usually greater in the standing position than in the supine position due to the adduction moment on the medial side of the knee [33] and because osteoarthritic varus knee may have other factors contributing to the deformity. Varus knees can be classified in three categories: primary varus (tibiofemoral bony alignment and deformity isolated), double varus (bony deformity plus soft tissue laxity), and triple varus (bony deformity plus severe laxity posterolateral structures and recurvatum in extension) [34].

DOI: http://dx.doi.org/10.5772/intechopen.1007398

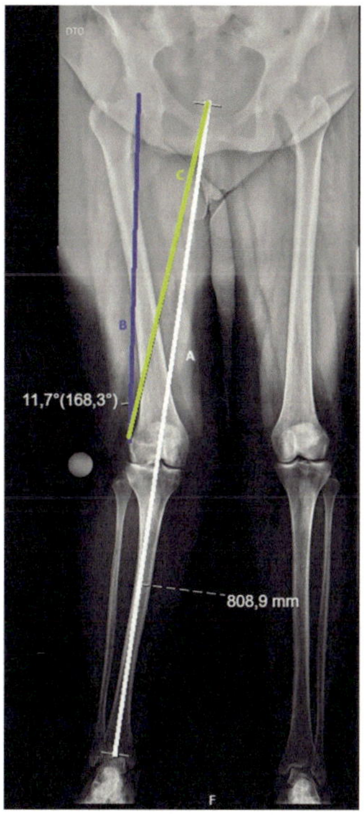

Figure 7.
Reverse Miniaci method.

Correcting a varus deformity involves not only addressing the bony deformity but also considering intra-articular deformities caused by cartilage wear and soft tissue laxity or contracture.

There are several methods used to predict the JLCA's effect on the final correction of limb alignment and balance this effect when planning the osteotomy, such as using a lateral wedge insole for valgus osteotomies [35], avoiding valgus MPTA corrections greater than 2°, and not allowing the WBL to pass over 57.5% of the width of the proximal tibia surface [36]. Equations such as the following can be used to predict postoperative JLCA and soft tissue correction:

- Soft tissue correction = 0.691 × JLCA −0.411 × valgus JLCA −0.399 [37]
- Postoperative JLCA = 0.478 + 0.188 x Preoperative JLCA (standing) +0.541 x Preoperative JLCA (supine) [33]

In the authors opinion, the easiest and most predictable method to avoid overcorrection is subtracting a value from the initial correction angle using the following equation:

- (JLCA – 2)/2 [38]

The joint line obliquity angle (JLO) should also be considered when planning an osteotomy. It is important to establish limits for single-bone corrections, and the surgeon must decide whether to slightly overcorrect or perform a double-level osteotomy. Historically, it was acceptable to obtain a JLO less than 10° [39], but recent evidence shows that a JLO greater than 5° doubles shear stress in one compartment and may lead to cartilage lost on postsurgical X-rays [38, 40]. Clinical and functional outcomes are poor with a JLO greater than 4°–5°, and in the majority of these cases a double-level osteotomy should be performed instead [24, 41]. Nowadays, we may conclude that an ideal JLO after osteotomy should not be greater than 4°.

Without appropriate software is it hard to plane and predict the exact vale of the JLO, but there are some signs that can alert the surgeon to the need for double-level osteotomy, such as preoperative JLO value greater than 3°, JLCA greater than 5°, hip-knee-ankle angle (HKA) greater than 10°, a predicted postoperative MPTA greater than 95°, and a gap correction of more than 15 mm [42]. There is no threshold for the MPTA overcorrection, but clinical outcomes are worse with postoperative MPTA greater than 94°. An equation to predict postoperative JLO has been described, which can be helpful to surgeons who do not have access to informatic tools:

- 1° increase in MPTA = 0.463° increase in JLO [43]

Double-level osteotomy may also help prevent leg length discrepancies after large corrections in only one bone, which is a potential complication and can cause gait changes and back pain [44].

In conclusion, double-level osteotomy should be considered when a large deformity exists in both the tibia and the femur, and the affected compartment cannot be unloaded without exceeding acceptable JLO limits. The goal is to achieve a postoperative JLO less than 4° and an MPTA less than 94°.

Patella height should also be evaluated when planning an osteotomy. There are several methods to measure patella height in a sagittal X-ray with a knee flexion of 30°. The most used are the Caton-Dechamps, Insall-Salvati, and Blackburne-Peel indices [45].

Nowadays, the majority of tibia osteotomies are supratubercle osteotomies, which may alter patella height: open-wedge tibial osteotomies tend to decrease patella height, while closing-wedge osteotomies tend to increase patella height [46]. Studies suggest that a valgus correction of 10° can decrease patella height by 2 mm [47]. These changes can increase patellofemoral joint contact pressure, leading to postoperative anterior knee pain and lower clinical and functional scores [48]. Distal tubercle osteotomies do not affect patellofemoral contact pressure or osteoarthritic progression [49] and may be preferable for large corrections [46]. A distal tibial tuberosity osteotomy or a biplanar tibial osteotomy with an L shape that is directed distal to the tibial tubercle are indicated in cases of patella baja, since these methods do not change patella height or patellofemoral joint contact pressure [50].

When planning a sagittal osteotomy or a slope-changing osteotomy, some considerations must be taken. Firstly, supratubercle anterior osteotomy may also change patella height. Secondly, slope-reducing osteotomy (anterior closing wedge) can increase hyperextension of the knee, and thus, a careful preoperative evaluation should be undertaken to exclude preexisting recurvatum [51]. This kind of osteotomy is more frequently performed in the sagittal plane. The interest in this method has grown over the years, especially in patients with ACL insufficiency or revision ACL surgery.

Small corrections in a patient with a normal patella height may be achieved through a supratubercle osteotomy. Most of the corrections require a biplanar osteotomy to ensure tibial tubercle and patellar tendon integrity.

When performing an infratubercle osteotomy the surgeon must plane it to be at least 3 cm distal to the tibial tubercle to decrease fracture avulsion risk [52]. The hinge points for these osteotomies should be placed at the level of the posterior cruciate ligament's (PCL) tibial insertion, which can be identified radiographically 1 cm distal do the tibial plateau in a sagittal plane [52].

In some patients, both the coronal and sagittal planes must be corrected, for example, in case of an ACL reversion surgery in a patient with a tibial slope greater than 12°.

Planning a biplanar osteotomy is particularly difficult without specialized software because even minor adjustments in the placement of the hinge point can produce an undesired correction. We will focus on the most common biplanar osteotomy: the valgus-producing, slope-decreasing osteotomy.

The natural tendency of a closing-wedge tibial osteotomy is to reduce the tibial slope, which can be advantageous. However, this procedure allows less fine-tuning during surgery and, as will be discussed later in the chapter, tibial closing-wedge osteotomies have some disadvantages and are technically difficult to perform.

On the contrary, an open-wedge tibial osteotomy tends to increase tibial slope. To prevent this in a single-plane osteotomy, the gap created must be asymmetric, with the posterior side being larger, to maintain the slope [53]. In a biplanar osteotomy, which addresses both the sagittal and coronal planes, the hinge point must be placed far anteriorly on the lateral cortex. Studies have demonstrated that rotating the hinge point 8.7°externally and 21.6°proximally decreases the tibial slope by 1°in a 10 mm medial open-wedge osteotomy model [54]. Since most osteotomies involve corrections of less 10 mm, identifying exact hinge point for the desired correction is challenging. As a result, patient-specific instrumentation (PSI) and implants may be necessary to ensure a precise and successful procedure.

5. Patient-specific instruments and navigation

Patient-specific instruments (PSI), including cutting guides and implants, were developed to improve accuracy and simplify the planning and surgical process. In coronal plane osteotomies, however, PSI offers no significant advantage over the conventional freehand method when performed by an experienced surgeon. The literature has shown no statistically significant differences in correction parameters or clinical outcomes between the two methods [55, 56]. Although PSI demonstrates good reproducibility and accuracy, [57–59] some evidence suggests it may offer a slight advantage in accuracy of closing-wedge osteotomies [60].

PSI can be particularly advantageous in some cases requiring multiplanar corrections, where preexisting implants are present or when precise planning of screw and bone tunnel placement is necessary. The PSI method requires a CT scan of the limb and specialized software to determine where the hinge point will be, the location of the opening or closing gap, the placement and length of screws, and the position of the plate. Once these details are determined, cutting and drill guides for the osteotomy are created. Some guides also incorporate Kirschner wire (K-wire) guides to protect the hinge and avoid hinge fractures.

During the surgery, after verifying the position of the guide, the screw holes are drilled first, followed by the osteotomy with a saw blade. After opening the gap and fixing the plate, the holes of the plate should align with the predrilled holes of the guide. This is an extra step to confirm accurate correction. PSI also has the advantages of a short learning curve, reduced surgical time, and less radiation exposure during surgery [59, 61].

Navigation or computer-assisted surgery may reduce outlier results, but its increased accuracy is not statistically significant when compared with the traditional freehand technique [56]. However, some studies suggest that navigation offers better accuracy in controlling tibial slope than conventional surgery [62]. This technique demands the placement of bone trackers and the registration of bone landmarks, which are critical steps that, if not executed properly, can lead to errors. It is important to check changes in coronal alignment under varus and valgus stress because the values acquired via navigation may be different from those obtained by weight-bearing X-rays. It is advisable to apply varus force until the navigated preoperative value matches the radiographic value [63]. This technique has a longer learning curve and can increase operating time [64, 65], but it also provides real-time intraoperative information on the HKA axis and the coronal, sagittal, and transverse axes.

6. Advantages and disadvantages of different osteotomies in the coronal plane

When choosing between different osteotomy methods for achieving the same type of correction, several factors must be considered, including patient conditions and the pros and cons of each technique. This section focuses on the two most commonly performed osteotomies: proximal high tibial osteotomy for varus correction and distal femur osteotomy for valgus correction.

For varus corrections in the tibia, two methods can produce valgus: medial opening-wedge and lateral closing-wedge osteotomies.

Lateral closing-wedge osteotomy, popularized by Coventry, was the first method developed for varus correction [66, 67]. This type of osteotomy is more stable and allows immediate weight bearing, has lower nonunion rates, and has lower risk of increasing posterior slope and changing patella height. However, this technique involves removing a block of bone, which may limit future surgical options. It also requires a lateral dissection and a possible proximal peroneal osteotomy, increasing the risk of damaging the lateral collateral ligament, injuring the peroneal nerve, or causing anterior compartment syndrome. Besides these risks, lateral closing-wedge osteotomy is technically demanding and, as it is a closing osteotomy, there is less room for fine-tuning the correction.

Medial opening-wedge osteotomy has gained popularity with the development of new osteotomy plates and fixations techniques. This surgical approach is much easier than the lateral one, as it avoids the risks of lateral exposure. Opening-wedge osteotomy preserves bone stock and allows some intraoperative fine-tuning, which gives the surgeon more control. Because there is a gap created during this procedure, the nonunion rate may be higher than in closing-wedge osteotomies. There may also be postoperative pain due to bleeding. To avoid this, the gap can be filled with autologous bone graft, allograft, or synthetic bone graft. Opening-wedge osteotomy has a higher risk of increasing the posterior tibial slope and altering patella height.

For valgus corrections in the femur, two methods produce varus: medial closing-wedge and lateral opening-wedge osteotomies. The most used method is the lateral opening-wedge femur osteotomy, which may be more comfortable for surgeons as it allows fine-tuning, preserves bone stock, and requires a lateral femur approach, which most surgeons are familiar with for treating distal femur fractures. However, this technique is less stable and has a higher risk of delayed union or nonunion. The hardware required can irritate the iliotibial band, often necessitating a second surgery for hardware removal [68].

Medial closing-wedge femur osteotomy is less commonly used but offers several benefits. It is more stable, with higher union rates and the hardware is less likely to cause irritation, reducing the need for a second surgery. Most surgeons are less familiar with the medial approach, which requires elevating the vastus medialis muscle and exposing the posterior femoral cortex to protect the neurovascular bundle.

7. Surgical technique, pearls, and pitfalls

The most important step in performing an osteotomy is planning. After adequate planning and choosing the type of osteotomy to be performed, care must be taken to avoid common complications and guarantee an appropriate correction.

In both opening- and closing-wedge osteotomies, it is critical to avoid a hinge fracture. To do this, the surgeon must ensure that the sawblade and osteotomes advance to within 1 cm of the hinge cortex. Care must be taken to avoid cutting too close to the hinge, which could lead to a fracture.

In an opening-wedge osteotomy, the surgeon must confirm the posterior cortex cut is complete before gradually opening the wedge. A controlled, slow opening process using osteotomes or a spreader is essential to avoid sudden stress on the bone.

In a closing-wedge osteotomy, removal of the bone triangle must be accurately planned because fine-tuning corrections are more difficult in closing-wedge techniques. The bone piece should be removed in one piece, if possible, to make closure easier. Any remaining bone fragments can complicate closure and increase fracture risk. If closure is difficult, a curette should be used to check for bone fragments, and Kirschner wires (K-wires) can be used to create small holes in the hinge cortex, improving plasticity and facilitating closure.

In recent years, K-wires have been used to protect the osteotomy site. A K-wire should be placed at the intersection of the osteotomy plane, 1 cm from the hinge. This technique acts as a barrier to protect the osteotomy site and sawblade and increases the mechanical resistance to breakage. It also enhances the allowable displacement, thus reducing the risk of hinge fractures in both opening- and closing-wedge osteotomies that require large corrections [28, 69].

In opening-wedge osteotomies, the surgeon must always consider the thickness of the sawblade. When performing the bone cut, a "natural" gap corresponding to saw thickness is created, but at this point no correction is made. For example, if the planned correction gap is 5 mm and the sawblade is 2-mm thick, the final gap will be 7 mm. Surgeons must account for this in their preoperative planning to avoid under or overcorrection.

Although rare, neurovascular bundle injury is a serious complication [70]. To minimize risk, the posterior cortex of the femur and tibia must always be bluntly dissected and protected during the osteotomy. Proper protection of the neurovascular bundle during bone cuts is more important than flexing the knee. This can be difficult and can lead to a misplacement of the retractors.

8. Conclusion

Osteotomies are powerful surgical interventions *that must be carefully planned and adjusted for each patient*. With *survivorship* rates *reaching 90%,* they are especially appealing for younger patients. A comprehensive understanding of lower limb deformities and the effects of each type of osteotomy is essential for surgeons performing these procedures.

Recent advancements such as planning software, navigation systems, and the availability of PSI guides, developed in collaboration with engineers from various industries, have enhanced the ability to analyze deformities and predict surgical outcomes more effectively.

In the future, innovations in robotic surgery and artificial intelligence will bring about new tools to improve surgical techniques and clinical results.

Thanks

I would like to express my deepest gratitude to Dr. André Ramos, my mentor during orthopedic residency who is responsible for my interest in knee surgery. I will always remember how he helped me continuously improve and face greater challenges.

I am extremely grateful to be working with the GRIP team whose members have become great friends who encourage and support me to continue evolving.

Conflict of interest

The authors declare no conflict of interest.

Author details

Filipa Goncalves Pereira*, André Carvalho and Ricardo Sousa
Centro Hospitalar Universitário de Santo António, Oporto, Portugal

*Address all correspondence to: filipa.pereira@ymail.com

References

[1] Coventry MB. Proximal tibial varus osteotomy for osteoarthritis of the lateral compartment of the knee. Journal of Bone and Joint Surgery. 1 Jan 1987;**69**(1):32-38. DOI: 10.2106/00004623-198769010-00006

[2] Smith JO, Wilson AJ, Thomas NP. Osteotomy around the knee: Evolution, principles and results. Knee Surgery, Sports Traumatology, Arthroscopy. 2013;**21**(1):3-22. DOI: 10.1007/s00167-012-2206-0

[3] Cantivalli A, Rosso F, Bonasia DE, Rossi R. High tibial osteotomy and anterior cruciate ligament reconstruction/revision. Clinics in Sports Medicine. 2019;**38**(3):417-433. DOI: 10.1016/j.csm.2019.02.008

[4] Ollivier B, Berger P, Depuy C, Vandenneucker H. Good long-term survival and patient-reported outcomes after hight tibial osteotomy for medial compartment osteoarthritis. Knee Surgery, Sports Traumatology, Arthroscopy. 2020;**29**(11):3569-3584

[5] Krych AJ, Hevesi M, Desai VS, Camp CL, Stuart MJ, Saris DBF. Learning from failure in cartilage repair surgery: An analysis of the mode of failure of primary procedures in consecutive cases at a tertiary referral center. Journal of experimental orthopaedics. Feb 2019;**6**:10. DOI: 10.1177/2325967118773041

[6] Won HH, Chang CB, Je MS, Chang MJ, Kim TK. Coronal limb alignment and indications for high tibial osteotomy in patients undergoing revision ACL reconstruction. Clinical Orthopaedics and Related Research. 2013;**471**(11):3504-3511. DOI: 10.1007/s11999-013-3185-2

[7] Zaffagnini S, Bonanzinga T, Grassi A, Marcheggiani Muccioli GM, Musiani C, Raggi F, et al. Combined ACL reconstruction and closing-wedge HTO for varus angulated ACL-deficient knees. Knee Surgery, Sports Traumatology, Arthroscopy. 2013;**21**(4):934-941. DOI: 10.1007/s00167-013-2400-8

[8] Stride D, Wang J, Horner NS, Alolabi B, Khanna V, Khan M. Indications and outcomes of simultaneous high tibial osteotomy and ACL reconstruction. Knee Surgery, Sports Traumatology, Arthroscopy. 2019;**27**(4):1320-1331. DOI: 10.1007/s00167-019-05379-5

[9] Song GY, Ni QK, Zheng T, Zhang ZJ, Feng H, Zhang H. Slope-reducing tibial osteotomy combined with primary anterior cruciate ligament reconstruction produces improved knee stability in patients with steep posterior tibial slope, excessive anterior tibial subluxation in extension, and chronic meniscal posterior horn tears. The American Journal of Sports Medicine. 2020;**48**(14):3486-3494. DOI: 10.1177/0363546520963083

[10] Dan MJ, Cance N, Pineda T, Demey G, Dejour DH. Four to 6° is the target posterior tibial slope after tibial deflection osteotomy according to the knee static anterior tibial translation. Arthroscopy. 2024;**40**(3):846-854. DOI: 10.1016/j.arthro.2023.07.007

[11] Noyes R, Barber-Westin S, Albright J. An analyses of the causes of failure in 57 consecutive posterolateral operative procedures. The American Journal of Sports Medicine. 2006;**34**:1419-1430

[12] Müller S, Frosch KH, Frings J, Berninger M, Krause M. Biplanar high

tibial osteotomy for the combined correction of varus and posterior tibial slope malalignment. Orthopaedics & Traumatology, Surgery & Research. 2023;**109**(4):103339. DOI: 10.1016/j.otsr.2022.103339

[13] Paley D. Intra-articular osteotomies of the hip, knee, and ankle. Operative Techniques in Orthopaedics. 2011;**21**:184-196. DOI: 10.1053/j.oto.2011.01.009

[14] Kfuri M, Schatzker J. Corrective intra-articular osteotomies for tibial plateau malunion. The Journal of Knee Surgery. 2017;**30**:784-792

[15] Snow M, Jermain P, Vipul M, Murray J, Khakha R, McNicholas M, et al. A 2021 consensus statement on osteotomies around the knee by the UK knee osteotomy consensus group (KOG). The Knee. 2021;**33**:73-83. DOI: 10.1016/j.knee.2021.08.034

[16] Akizuki S, Shibakawa A, Takizawa T, Yamazaki I, Horiuchi H. The long-term outcome of high tibial osteotomy: A ten- to 20-year follow-up. Journal of Bone and Joint Surgery. British Volume (London). 2008;**90**(5):592-596. DOI: 10.1302/0301-620X.90B5.20386

[17] Elson DW, Dawson M, Wilson C, Risebury M, Wilson A. The UK knee osteotomy registry (UKKOR). The Knee. 2015;**22**(1):1-3. DOI: 10.1016/j.knee.2014.10.004

[18] Pearson RG, Clement RGE, Edwards KL, et al. Do smokers have greater risk of delayed and non-union after fracture, osteotomy and arthrodesis? A systematic review with meta-analysis. BMJ Open. 2016;**6**:e010303. DOI: 10.1136/bmjopen-2015-010303

[19] Paley D. Radiographic assessment of lower limb deformities. In: Principles of Deformity Correction. Berlin, Heidelberg: Springer Berlin Heidelberg; 2002. pp. 31-60. DOI: 10.1007/978-3-642-59373-4

[20] Bowd J, Van Rossom S, Williams D, Elson D, Wilson C, Whatling G, et al. Using musculoskeletal modelling to estimate knee joint loading pre and post high tibial osteotomy. Clinical Biomechanics (Bristol, Avon). 2023;**101**:105855. DOI: 10.1016/j.clinbiomech.2022.105855

[21] Kloos F, Becher C, Fleischer B, Ettinger M, Bode L, Schmal H, et al. Discharging the medial knee compartment: Comparison of pressure distribution and kinematic shifting after implantation of an extra-capsular absorber system (ATLAS) and open-wedge high tibial osteotomy-a biomechanical *in vitro* analysis. Archives of Orthopaedic and Trauma Surgery. 2023;**143**(6):2929-2941. DOI: 10.1007/s00402-022-04496-0

[22] Kuriyama S, Watanabe M, Nakamura S, Nishitani K, Tanaka Y, Sekiguchi K, et al. Large medial proximal tibial angles cause excessively medial tibiofemoral contact forces and abnormal knee kinematics following open-wedge high tibial osteotomy. Clinical Biomechanics (Bristol, Avon). 2020;**80**(105190):105190. DOI: 10.1016/j.clinbiomech.2020.105190

[23] Eberbach H, Mehl J, Feucht MJ, Bode G, Sudkamp NP, Niemeyer P. Geometry of the valgus knee: Contradicting the dogma of a femoral-based deformity. The American Journal of Sports Medicine. 2017;**45**(4):909-914. DOI: 10.1177/0363546516676266

[24] Feucht MJ, Winkler PW, Mehl J, Bode G, Forkel P, Imhoff AB, et al. Isolated high tibial osteotomy is appropriate in less than two-thirds of

varus knees if excessive overcorrection of the medial proximal tibial angle should be avoided. Knee Surgery, Sports Traumatology, Arthroscopy. 2021;**29**(10):3299-3309. DOI: 10.1007/s00167-020-06166-3

[25] Otsuki S, Ikeda K, Ishitani T, Okamoto Y, Wakama H, Matsuyama J, et al. Impact of the weightbearing line on cartilage regeneration of the medial knee compartment after open-wedge high tibial osteotomy, based on second-look arthroscopy. Cartilage. 2022;**13**(4):87-93. DOI: 10.1177/19476035221137724

[26] Martay JL, Palmer A Jr, Bangerter NK, Clare S, Monk AP, Brown CP, et al. A preliminary modeling investigation into the safe correction zone for high tibial osteotomy. The Knee. 2018;**25**(2):286-295. DOI: 10.1016/j.knee.2017.12.006

[27] Tripon M, Sautet P, Argenson JN, Jacquet C, Martz P, Ollivier M. Is the lateral tibial spine a reliable landmark for planning tibial or femoral valgus osteotomies? Orthopaedics & Traumatology, Surgery & Research. 2022;**108**(3):103253. DOI: 10.1016/j.otsr.2022.103253

[28] An J, Kley Kristian, Jacquet C., Reina F. L.,Ollivier M. "Closing wedge femoral osteotomy for knee valgus: Indications, technique, rehabilitation and outcomes", Journal of Cartilage & Joint Preservation 2023; 3(1):100110

[29] Dugdale TW, Noyes FR, Styer D. Preoperative planning for high tibial osteotomy. The effect of lateral tibiofemoral separation and tibiofemoral length. Clinical Orthopaedics and Related Research. 1992;**274**:248-264

[30] Micicoi G, Martz P, Jacquet C, Fernandes LR, Khakha R, Ollivier M. High tibial osteotomy with Miniaci planning using manual and semiautomated digital measures. Video Journal of Sports Medicine. 2021;**1**(6):263502542110329. DOI: 10.1177/263502542110329

[31] Leedh P, Han SB. Effect of soft tissue laxity of the knee joint on limb alignment correction in open-wedge high tibial osteotomy. Knee Surgery, Sports Traumatology, Arthroscopy. 2016;**24**(12):3704-3712

[32] Na YG, Lee BK, Choi JU, Lee BH, Sim JA. Change of joint-line convergence angle should be considered for accurate alignment correction in high tibial osteotomy. Knee Surgery & Related Research. 2021;**33**(1):4. DOI: 10.1186/s43019-020-00076-x

[33] Specogna AV, Birmingham TB, Hunt MA, Jones IC, Jenkyn TR, Fowler PJ, et al. Radiografic measures of knee alignment in patients with varus gonarthrosis: Effect of weightbearing status and associations with dynamic joint load. The American Journal of Sports Medicine. 2007;**35**(1):65-67

[34] Noyes FR, Barber-Westin SD, Hewwett TE. High tibial osteotomy and ligament reconstruction for varus angulated anterior cruciate ligament-deficient knees. The American Journal of Sports Medicine. 2000;**28**:282-296. DOI: 10.1177/03635465000280030201

[35] Akasaki Y, Mizu-Uchi H, Hamai S, Tsushima H, Kawahara S, Horikawa T, et al. Patient-specific prediction of joint line convergence angle after high tibial osteotomy using a whole-leg radiograph standing on lateral-wedge insole. Knee Surgery, Sports Traumatology, Arthroscopy. 2020;**28**:3200-3206. DOI: 10.1007/s00167-019-05821-8

[36] Lee DK, Wang JH, Won Y, Min YK, Jaiswal S, Lee BH, et al. Preoperative

latent medial laxity and correction angle are crucial factors for overcorrection in medial open-wedge high tibial osteotomy. Knee Surgery, Sports Traumatology, Arthroscopy. 2020;**28**:1411-1418. DOI: 10.1007/s00167-019-05502-6

[37] Takagawa S, Kobayashi N, Yukizawa Y, Oishi T, Tsuji M, Inaba Y. Preoperative soft tissue laxity around knee was associated with less accurate alignment correction after hybrid closed-wedge high tibial osteotomy. Knee Surgery, Sports Traumatology, Arthroscopy. 2020;**28**:3022-3030. DOI: 10.1007/s00167-019-05762-2

[38] Micicoi G, Khakha R, Kley K, Wilson A, Cerciello S, Ollivier M. Managing intra-articular deformity in high tibial osteotomy: A narrative review. Journal of Experimental Orthopaedics. 2020;**7**(1):65. DOI: 10.1186/s40634-020-00283-1

[39] Coventry MB. Proximal tibial varus osteotomy for osteoarthritis of the lateral compartment of the knee. The Journal of Bone and Joint Surgery. American Volume. 1987;**69**(1):32-38. DOI: 10.2106/00004623-198769010-00006

[40] Song JH, Bin SI, Kim JM, Lee BS. What is an acceptable limit of joint-line obliquity after medial open wedge high tibial osteotomy? Analysis based on midterm results. The American Journal of Sports Medicine. 2020;**48**(12):3028-3035. DOI: 10.1177/0363546520949552

[41] Babis GC, Dsc An K-N, Phd CEYS, Rand JA, Sim FH. Double level osteotomy of the knee: A method to retain joint-line obliquity: Clinical results. The Journal of Bone & Joint Surgery. 2002;**84**(8):1380-1388

[42] Nakayama H, Schröter S, Yamamoto C, Iseki T, Kanto R, Kurosaka K, et al. Large correction in opening wedge high tibial osteotomy with resultant joint-line obliquity induces excessive shear stress on the articular cartilage. Knee Surgery, Sports Traumatology, Arthroscopy. 2018;**26**(6):1873-1878. DOI: 10.1007/s00167-017-4680-x

[43] Park J-Y, Chang CB, Kang D-W, Oh S, Kang S-B, Lee MC. Development and validation of a prediction model for knee joint line orientation after high tibial osteotomy. BMC Musculoskeletal Disorders. 2019;**20**(1):434. DOI: 10.1186/s12891-019-2820-9

[44] Iseki T, Onishi S, Kanto M, Kanto R, Kambara S, Yoshiya S, et al. Double-level osteotomy for severe varus osteoarthritic knees can prevent change in leg length and restore physiological joint geometry. The Knee. 2021;**31**:136-143. DOI: 10.1016/j.knee.2021.04.011

[45] Seil R, Müller B, Georg T, Kohn D, Rupp S. Reliability and interobserver variability in radiological patellar height ratios. Knee Surgery, Sports Traumatology, Arthroscopy. 2000;**8**(4):231-236. DOI: 10.1007/s001670000121

[46] Brinkman J-M, Lobenhoffer P, Agneskirchner JD, Staubli AE, Wymenga AB, van Heerwaarden RJ. Osteotomies around the knee: Patient selection, stability of fixation and bone healing in high tibial osteotomies. Journal of Bone and Joint Surgery. British Volume (London). 2008;**90-B**(12):1548-1557. DOI: 10.1302/0301-620x.90b12.21198

[47] Lobenhoffer P, Agneskirchner JD. Improvements in surgical technique of valgus high tibial osteotomy. Knee Surgery, Sports Traumatology, Arthroscopy. 2003;**11**(3):132-138. DOI: 10.1007/s00167-002-0334-7

[48] Stoffel K, Willers C, Korshid O, Kuster M. Patellofemoral contact pressure following high tibial osteotomy: A cadaveric study. Knee Surgery, Sports Traumatology, Arthroscopy. 2007;**15**(9):1094-1100. DOI: 10.1007/s00167-007-0297-9

[49] Kurien T, East J, Mandalia V. The effects of open wedge high tibial osteotomy for knee osteoarthritis on the patellofemoral joint. A systematic review. The Knee. 2023;**40**:201-219. DOI: 10.1016/j.knee.2022.11.023

[50] Erquicia J, Gelber PE, Perelli S, Ibañez F, Ibañez M, Pelfort X, et al. Biplane opening wedge high tibial osteotomy with a distal tuberosity osteotomy, radiological and clinical analysis with minimum follow-up of 2 years. Journal of Experimental Orthopaedics. Feb 2019;**6**:10. DOI: 10.1186/s40634-019-0176-6

[51] Alaia MJ, Kaplan DJ, Mannino BJ, Strauss EJ. Tibial sagittal slope in anterior cruciate ligament injury and treatment. The Journal of the American Academy of Orthopaedic Surgeons. 2021;**29**(21):e1045-e1056. DOI: 10.5435/JAAOS-D-21-00143

[52] Ollivier M et al. Infratuberosity anterior closing-wedge high tibial osteotomy for slope correction in anterior cruciate ligament–deficient knees. Arthroscopy Techniques. 2024:103153. DOI: 10.1016/j.eats.2024.103153

[53] Nha KW, Kim HJ, Ahn HS, Lee DH. Change in posterior tibial slope after open-wedge and closed-wedge high tibial osteotomy: A meta-analysis. The American Journal of Sports Medicine. 2016;**44**:3006-3013. DOI: 10.1177/0363546515626172

[54] Eliasberg CD, Hancock KJ, Swartwout E, Robichaud H, Ranawat AS. Theideal hinge axis position to reduce tibial slope in opening-wedge hightibial osteotomy includes proximalization-extension and internal rotation. Arthroscopy. 2021;**37**:1577-1584

[55] Abdelhameed MA, Yang CZ, AlMaeen BN, Jacquet C, Ollivier M. No benefits of knee osteotomy patient's specific instrumentation in experienced surgeon hands. Knee Surgery, Sports Traumatology, Arthroscopy. 2023;**31**(8):3133-3140. DOI: 10.1007/s00167-022-07288-6

[56] Cerciello S, Ollivier M, Corona K, Kaocoglu B, Seil R. CAS and PSI increase coronal alignment accuracy and reduce outliers when compared to traditional technique of medial open wedge high tibial osteotomy: A meta-analysis. Knee Surgery, Sports Traumatology, Arthroscopy. 2022;**30**(2):555-566. DOI: 10.1007/s00167-020-06253-5

[57] Noyes FR, Goebel SX, West J. Opening wedge tibial osteotomy: The 3-triangle method to correct axial alignment and tibial slope. The American Journal of Sports Medicine. 2005;**33**(3):378-387. DOI: 10.1177/0363546504269034

[58] Bae DK, Song SJ, Yoon KH. Closed-wedge high tibial osteotomy using computer-assisted surgery compared to the conventional technique. The Journal of Bone and Joint Surgery British volume [Internet]. 2009;**91-B**(9):1164-1171. DOI: 10.1302/0301-620X.91B9.22058

[59] Aman ZS, DePhillipo NN, Peebles LA, Familiari F, LaPrade RF, Dekker TJ. Improved accuracy of coronal alignment can be attained using 3D-printed patient-specific instrumentation for knee osteotomies: A systematic review of level III and IV studies. Arthroscopy. 2022;**38**(9):2741-2758. DOI: 10.1016/j.arthro.2022.02.023

[60] Jacquet C, Chan-Yu-Kin J, Sharma A, Argenson J-N, Parratte S, Ollivier M. More accurate correction using "patient-specific" cutting guides in opening wedge distal femur varization osteotomies. International Orthopaedics. 2019;**43**(10):2285-2291. DOI: 10.1007/s00264-018-4207-1

[61] Pang R, Jiang Z, Xu C, Shi W, Zhang X, Wan X, et al. Is patient-specific instrumentation accurate and necessary for open-wedge high tibial osteotomy? A meta-analysis. Orthopaedic Surgery. 2023;**15**(2):413-422. DOI: 10.1111/os.13483

[62] Ribeiro CH, Severino NR, de Barros M, Fucs PM. Opening wedge high tibial osteotomy: Navigation system compared to the conventional technique in a controlled clinical study. International Orthopaedics. 2014;**38**(8):1627-1631. DOI: 10.1007/s00264-014-2341-y

[63] Kendoff DO, Fragomen AT, Pearle AD, Citak M, Rozbruch SR. Computer navigation and fixator-assisted femoral osteotomy for correction of malunion after periprosthetic femur fracture. The Journal of Arthroplasty. 2010;**25**(2):333.e13-333.e19. DOI: 10.1016/j.arth.2008.11.102

[64] Young SW, Safran MR, Clatworthy M. Applications of computer navigation in sports medicine knee surgery: An evidence-based review. Current Reviews in Musculoskeletal Medicine. 2013;**6**(2):150-157. DOI: 10.1007/s12178-013-9166-y

[65] Gebhard F, Krettek C, Hüfner T, Grützner PA, Stöckle U, et al. Reliability of computer-assisted surgery as an intraoperative ruler in navigated high tibial osteotomy. Archives of Orthopaedic and Trauma Surgery. 2011;**131**(3):297-302. DOI: 10.1007/s00402-010-1145-9

[66] Coventry MB. Upper tibial osteotomy for gonarthrosis. The evolution of the operation in the last 18 years and long term results. The Orthopedic Clinics of North America. 1979;**10**(1):191-210

[67] Coventry MB, Bowman PW. Long-term results of upper tibial osteotomy for degenerative arthritis of the knee. Acta Orthopaedica Belgica. 1982;**48**(1):139-156

[68] Peng H, Ou A, Huang X, Wang C, Wang L, Yu T, et al. Osteotomy around the knee: The surgical treatment of osteoarthritis. Orthopaedic Surgery. 2021;**13**(5):1465-1473. DOI: 10.1111/os.13021

[69] Gulagaci F, Jacquet C, Ehlinger M, Sharma A, Kley K, Wilson A, et al. A protective hinge wire, intersecting the osteotomy plane, can reduce the occurrence of perioperative hinge fractures in medial opening wedge osteotomy. Knee Surgery, Sports Traumatology, Arthroscopy. 2020;**28**(10):3173-3182. DOI: 10.1007/s00167-019-05806-7

[70] Miltenberg B, Puzzitiello RN, Ruelos VCB, Masood R, Pagani NR, Moverman MA, et al. Incidence of complications and revision surgery after high tibial osteotomy: A systematic review. The American Journal of Sports Medicine. 2024;**52**(1):258-268. DOI: 10.1177/03635465221142868

Chapter 2

High Tibial Osteotomy within the Knee Health Promotion Option for Knee Osteoarthritis

Jung-Pin Hung, Li-Chan Chou and Shaw-Ruey Lyu

Abstract

This chapter explores the utilization of High Tibial Osteotomy (HTO) within the framework of the Knee Health Promotion Option (KHPO) for treating knee osteoarthritis (OA). HTO serves as a fundamental treatment approach, especially in advanced OA cases, showcasing initial success. However, this chapter delves into the comprehensive analysis of HTO, examining survivorship rates, patient-reported outcomes, long-term implications, concerns regarding revision surgeries, and comparisons with other treatment modalities like unicompartmental knee arthroplasty (UKA). Additionally, the chapter discusses advancements in technology, such as patient-specific instrumentation (PSI), and the synergistic effects of the Arthroscopic Cartilage Regeneration Facilitating Procedure (ACRFP) with HTO in optimizing knee health management. The study emphasizes the crucial need for ongoing research efforts to enhance the efficacy of HTO while navigating its limitations in managing knee OA. Through a multidisciplinary approach encompassing surgical advancements, tailored treatment plans, and precise assessments, this chapter provides a roadmap for healthcare practitioners to optimize patient outcomes and revolutionize the management of knee OA within the realm of the KHPO.

Keywords: knee osteoarthritis, cartilage regeneration, high tibial osteotomy, knee health promotion option, medial plica, medial abrasion phenomenon, arthroscopic cartilage regeneration facilitating procedure

1. Introduction

High Tibial Osteotomy (HTO) is a surgical procedure commonly used in the treatment of knee osteoarthritis (OA). This procedure involves realigning the weight-bearing axis of the knee joint to relieve pressure on damaged areas of the joint, thereby addressing symptoms and potentially delaying or avoiding the need for Total Knee Arthroplasty (TKA). HTO has shown promising outcomes in providing pain relief, improving knee function, and slowing down the progression of joint degeneration, particularly in younger and active patients. Recent advancements in surgical techniques and technologies, such as intraoperative navigation and 3-D printing, have enhanced the precision and effectiveness of HTO procedures. However, challenges persist, including the potential need for conversion to TKA in some cases and the long-term effects of HTO on joint health. Future research directions in HTO focus on biomechanics, combination with cartilage repair techniques, postoperative outcomes, and further advancements in surgical methods to optimize patient outcomes and quality of life. Overall, HTO remains a pivotal treatment option for knee OA, particularly in younger and more active demographics, ongoing research endeavors are essential to maximize patient benefits. Continued enhancements in surgical methodologies, precise assessment tools, and individualized treatment strategies hold the potential in optimizing HTO's effectiveness while addressing its inherent limitations in managing knee OA.

This chapter explores the relationship between the medial abrasion phenomenon (MAP) and knee OA, emphasizing MAP's role in the condition's progression. Characterized by repetitive abrasion between the medial plica and femoral condyle, MAP causes physical and chemical damage in the knee joint, leading to cartilage degradation and inflammation. Research highlights the biochemical and histological changes linked to MAP, revealing its impact on cartilage integrity through the expression of matrix metalloproteinases and cytokines.

The proposed Knee Health Promotion Option (KHPO) incorporates findings from MAP research into a comprehensive treatment protocol for managing knee OA. It offers clinical staging and personalized treatment recommendations, starting with Smart Knee Care (SKC), which emphasizes patient education and customized rehabilitation exercises. For more advanced cases, combining the Arthroscopic Cartilage Regeneration Facilitating Procedure (ACRFP) with High Tibial Osteotomy (HTO) provides a promising strategy for preserving knee function and potentially avoiding prosthetic replacements by addressing MAP-related etiological factors and promoting cartilage regeneration.

Recent outcome studies show that these combined treatments lead to high patient satisfaction and observable cartilage regeneration post-surgery. This tailored approach emphasizes the importance of early intervention and personalized care in slowing the progression of knee OA. Overall, the chapter highlights MAP's critical role in knee OA and the effectiveness of targeted interventions such as ACRFP and HTO within the KHPO framework, ultimately aiming to enhance patient outcomes and improve the quality of life for those affected by this debilitating condition.

2. The status and limitation of High Tibial Osteotomy in knee OA treatment

High Tibial Osteotomy (HTO) stands as a fundamental treatment approach for knee osteoarthritis (OA), particularly in advanced cases. While HTO showcases initial success, several aspects and implications must be carefully analyzed for a complete understanding of its status and limitations.

Survivorship and patient-reported outcomes constitute primary evaluation metrics for HTO efficacy. Systematic reviews and meta-analyses [1, 2] have revealed promising results, showing an average survivorship rate of 74.6% at 10-year follow-up, although outcomes may deteriorate over time. Maintaining high functional scores while preserving knee health presents a challenge, especially considering the natural progression of the disease. While HTO is favored among younger patients for its potential to delay or avoid total knee arthroplasty (TKA), the long-term implications raise concerns for both practitioners and patients.

Concerns regarding revision surgeries after HTO failure add further complexity to the debate [3, 4]. Competing analyses suggest that transitioning from HTO to TKA after a failed osteotomy poses challenges, including longer operative times, impacts on postoperative function, and heightened risks of infection and revision compared to primary TKA. This underscores the critical need for thorough research into the effectiveness of osteotomies to ensure significant improvements in patient quality of life.

Comparative studies between HTO and Unicompartmental Knee Arthroplasty (UKA) present differing advantages and outcomes [5, 6]. While UKA may surpass HTO in reducing complications and enhancing postoperative functional scores, choosing between the two remains a nuanced decision. The ongoing debate between HTO and UKA continues, emphasizing the need for tailored treatments based on patient demographics and condition severity.

Emerging technologies like patient-specific instrumentation (PSI) and computer-assisted surgery (CAS) aim to enhance precision and reduce complications in high tibial osteotomies (HTOs) [7–10]. These advancements offer higher accuracy in alignment correction and align with modern trends in improving surgical outcomes. Complementary approaches such as mesenchymal stem cell (MSC) augmentation [11, 12] and cartilage repair techniques [13, 14] showcase potential benefits, albeit with limited data on improved knee function post-surgery [11, 12].

In conclusion, while HTO remains a significant treatment option for knee osteoarthritis, especially in the younger, more active patient population, continued research efforts are vital to optimize patient outcomes. Ongoing advancements in surgical techniques, accurate assessment tools, and tailored treatment plans demonstrate promising prospects in enhancing the efficacy of HTO while addressing its limitations in the management of knee OA.

3. What is a Knee Health Promotion Option?

Knee Health Promotion Option (KHPO) provides a comprehensive approach to managing knee osteoarthritis (OA) through a multidisciplinary treatment plan. This option encompasses prevention to treatment and addresses the medial abrasion phenomenon (MAP) as a contributing factor to knee OA.

3.1 Medial abrasion phenomenon as a cause of knee osteoarthritis

Knee osteoarthritis (OA) poses a significant challenge in the medical field, prompting extensive research to understand its complex mechanisms and potential causes. One prevailing factor under scrutiny is the medial abrasion phenomenon (MAP), speculated to play a crucial role in the pathogenesis and progression of knee OA.

In knees with medial plica and MAP, the repetitive abrasion and impingement between the medial plica and medial femoral condyle result in both physical and chemical damages to adjacent cartilage and the plica itself. Studies have unveiled that most patients with chronic knee pain harbor signs of medial plica, often leading to knee OA diagnoses [15]. Subtle cartilage lesions, known as "hidden lesions," often remain unseen during routine examinations but become apparent post-medial release. These findings underscore the interplay between medial plica and knee degeneration [16].

Notable experimental studies on the tensile strength and histomorphology of the medial plica have provided valuable insights. Investigations into Young's modulus of the plica and topographic changes during knee motion offer a deeper understanding of cartilage stresses and lesions in OA knees. Finite element models have bolstered these findings, showcasing the damaging effects of advanced medial plica on chondrocytes and cartilage [17–19]. Histological analyses further underline the relationship between medial plica and cartilage degradation, reinforcing the critical role of MAP in knee OA development [20].

Examinations into the expression of matrix metalloproteinases (MMPs), interleukins, and tumor necrosis factors in the plica and accompanying tissues elucidate the biochemical underpinnings of knee OA pathogenesis. Elevated levels of cytokines and extracellular matrix degradation enzymes in the plicae of OA knees underscore their

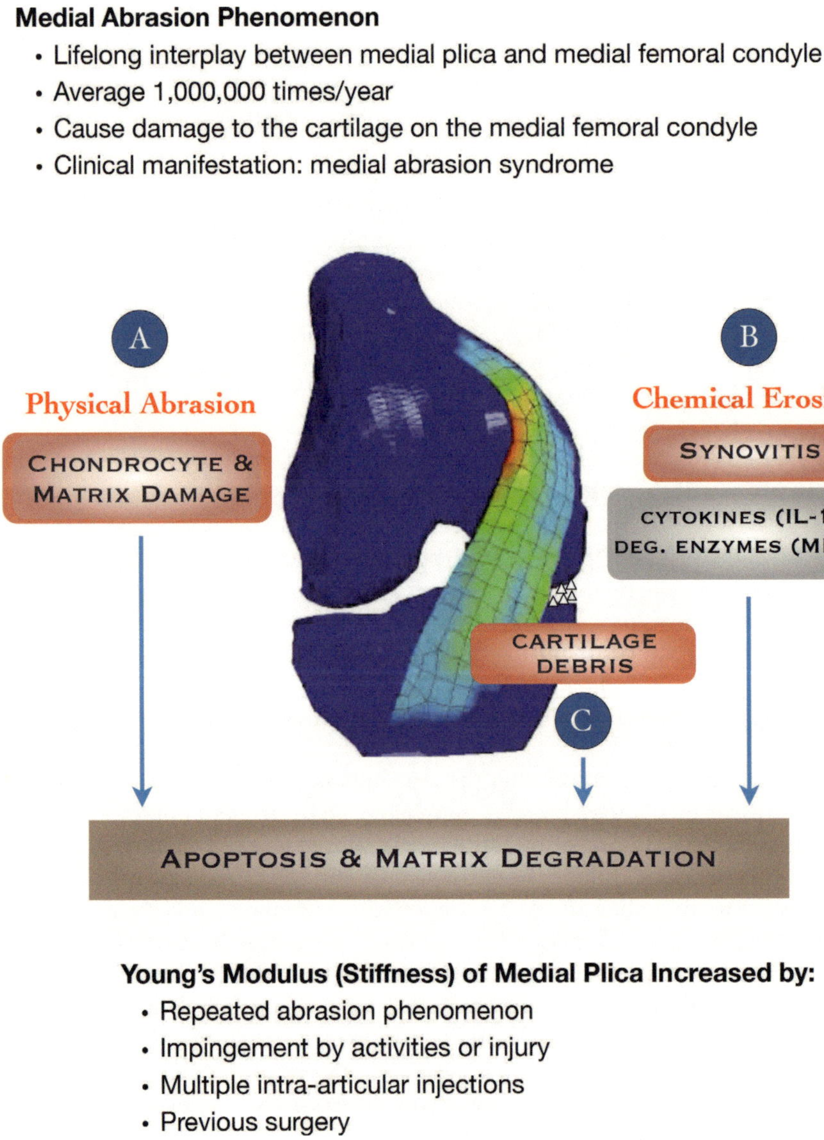

Figure 1.
Medial abrasion phenomenon as a cause of knee osteoarthritis.

contributory role in cartilage breakdown and pathology progression, highlighting the significance of MAP in these processes [21, 22].

The comprehensive synthesis of clinical observations, experimental data, and biochemical profiling underscores the intricate relationship between MAP and knee OA (**Figure 1**) [23]. These insights shed light on the multifaceted mechanisms of OA development and progression, emphasizing the need for targeted therapeutic interventions addressing MAP-induced pathology. Personalized treatment strategies and disease management are warranted to alleviate the burden of knee OA and enhance patient outcomes.

3.2 The conceptualization of Knee Health Promotion Option

The integrated treatment protocol for knee osteoarthritis (OA), illustrated in **Figure 2**, has been designated as the "Knee Health Promotion Option (KHPO)." This

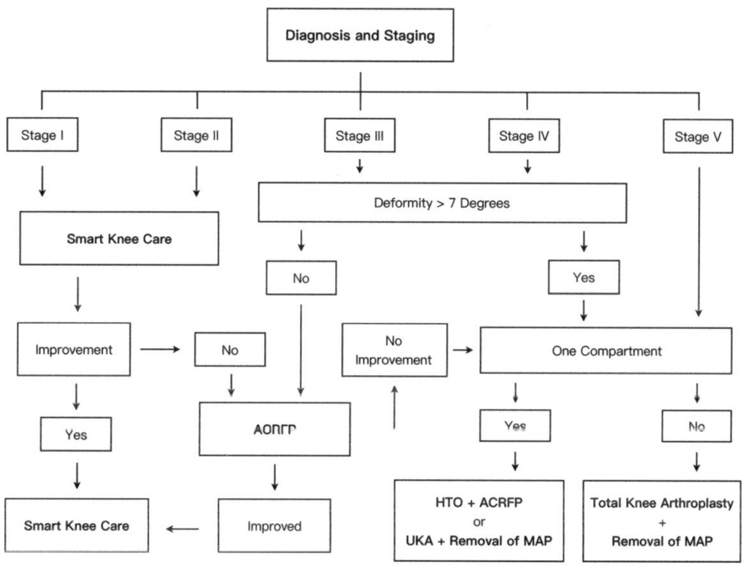

Figure 2.
Protocol of Knee Health Promotion Option for knee OA. ACRFP: arthroscopic cartilage regeneration facilitating procedure; HTO: high tibial osteotomy; UKA: unicompartmental knee arthroplasty; MAP: medial abrasion phenomenon.

Stage	Roentgenographic findings		Clinical findings	
	Joint space narrowing	Osteophyte	Deformity	Stability
I	Doubtful	No	Normal	Stable
II	Definite, less than 1/2	Doubtful	< 5°	Stable
III	Marked, more than 1/2	Definite	> 5°	Stable
IV	Complete obliterated	Marked	> 5°	Stable
V	Complete obliterated	Marked	> 5°	Unstable

Table 1.
Clinical staging for OA of individual compartments based on roentgenographic and clinical findings.

protocol is applied in the management of OA knees, incorporating the insights from our research on the medial abrasion phenomenon (MAP) as a contributing factor to knee OA [24].

In the KHPO protocol, the initial step involved determining the clinical stage for each compartment of the knee through roentgenographic examination, which included standing anteroposterior, lateral, and Merchant's views. The assessment focused on parameters such as the degree of joint space narrowing, the presence of osteophytes, and the alignment measured by the femorotibial angle, as outlined in **Table 1**. The most advanced stage identified among the three compartments was considered the diagnosed stage of osteoarthritis for the entire knee.

Upon determining the clinical stage of the knee, the appropriate treatment option can be selected based on the guidelines provided in **Table 2**. For patients in stages I–II, Smart Knee Care (SKC) is the preferred choice. Stage III patients are best suited for Arthroscopic Cartilage Regeneration Facilitating Procedure (ACRFP). In the case of stage IV patients, while arthroplasty is typically recommended, ACRFP remains a valuable option depending on the patient's biopsychosocial circumstances and preferences. Unicompartmental Knee Arthroplasty (UKA) is recommended as the primary choice for stage IV or V OA affecting a single compartment. Total Knee Arthroplasty (TKA) is advised for stage IV or V OA involving multiple compartments. In some

Stage	SKC	ACRFP	HTO	UKA	TKA
I	++++	—	—	—	—
II	++++	+++	—	—	—
III	+++	++++	+	++	—
IV	+++	++	+	++++	+++
V	+++	—	—	+++	++++

SKC: smart knee care; ACRFP: arthroscopic cartilage regeneration facilitating procedure; HTO: high tibial osteotomy; UKA: unicompartmental knee arthroplasty; TKA: total knee arthroplasty.

Table 2.
Treatment guidelines for knee OA.

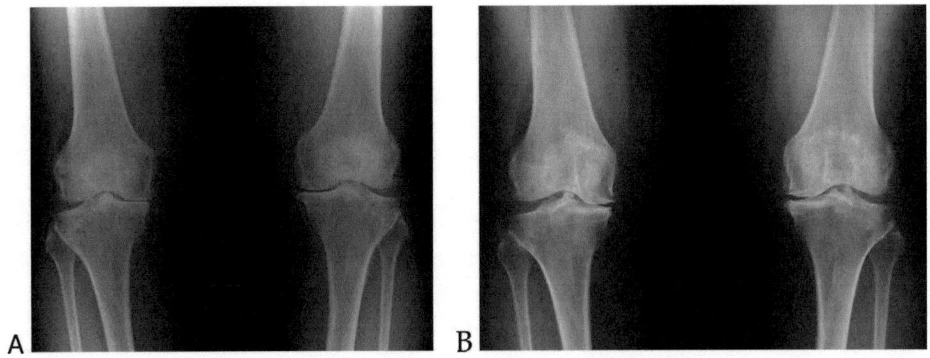

Figure 3.
An illustration of the effects of SKC on halting knee cartilage degeneration and promoting its regeneration. (A) Anteroposterior standing view of a 65-year-old female patient diagnosed with stage III osteoarthritis in the medial compartment of both knees, for which SKC was recommended and performed; and (B) one year later, significant radiographic improvements were observed in both knees.

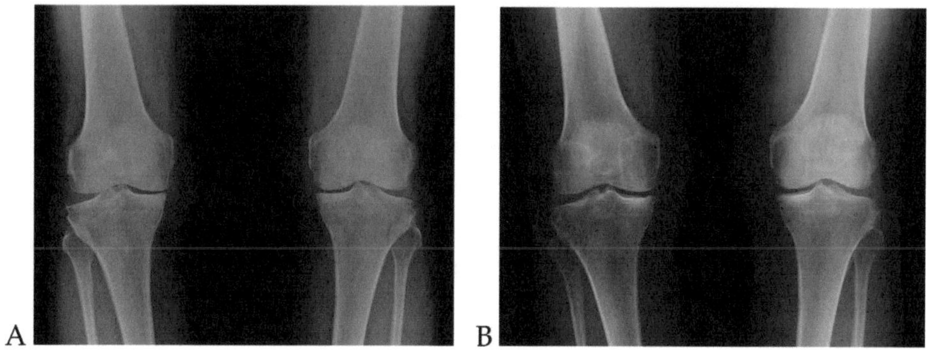

Figure 4.
Another illustration of the impact of SKC on halting knee cartilage degeneration and promoting its regeneration. (A) Anteroposterior standing view of a 61-year-old male patient diagnosed with stage III osteoarthritis in the medial compartment of both knees, for which SKC was recommended and performed; and (B) one year later, significant radiographic improvements were noted in both knees.

instances, High Tibial Osteotomy (HTO) may be recommended for younger, active patients with stage III or IV OA.

Patients are advised to undergo supervised conservative treatment, known as "Smart Knee Care (SKC)", for a minimum of 3 months before considering surgery, as an integral part of the Knee Health Promotion Option (KHPO). The success of SKC hinges on ensuring that patients and their families grasp the essence of KHPO, with a specific focus on understanding the role of the medial abrasion phenomenon (MAP) as a key contributor to knee issues.

Tailored adjustments to daily routines, work tasks, and exercise regimens are personalized for each patient to mitigate the impact of MAP. Activities or exercises that entail repetitive or swift knee bending are generally discouraged to prevent exacerbating MAP. Home-based rehabilitation exercises, incorporating muscle strengthening and soft tissue stretching around the knee are prescribed. The adherence of patients to the exercise plan is vigilantly overseen by our case managers and nursing specialists.

Promising outcomes, including evidence of cartilage regeneration post-SKC, are visually emphasized in **Figures 3** and **4**, underscoring the beneficial impact of this tailored care approach on patient recovery and knee health.

In adherence to the KHPO protocol, if Smart Knee Care (SKC) does not yield the desired results, the next step involves exploring knee preservation options such as Arthroscopic Cartilage Regeneration Facilitating Procedure (ACRFP), High Tibial Osteotomy (HTO), and Unicompartmental Knee Arthroplasty (UKA) before considering Total Knee Arthroplasty (TKA) as a potential treatment.

4. High Tibial Osteotomy under Knee Health Promotion Option

Within the framework of the Knee Health Promotion Option (KHPO), the combined approach of Arthroscopic Cartilage Regeneration Facilitating Procedure (ACRFP) and High Tibial Osteotomy (HTO) has the potential to yield favorable long-term results. This combined strategy aims to address the etiological factors associated with the medial abrasion phenomenon (MAP) by employing ACRFP, thereby enhancing the overall effectiveness of HTO within a comprehensive knee health management paradigm.

4.1 Arthroscopic Cartilage Regeneration Facilitating Procedure

Arthroscopic Cartilage Regeneration Facilitating Procedure (ACRFP) [25, 26], a minimally invasive arthroscopic procedure, plays a pivotal role in the clinical effectiveness of the Knee Health Promotion Option (KHPO) protocol. What sets ACRFP apart from traditional arthroscopic knee OA procedures is its unique ability to address the root cause of the condition. Unlike mainstream techniques, ACRFP specifically targets and removes the problematic and abrasive medial plica along with the consequences of the medial abrasion phenomenon. By eliminating these factors, ACRFP creates a more conducive environment within the joint, allowing damaged articular cartilage to regenerate. This distinction is crucial as it addresses the underlying cause of knee OA, unlike other procedures that often leave this factor unaddressed, perpetuating the medial abrasion phenomenon (MAP) and associated knee discomfort. Additionally, the anabolic effects of ACRFP go beyond physical abrasion damage and chemical erosion of inflammatory tissues. The procedure also relieves increased static pressure in the patellofemoral joint, a result of chronic inflammation triggered by MAP. These beneficial effects create optimal conditions for cartilage regeneration not only in the medial compartment but also in the lateral and patellofemoral compartments, enhancing the overall success of the treatment.

In our study involving 369 patients with a total of 634 knees who underwent ACRFP and were followed up for over 3 years, we observed an impressive overall satisfaction rate of 91.1% among our patients. Notably, there was a discernible reversal of cartilage degeneration in 80.1% of the entire patient cohort as illustrated in **Figure 5**.

4.2 Surgical procedure of High Tibial Osteotomy combined with ACRFP

When conducting High Tibial Osteotomy (HTO) within the framework of the Knee Health Promotion Option (KHPO), whether utilizing traditional methods or

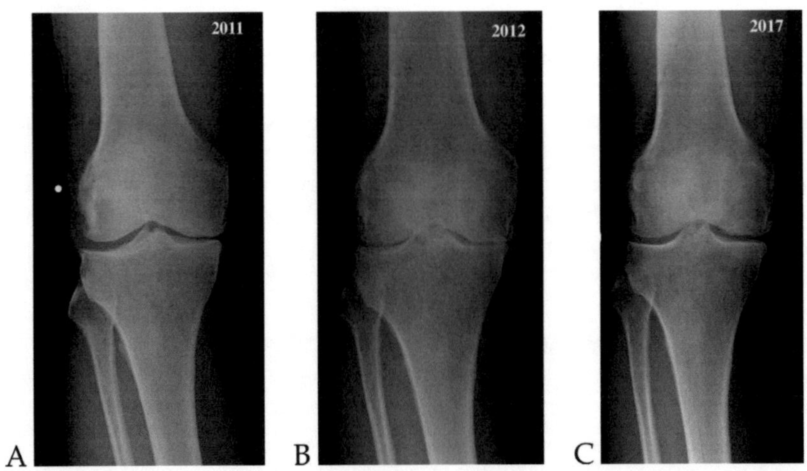

Figure 5.
An example of the effect of ACRFP on halting knee cartilage degeneration and promoting its regeneration. (A) Anteroposterior standing view of a 69-year-old female patient diagnosed with stage III osteoarthritis in the medial compartment of her right knee; (B) following one year of conservative treatment, the condition worsened; and (C) five years after undergoing ACRFP, X-ray images reveal significant improvements in her knee.

patient-specific instrumentation (PSI), the protocol involves initiating the treatment pathway with Arthroscopic Cartilage Regeneration Facilitating Procedure (ACRFP). This step is crucial in addressing the detrimental factors within the joint cavity before proceeding with the HTO, ensuring a comprehensive approach to optimizing the outcomes of the surgical intervention.

4.2.1 Arthroscopic cartilage regeneration facilitating procedure

The arthroscopic procedure commences with examination through the infero-lateral portal to assess the presence of medial abrasive phenomenon (MAP) related to the medial plica. Medial release involves removing inflammatory synovium and the obstructing medial plica in the inferomedial patella region and medial gutter. Subsequently, the constrained medial facet of the patellofemoral joint is freed by the precise severing of the medial retinaculum. Verification of the release's adequacy is ensured by passing an arthroscope under the patella, confirming increased space, and visualizing the medial retinaculum. Post-release, the patella shifts laterally. A sharp dissection aids in the lateral release by percutaneously cutting the lateral retinaculum with a No. 11 scalpel through the inferolateral portal. Assessment of the release's effectiveness is visually confirmed *via* arthroscopy. Any focal synovitis or chondral flaps on the cartilage surface are addressed through standard arthroscopic debridement, without involving bone procedures like drilling or microfracture. Postoperative care focuses on activating the degenerated cartilage's innate repair capabilities, aiming to prevent scar contracture and the recurrence of the medial abrasion phenomenon during the initial 3 months. Rehabilitation includes gentle exercises, avoidance of repetitive knee bending, and following strict guidelines on daily activities and exercises for optimal cartilage regeneration throughout the first year post-surgery.

4.2.2 High Tibial Osteotomy utilizing traditional methods

The surgical procedure for High Tibial Osteotomy (HTO) utilizing the traditional open wedge method involves a systematic approach to realign the knee joint and alleviate pressure on the damaged or worn-out area. In this method, a surgical incision is made along the front of the knee to access the tibia bone. The bone is then carefully cut to create a wedge-shaped opening, enabling the alignment of the leg to be adjusted as per the preoperative planning. Once the correction is achieved, the gap created in the tibia bone is typically filled with bone graft material to support the realigned position. Fixation hardware, such as plates and screws, is used to secure the bone in its new position, allowing for proper healing and stability. Postoperatively, patients undergo a structured rehabilitation program to facilitate recovery, regain strength, and improve the functionality of the knee joint.

4.2.3 High Tibial Osteotomy utilizing patient-specific instrumentation

The surgical procedure for High Tibial Osteotomy (HTO) with Patient-Specific Instrumentation (PSI) involves comprehensive preoperative planning, utilizing imaging studies to create a 3D knee model for precise correction assessment. Custom cutting guides are then designed based on this model to ensure accurate realignment during the surgery. Under appropriate anesthesia, an incision is made, and with the assistance of the custom guides, the surgeon performs the osteotomy on the tibia bone, shifting weight-bearing forces as planned. Following successful realignment, fixation devices are used to secure the bone. Postoperatively, the incision is closed, and patients are provided with care instructions, such as weight-bearing limitations and physical therapy, for optimal healing and rehabilitation progress. This tailored approach with PSI enhances surgical precision, alignment, and potential outcomes in knee osteoarthritis management.

4.2.4 Outcome

In 2013, 521 patients underwent surgical treatments based on the Knee Health Promotion Option (KHPO) protocol for various stages of knee osteoarthritis (OA), totaling 872 knees (**Table 3**). These patients were monitored for over 5 years in an outcome study. After the final review, a subjective assessment indicated a satisfactory outcome in 812 knees, representing 93.1% of the cases as per **Table 4**. Specifically, within the High Tibial Osteotomy (HTO) group utilizing the traditional open wedge

	ACRFP	AMR	HTO	UKA	TKA	Total
Age (SD) No.	68.1 (9.5) 649	76.3* (5.7) 16	54.3* (8.4) 11	72.1* (7.8) 80	74.0* (6.6) 116	69.4 (9.3) 872
F/M (Ratio)	491/158 (3.1)	15/1 (15)	5/6 (0.8)	53/27 (2.0)	95/21 (4.5)	659/213 (3.2)
M/L (Ratio)	608/41 (14.8)	16/0 –	11/0 –	80/0 –	104/12 (8.7)	819/53 (14.9)

**Statistically significant compared to that of the ACRFP group by comparisons for each pair using paired t-test ($p < 0.05$).*

Table 3.
Age, sex, and main involved compartment distribution in different types of surgery.

Operation (N)	E	G	F	P	Sat. (%)
ACRFP (649)	390 (60.1)	201 (31.0)	28 (4.3)	30 (4.6)	91.1
AMR (16)	10 (62.5)	6 (37.5)	0	0	100.0
HTO (11)	9 (81.8)	2 (18.2)	0	0	100.0
UKA (80)	74 (92.5)	5 (6.3)	0	1 (1.2)	98.8
TKA (116)	108 (93.1)	7 (6.0)	0	1 (0.9)	99.1
Total (872)	591 (67.8)	221 (25.3)	28 (3.2)	32 (4.0)	93.1

† E: excellent; G: good; F: fair; P: poor; Sat.: satisfied = E + G.
** Statistically significant by comparisons for each pair using a paired t-test ($p < 0.05$).*

Table 4.
Comparison of satisfactory rates in different surgical groups.

Evaluation metric	Preoperation (SD)	Postoperation (SD)	p-value
OKS	24.1 (3.7)	40.4 (2.5)	<0.001
KSS (pain)	57.0 (5.4)	80.3 (4.6)	<0.001
KSS (function)	57.7 (5.9)	80.6 (5.0)	<0.001

OKS: oxford knee score; KSS: knee society score.

Table 5.
Outcome evaluation of HTO using PSI within the KHPO.

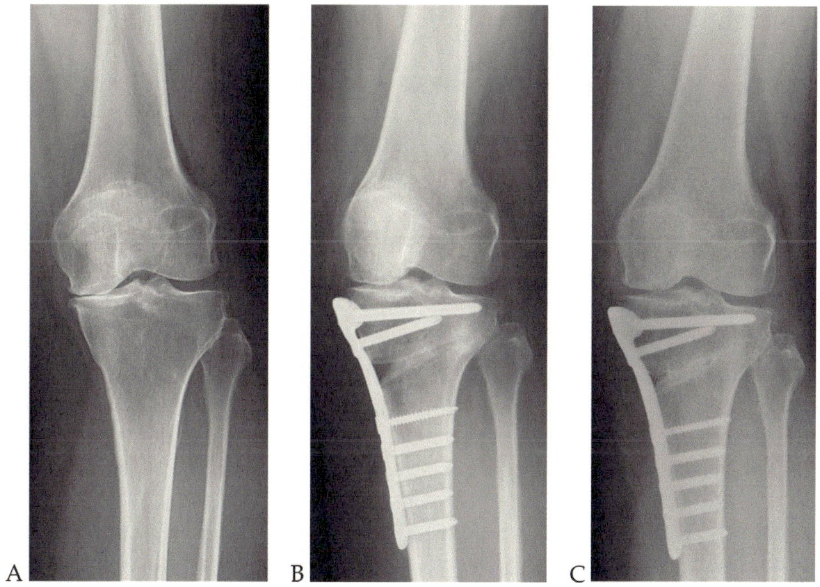

Figure 6.
(A) the preoperative radiograph reveals complete obliteration of the medial compartment; (B) and (C), illustrate progressive cartilage regeneration and the reopening of the joint space in radiographs captured at 3 months and 1 year postoperation, respectively.

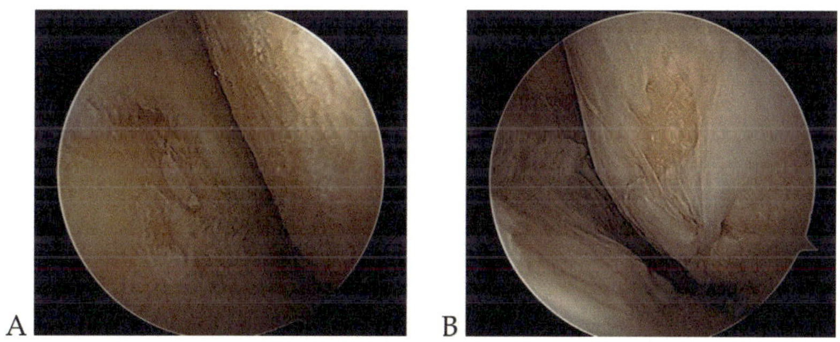

Figure 7.
(A) this arthroscopic image displays complete cartilage loss with bone exposure on both medial femoral condyle and medial tibial plateau, the ACRFP and HTO were performed; and (B) 1 year later, during the same operation when the plate was removed, the second-look arthroscopy reveals substantial cartilage regeneration.

method following the Arthroscopic Cartilage Regeneration Facilitating Procedure (ACRFP), the satisfaction rate stood at a notable 100%, highlighting the effectiveness of this combined approach in managing knee OA.

In the period from 2021 to 2022, 14 patients, aged between 48 and 67 with an average of 58, underwent HTO with Patient-Specific Instrumentation (PSI) following ACRFP. After a follow-up period of over 2 years, all patients reported satisfaction with the outcomes of the procedures. Notable enhancements were seen in both the Oxford Knee Score (OKS) and the Knee Society Score (KSS) across all patients, as outlined in **Table 5**. The success of the treatment was further validated through visible cartilage regeneration observed *via* radiographic examination (**Figure 6**) and second-look arthroscopy (**Figure 7**).

5. Conclusion

This chapter highlights the crucial role of High Tibial Osteotomy (HTO) as an effective intervention for knee OA within the KHPO framework. HTO is particularly beneficial for younger, more active patients and represents a contemporary approach to managing knee osteoarthritis (OA) by tackling the Medial Abrasion Phenomenon (MAP), a significant cause of cartilage degeneration. When combined Arthroscopic Cartilage Regeneration Facilitating Procedure (ACRFP), this approach has led to substantial improvements in patient-reported outcomes and overall satisfaction, underscoring the need to address the underlying factors of knee OA to enhance functionality and quality of life. Although there are promising advancements, challenges remain regarding the long-term success of HTO and the risk of conversion to total knee arthroplasty, calling for further research into its biomechanics, patient outcomes, and conservative management strategies. Ultimately, this chapter advocates for a holistic approach that integrates surgical interventions, innovative technologies, and personalized rehabilitation programs to optimize knee health. By recognizing and addressing factors like MAP, healthcare providers can better manage knee osteoarthritis, improve recovery trajectories, and enhance the quality of life for those affected by this prevalent condition. Through a sustained commitment to research and patient-centered care, the management of knee OA can become increasingly effective and impactful.

Author details

Jung-Pin Hung, Li-Chan Chou and Shaw-Ruey Lyu*
Tzu-Chi Dalin General Hospital, Tzu-Chi University, Taiwan

*Address all correspondence to: srlyu@mac.com

References

[1] Virolainen P, Aro HT. High tibial osteotomy for the treatment of osteoarthritis of the knee: A review of the literature and a meta-analysis of follow-up studies. Archives of Orthopaedic and Trauma Surgery. 2004;**124**(4):258-261. DOI: 10.1007/s00402-003-0545-5

[2] Dal Fabbro G, Grassi A, Agostinone P, Lucidi GA, Fajury R, Ravindra A, et al. High survivorship rate and good clinical outcomes after high tibial osteotomy in patients with radiological advanced medial knee osteoarthritis: A systematic review. Archives of Orthopaedic and Trauma Surgery. 2 Mar 2024. DOI: 10.1007/s00402-024-05254-0. PMID: 38430233 [Epub ahead of print]

[3] Chen X, Yang Z, Li H, Zhu S, Wang Y, Qian W. Higher risk of revision in total knee arthroplasty after high tibial osteotomy: A systematic review and updated meta-analysis. BMC Musculoskeletal Disorders. 2020;**21**(1):153. DOI: 10.1186/s12891-020-3177-9

[4] Sun X, Wang J, Su Z. A meta-analysis of total knee arthroplasty following high tibial osteotomy versus primary total knee arthroplasty. Archives of Orthopaedic and Trauma Surgery. 2020;**140**(4):527-535. DOI: 10.1007/s00402-020-03333-6

[5] Huang L, Xu Y, Wei L, Yuan G, Chen W, Gao S, et al. Unicompartmental knee arthroplasty is superior to high tibial osteotomy for the treatment of medial unicompartmental osteoarthritis: A systematic review and meta-analysis. Medicine (Baltimore). 2022;**101**(30):e29576. DOI: 10.1097/MD.0000000000029576

[6] Santoso MB, Wu L. Unicompartmental knee arthroplasty, is it superior to high tibial osteotomy in treating unicompartmental osteoarthritis? A meta-analysis and systemic review. Journal of Orthopaedic Surgery and Research. 2017;**12**(1):50. DOI: 10.1186/s13018-017-0552-9

[7] Wu ZP, Zhang P, Bai JZ, Liang Y, Chen PT, He JS, et al. Comparison of navigated and conventional high tibial osteotomy for the treatment of osteoarthritic knees with varus deformity: A meta-analysis. International Journal of Surgery. 2018;**55**:211-219. DOI: 10.1016/j.ijsu.2018.03.024

[8] Pang R, Jiang Z, Xu C, Shi W, Zhang X, Wan X, et al. Is patient-specific instrumentation accurate and necessary for open-wedge high Tibial osteotomy? A Meta-Analysis. Journal of Orthopaedic Surgery. 2023;**15**(2):413-422. DOI: 10.1111/os.13483

[9] Cerciello S, Ollivier M, Corona K, Kaocoglu B, Seil R. CAS and PSI increase coronal alignment accuracy and reduce outliers when compared to traditional technique of medial open wedge high tibial osteotomy: A meta-analysis. Knee Surgery, Sports Traumatology, Arthroscopy. 2022;**30**(2):555-566. DOI: 10.1007/s00167-020-06253-5

[10] Dasari SP, Hevesi M, Mameri E, Ferrer-Rivero R, Fortier LM, Jackson GR, et al. Patient-specific instrumentation for medial opening wedge high tibial osteotomies in the management of medial compartment osteoarthritis yields high accuracy and low complication rates: A systematic review. Journal of ISAKOS. 2023;**8**(3):163-176. DOI: 10.1016/j.jisako.2023.02.001

[11] Tan SHS, Kwan YT, Neo WJ, Chong JY, Kuek TYJ, See JZF, et al.

Outcomes of high Tibial osteotomy with versus without mesenchymal stem cell augmentation: A systematic review and meta-analysis. Orthopaedic Journal of Sports Medicine. 2021;**9**(6):23259671211014840. DOI: 10.1177/23259671211014840

[12] Jin L, Yang G, Men X, Zhang J, Chen Z, Li Z, et al. Intra-articular injection of mesenchymal stem cells after high Tibial osteotomy: A systematic review and meta-analysis. Orthopaedic Journal of Sports Medicine. 2022;**10**(11):23259671221133784. DOI: 10.1177/23259671221133784

[13] Lee OS, Ahn S, Ahn JH, Teo SH, Lee YS. Effectiveness of concurrent procedures during high tibial osteotomy for medial compartment osteoarthritis: A systematic review and meta-analysis. Archives of Orthopaedic and Trauma Surgery. 2018;**138**(2):227-236. DOI: 10.1007/s00402-017-2826-4

[14] Yao RZ, Liu WQ, Sun LZ, Yu MD, Wang GL. Effectiveness of high Tibial osteotomy with or without other procedures for medial compartment osteoarthritis of knee: An update meta-analysis. The Journal of Knee Surgery. 2021;**34**(9):952-961. DOI: 10.1055/s-0039-1700978

[15] Lyu SR, Lee CC, Hsu CC. Medial abrasion syndrome: A neglected cause of knee pain in middle and old age. Medicine (Baltimore). 2015;**94**(16):e736. DOI: 10.1097/MD.0000000000000736

[16] Lyu SR, Hsu CC. Medial plicae and degeneration of the medial femoral condyle. Arthroscopy. 2006;**22**(1):17-26. DOI: 10.1016/j.arthro.2005.08.039

[17] Lyu SR, Tzeng JE, Kuo CY, Jian AR, Liu DS. Mechanical strength of mediopatellar plica--the influence of its fiber content. Clinical Biomechanics (Bristol, Avon). 2006;**21**(8):860-863. DOI: 10.1016/j.clinbiomech.2006.03.010

[18] Lyu SR. Relationship of medial plica and medial femoral condyle during flexion. Clinical Biomechanics (Bristol, Avon). 2007;**22**(9):1013-1016. DOI: 10.1016/j.clinbiomech.2007.08.001

[19] Liu DS, Zhuang ZW, Lyu SR. Relationship between medial plica and medial femoral condyle--a three-dimensional dynamic finite element model. Clinical Biomechanics (Bristol, Avon). 2013;**28**(9-10):1000-1005. DOI: 10.1016/j.clinbiomech.2013.09.012

[20] Lyu SR, Chiang JK, Tseng CE. Medial plica in patients with knee osteoarthritis: A histomorphological study. Knee Surgery, Sports Traumatology, Arthroscopy. 2010;**8**(6):769-776. DOI: 10.1007/s00167-009-0946-2

[21] Wang HS, Kuo PY, Yang CC, Lyu SR. Matrix metalloprotease-3 expression in the medial plica and pannus-like tissue in knees from patients with medial compartment osteoarthritis. Histopathology. 2011;**58**(4):593-600. DOI: 10.1111/j.1365-2559.2011.03783.x

[22] Yang CC, Lin CY, Wang HS, Lyu SR. Matrix metalloproteases and tissue inhibitors of metalloproteinases in medial plica and pannus-like tissue contribute to knee osteoarthritis progression. PLoS One. 2013;**8**(11):e79662. DOI: 10.1371/journal.pone.0079662

[23] Lyu SR, Chiang CY, Cherng JY, Huang YC, Li CH, Lin YJ, et al. Role of medial abrasion phenomenon in the pathogenesis of knee osteoarthritis. Medical Hypotheses. 2015;**85**(2):207-211. DOI: 10.1016/j.mehy.2015.04.028

[24] Lyu S-R. Knee health promotion option for knee osteoarthritis: A

preliminary report of a concept of multidisciplinary management. Healthy Aging Research (www.har-journal.com). 2015;**4**:34

[25] Lyu SR, Hsu CC, Lin CW. Arthroscopic cartilage regeneration facilitating procedure for osteoarthritic knee. BMC Musculoskeletal Disorders. 2012;**21**(13):226. DOI: 10.1186/1471-2474-13-226

[26] Lyu SR, Hsu CC, Hung JP, Chou LC, Chen YR, Lin CW. Arthroscopic cartilage regeneration facilitating procedure: A decompressing arthroplasty for knee osteoarthritis. Medicine (Baltimore). 2022;**101**(39):e30895. DOI: 10.1097/MD.0000000000030895

Chapter 3

Concomitant High Tibial Osteotomy with Medial Meniscus Posterior Root Repair in Medial Knee Joint Osteoarthritis

Kyun-Ho Shin and Seung-Beom Han

Abstract

Medial knee joint osteoarthritis with varus alignment significantly impairs mobility and quality of life. Combining high tibial osteotomy (HTO) with medial meniscus posterior root tear (MMPRT) repair offers a comprehensive solution. This chapter reviews the anatomical, biomechanical, and clinical aspects of MMPRTs and varus malalignment, discussing diagnostic imaging techniques, treatment options, and outcomes of HTO and MMPRT repair both individually and in combination. Detailed surgical techniques for concurrent HTO and MMPRT repair are outlined. The combination of HTO and MMPRT repair corrects malalignment, restores meniscal function, and redistributes joint load, thereby improving meniscal healing and patient outcomes compared to HTO alone. While short-term benefits are noted, the long-term benefits on cartilage status and overall outcomes remain to be clarified, necessitating further research to confirm these advantages and optimize surgical methods.

Keywords: meniscal root tears, varus knee deformities, high tibial osteotomy, meniscus repair, osteoarthritis, knee

1. Introduction

Medial meniscal posterior root tears (MMPRTs) can lead to osteoarthritis (OA) progression, as the loss of meniscal hoop tension results in elevated contact pressure within the medial compartment [1, 2]. The goal of arthroscopic MMPRT repair is to restore the hoop tension and prevent further denudation of the medial tibiofemoral cartilage. Meniscal healing and long-term success following MMPRT repair are significantly influenced by varus deformity in the lower limbs, a common condition in medial knee OA [3–7]. Alleviating the medial compartment overload requires not only MMPRT repair but also correction of the varus deformity for optimal outcomes.

Medial open-wedge high tibial osteotomy (HTO) is a joint preserving surgery used to treat medial compartment OA associated with varus malalignment. The procedure works by redistributing the weight-bearing load away from the medial compartment, which helps to increase the medial proximal tibial angle and lower the pressure in the medial compartment [8–10]. While this procedure can help cover damaged articular cartilage and slow the progression of OA, the fibrous cartilage that forms may not be as high-quality as the original hyaline cartilage [11–15]. Furthermore, second-look arthroscopy after HTO alone frequently reveals that MMPRTs have either incompletely healed or show laxity [16–18].

The primary objective of joint preservation surgeries is to delay the necessity of total knee arthroplasty. Consequently, combining MMPRT repair with HTO may be an optimal strategy to slow OA progression by restoring medial meniscal hoop tension and reducing tibiofemoral contact pressure. Despite the absence of randomized controlled trials or large-scale cohort studies, systematic reviews present conflicting evidence on whether MMPRT repair by itself or in combination with HTO provides superior patient outcomes [19, 20]. This chapter comprehensively reviews current knowledge on concurrent MMPRT repair with high tibial osteotomy, including cutting-edge techniques and clinical, radiological, and arthroscopic outcomes.

2. Anatomical and biomechanical understanding of MMPRT

The medial meniscus posterior root (MMPR), where the posterior horn of the medial meniscus attaches to the tibia, acts as a ligament-like structure that secures the meniscus to the tibia. The shift in structure from the fibrocartilaginous body of the meniscus to a ligament-like form plays a crucial role in facilitating the effective transfer of load from the meniscus to the bone [21]. These mechanical properties enable the MMPR to stabilize the meniscus between the femoral condyle and the tibial plateau, ensuring efficient load transfer [1]. The MMPR attaches approximately 9.6 mm posterior and 0.7 mm lateral to the apex of the medial tibial eminence, covering an area of approximately 30.4 mm^2 [22]. According to Pagnani et al., MMPRTs are the most common type of meniscal root tears, which typically occur within 1 cm of the root attachment and can manifest as either radial tears or avulsion injuries [23, 24].

According to the classification system by LaPrade et al., these injuries can be categorized as follows: (1) type 1, partial stable tear; (2) type 2, complete radial tear; (3) type 3, bucket-handle tear with meniscus root detachment; (4) type 4, complex oblique tear extending into the root attachment; and (5) type 5, avulsion fracture of the root attachment [25]. Types 1, 2, and 4 are associated with both acute and chronic MMPRTs, while types 3 and 5 are typically seen in acute traumatic injuries, helping to predict the tear's chronicity. Among these, type 2 is the most common [25, 26].

3. Epidemiology and clinical presentation

By disrupting the meniscal hoop structure, MMPRTs greatly elevate the likelihood of developing knee osteoarthritis, representing 10–21% of all meniscus injuries [19, 27–30]. These tears can arise from either degenerative changes or acute traumatic incidents [31]. Degenerative MMPRTs typically develop during routine activities, such as walking or descending stairs, and often occur without any accompanying acute injuries to other knee structures [32].

The risk factors for degenerative MMPRT include advanced age, female gender, a sedentary lifestyle, obesity, and varus knee alignment [27, 32]. An increased medial tibial slope also raises the risk for degenerative MMPRT [28]. Degenerative MMPRTs occur more frequently than traumatic tears and are more prone to rupture compared to root tears in other areas [31]. The medial meniscus posterior horn bears a substantial amount of the load applied to the knee joint, including both compressive and shear forces [33]. Furthermore, the MMPR exhibits the least mobility compared to other meniscus roots, making it especially susceptible to degenerative tears [34]. According to Park et al., there is a significant relationship between the extent of MMPR degeneration and the severity of MMPRT. They also observed that degeneration, often marked by fibrocartilage metaplasia or calcification, may precede the occurrence of MMPRT [35]. MMPRTs often happen during simple movements like squatting, standing up from a chair, or climbing stairs [3, 36]. Unlike other types of meniscus tears, MMPRTs are usually marked by a distinct onset of symptoms, often described as a painful popping sensation. In fact, about 85–91% of patients are able to pinpoint the exact moment their symptoms began [5, 37]. Bae et al. reported that experiencing a single painful popping sensation is a strong clinical indicator for diagnosing MMPRTs, with a positive predictive value of 96.5% [38].

The majority of traumatic MMPRTs is typically associated with knee ligament injuries, especially involving the anterior cruciate ligament [39]. These tears are especially common in instances of multi-ligament injuries [40–42], and the presence of varus injury patterns heightens the risk of these tears [41]. The occurrence of traumatic MMPRTs in conjunction with knee ligament injuries is reported to be between 3 and 14% [40–42].

During a physical examination, indicators like pain during full flexion, joint line tenderness, and a positive McMurray test may be assessed; however, none of these findings are definitive for diagnosing MMPRTs [36, 43]. The Akmese sign, defined by severe medial joint line tenderness when the knee is nearly extended and minimal tenderness during hyperflexion, has been proposed as a novel approach to differentiate MMPRTs from other medial meniscus injuries. It has shown high levels of sensitivity and specificity [44].

4. Diagnostic imaging

Magnetic resonance imaging (MRI) remains the most reliable method for diagnosing MMPRTs, offering excellent sensitivity, specificity, and overall accuracy (**Figure 1**) [45]. T2-weighted sequences are especially effective in detecting MMPRTs [45]. Key MRI indicators include vertical high-intensity signals at the MMPR on coronal and axial views, along with the appearance of the "ghost sign" on sagittal images [46–48]. Medial meniscus extrusion seen on the coronal plane, which reflects medial displacement of the meniscus in relation to the tibial plateau, can serve as a predictor of MMPRTs [49–51]. According to Choi et al., an extrusion of more than 3 mm is linked to a higher likelihood of MMPRT occurrence [49]. Comprehensive evaluation of these MRI findings allows for accurate MMPRT diagnosis [46, 48]. Preoperative radiographic evaluation should consist of weight-bearing anteroposterior, lateral, and skyline views. The Rosenberg view (a 45-degree flexion, weight-bearing postero-anterior view) is more effective at detecting joint space narrowing compared to standard weight-bearing AP radiographs [52]. In patients with MMPRTs, weight-bearing knee radiographs often reveal reduced medial joint space, likely resulting from osteoarthritis and medial meniscus subluxation [53–55].

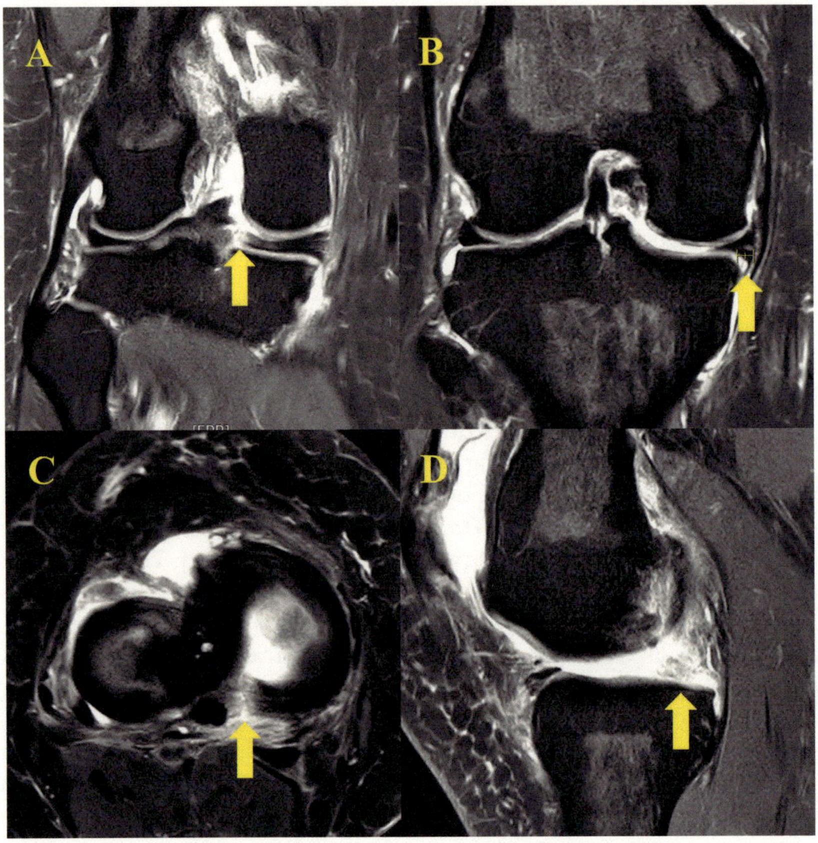

Figure 1.
Characteristic magnetic resonance imaging findings indicating a medial meniscus posterior root tear (A) Coronal image showing a vertical high signal, also known as the truncation or cleft sign (yellow arrow). (B) Coronal image displaying meniscus extrusion (yellow arrow). (C) Axial image highlighting a vertical high signal (yellow arrow). (D) Sagittal image demonstrating the loss of a clearly identifiable medial meniscus posterior root, referred to as the ghost sign (yellow arrow).

Bilateral weight-bearing long leg radiographs (LLR) are widely recognized as the gold standard for evaluating coronal plane alignment of the lower limbs. To ensure reliable and accurate measurements, it is important to use standardized imaging techniques. Detecting deformities such as malrotation or fixed flexion is essential, as they can greatly affect the accuracy and utility of the LLR [56]. Identifying these problems preoperatively is crucial for minimizing potential errors. The joint line congruence angle, typically 2° or less, can highlight intra-articular deformities stemming from medial compartment cartilage damage or increased lateral soft tissue laxity. Detecting lateral joint space widening before surgery is vital, as it tends to reduce after osteotomy. Failure to consider this can result in significant over-correction [57, 58]. When the lateral joint space opening exceeds 5 mm on a weight-bearing LLR, it signals a significant varus deformity that should be factored into surgical planning [59]. One simple method to account for this is by using supine non-weight-bearing long leg radiographs to determine the correction angle, or by comparing the lateral joint space width between the affected and contralateral limbs and subtracting this difference from the calculated opening gap [58].

5. Treatment options and outcomes

Treatment strategies for MMPRTs with varus malalignment include non-surgical management, MMPRT repair alone, HTO alone, or a combination of MMPRT repair and HTO. While non-operative methods and partial meniscectomy were historically more prevalent, the emphasis on surgical repair has grown as the biomechanical significance of the MMPR has become clearer [1, 2, 60, 61]. Patients with varus alignment exceeding 5° tend to have less favorable outcomes after MMPRT repair [6, 7]. Previous research has shown that individuals with varus alignment greater than 5° fare worse compared to those with less severe varus deformities [7]. A long-term study following 37 patients who underwent pullout repair found that 8 eventually progressed to total knee arthroplasty over a period of more than 10 years [6]. These 8 patients who required total knee arthroplasty had greater degrees of varus alignment, larger affected areas, and greater progression in meniscus extrusion compared to the others. The researchers proposed that a varus alignment of 5 degrees and a 0.7 mm increase in meniscus extrusion between preoperative and 1-year postoperative measurements could be used as cutoff values to predict MMPRT repair failure.

Theoretically, HTO can correct the malalignment of the lower limb, thereby improving stress distribution on the meniscus and accelerating its healing. HTO corrects the mechanical axis of the lower limb, which improves stress distribution and supports meniscal healing. This alignment correction is crucial for redistributing load away from the damaged meniscus, thus facilitating better healing outcomes.

HTO addresses lower limb malalignment by realigning the mechanical axis, which optimizes stress distribution across the meniscus and promotes its healing. By shifting the load away from the injured meniscus, HTO plays a pivotal role in enhancing the meniscal healing process and improving overall outcomes. Proper alignment correction is key to reducing the strain on the damaged area, allowing for more effective recovery. While combining MMPRT repair with HTO may enhance healing, research indicates no significant short-term advantage over HTO alone regarding cartilage health or patient-reported outcomes. According to studies, all-inside repair methods for MMPRT, along with medial open-wedge HTO, have shown higher healing rates and cartilage regeneration in the medial condyles. However, improved healing of MMPRTs did not correlate with better clinical results, as reflected by Hospital for Special Surgery scores and the Lysholm score scale [62]. In a similar study, researchers reported higher MMPRT healing rates but no significant differences were found in radiological and clinical outcomes. These included medial meniscal extrusion, medial joint space width, Kellgren-Lawrence grade, hip-knee-ankle angle, weight-bearing line ratio, Knee Society score, and Western Ontario and McMaster University score [63]. Similarly, other research have observed no significant clinical advantages of combining MMPRT repairs with HTO, as indicated by the Lysholm score, Hospital for Special Surgery score, hip-knee-ankle angle, and weight-bearing line ratio. The primary benefit observed was an increase in meniscal healing rates [64]. Another study suggests that performing MMPRT repair together with HTO may improve arthroscopic findings, showing better healing of the MMPR and signs of cartilage regeneration during second-look procedures [65]. Despite these arthroscopic improvements, the combined approach does not lead to significant improvements in clinical or radiologic outcomes in the short term. Evaluated metrics, such as the Lysholm score, International Knee Documentation Committee subjective score, Tegner activity scale, and Kellgren-Lawrence grade, showed no notable differences [65]. A previous systematic review also concluded that concurrent MMPRT repair during HTO has minimal benefits on clinical, radiological, and arthroscopic outcomes in the short term [19].

Most second-look arthroscopies show no difference in cartilage recovery between patients with and without concurrent MMPRT repair. Jing et al. reported complete coverage of preoperative cartilage defects in the medial femoral condyles on second-look arthroscopy [62]. Kim et al. reported improved Outerbridge grades of the medial femoral condyle after HTO with concurrent MMPRT repair [66]. Lee et al. and Ke et al. reported favorable medial compartment coverage with no significant intergroup differences assessed by ICRS and Outerbridge grading systems, respectively [64, 65]. Long-term benefits of concurrent MMPRT repair during HTO, particularly in cartilage recovery and disease progression, require reassessment in long-term follow-up studies.

Most second-look arthroscopies reveal no significant difference in cartilage recovery between patients who underwent concurrent MMPRT repair and those who did not. One study observed complete coverage of preoperative cartilage defects in the medial femoral condyles during second-look arthroscopy [62]. Another reported improvement in the Outerbridge grades of the medial femoral condyle following HTO combined with MMPRT repair [66]. Further research also indicated favorable medial compartment coverage, though no significant differences were found between groups based on ICRS and Outerbridge grading systems [64, 65]. The potential long-term advantages of performing MMPRT repair alongside HTO, especially regarding cartilage restoration and slowing disease progression, need further investigation in long-term follow-up studies.

6. Surgical techniques

For patients diagnosed with MMPRTs and varus malalignment, surgical repair is essential to avoid meniscectomy. The criteria for concurrent surgical repair of MMPRTs and HTO include patients typically under the age of 70 years, radiographic osteoarthritis grade ≤ 3 according to the Kellgren-Lawrence grading system, pathologic varus alignment of the lower extremity (hip-knee-ankle angle $>5°$), and willingness to adhere to a strict postoperative rehabilitation program. If these criteria are not met, non-operative treatment should be considered based on the patient's knee pathology, characteristics, comorbidities, and treatment preferences.

The repair methods for MMPRTs include suture anchor repair and transtibial pull-out repair. Suture anchor repair involves placing a suture anchor on the MMPRT region above the posterior tibial plateau [3, 67–70]. It reduces risks associated with long meniscus-suture constructs, such as the bungee effect, micromotion, and suture material abrasion [71, 72]. This method is technically demanding and requires a high posteromedial working portal and specialized instruments [73].

In transtibial pull-out repair, suture strands are stitched on the torn edge of the MMPRT and pulled through a transosseous tunnel from the MMPRT footprint to the tibia's outer cortex, with fixation above the anterior tibial cortex. This method may face issues like micromotion and suture abrasion, but it is widely used [71, 72, 74]. Studies indicate no significant differences in outcomes between suture anchor and transtibial pull-out repairs [3].

Proper handling of the medial collateral ligament (MCL) is crucial to prevent insufficiency. Two approaches are commonly used: MCL transection or subperiosteal elevation during HTO and MCL pie crusting at the joint line during MMPRT repair. Performing MCL release twice can lead to MCL insufficiency and valgus instability, complicating future revision of total knee arthroplasty. Therefore, MCL handling should be done only once, typically during the HTO approach. The medial approach for proximal tibia is performed first, followed by arthroscopic procedures for MMPRT repair with a widened medial joint space.

To avoid interference between locking screws of the HTO plate and tibial bone tunnels required for MMPRT repair, suture anchor repair is preferred. Although technically demanding, it prevents conflicts between locking screws and tibial bone tunnels. If bone quality is low, suture anchor repair is abandoned in favor of transosseous repair via a tibial bone tunnel. Avoiding the anteromedial tibial cortex position is crucial to prevent interference with locking screws [75]. For the posteromedial tibial cortex position, anterior placement of the locking plate can help avoid interference. When positioning the tibial tunnel in the anterolateral cortex, attention is needed to avoid interference with most proximal screws.

The detailed surgical steps are as follows: First, a diagnostic arthroscopy is performed via the parapatellar high anterolateral portal to evaluate

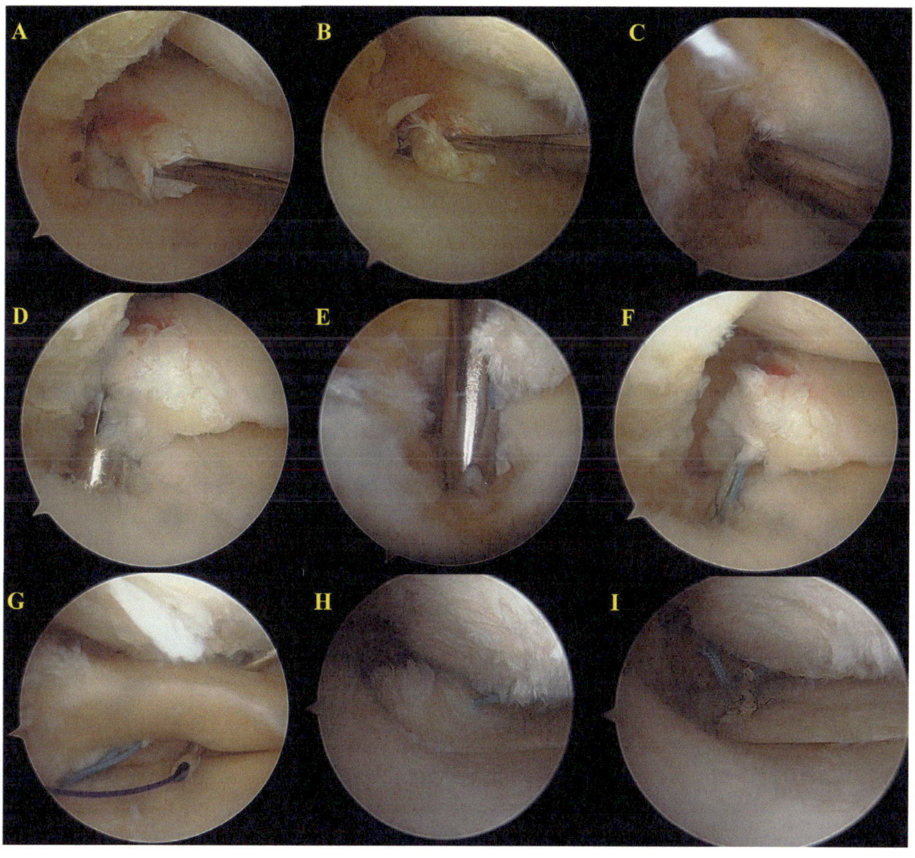

Figure 2.
Arthroscopic suture anchor repair of a medial meniscus posterior root tear (MMPRT) (A, B, C) The MMPRT is confirmed, the anatomical footprint of the medial meniscus posterior root is identified, and the bone bed is decorticated (view from the high anterolateral portal). (D, E, F) A curved anchor guide is introduced through the high posteromedial portal, ensuring the trajectory is perpendicular to the tibial plateau, and the anchor is inserted (view from the anterolateral portal). (G, H, I) The sutures are passed through the medial meniscus using shuttle relays and tied to form modified Mason-Allen stitches (view from the anterolateral portal).

accompanying lesions. The frayed portion of the MMPRT's torn edge is gently debrided using an arthroscopic shaver to prepare for the subsequent repair (**Figure 2A**). Next, the decortication of the MMPR footprint is performed. The MMPR footprint is identified through the anterolateral portal, and an arthroscopic rasp or curette is used to decorticate the bone bed, promoting meniscus-to-bone healing (**Figure 2B**).

Following this, anchor insertion is carried out. Following this, the anchor is inserted. A high posteromedial portal is created, through which the anchor guide is inserted to confirm the proper insertion trajectory (**Figure 2C** and **D**). Using a crescent-shaped suture hook or an antegrade suture passer through the anteromedial or accessory medial working portal, the surgeon sutures approximately 3–5 mm medial to the torn edge of the MMPR (**Figure 2E** and **F**). These sutures are then tied to complete the MMPRT repair (**Figure 2G** and **H**).

In cases where bone marrow density and quality are low, suture anchor repair is not feasible. Instead, transosseous repair via a tibial bone tunnel is selected. This approach requires careful planning to avoid interference with locking screws. The anteromedial tibial cortex position is avoided to prevent inevitable conflicts with the screws. If the tibial tunnel is created in the posteromedial position, interference with proximal-posterior screw must be managed, potentially using an anterior placement of the locking plate. When positioning the tibial tunnel in the anterolateral cortex, attention is needed to avoid interference with proximal screws. The guide wire is drilled from the anterolateral proximal tibia to the posterior MMPR footprint using a low-profile aiming device. After drilling to the subchondral bone meniscus footprint, over-reaming is performed with round curettage to protect the cartilage during joint penetration. During the osteotomy, suture protection is crucial. All suture strands are reinserted into the drill bit and pulled into the tibial tunnel [76]. Arthroscopy confirms the drill bit's position beneath the meniscus root, protecting the sutures from being damaged by the sawing bone at the osteotomy site. Final suture tightening and securing are performed after HTO and plate fixation. Sutures are then secured to the anterolateral tibial cortex using suspensory fixation. This comprehensive approach ensures proper alignment correction, meniscal repair, and joint load redistribution, leading to improved clinical outcomes and delayed progression of osteoarthritis.

7. Summary

Combining HTO with MMPRT repair provides an effective treatment for medial knee joint osteoarthritis with varus alignment. This dual procedure corrects lower limb alignment, restores meniscal hoop tension, and redistributes knee joint load, thereby reducing pain, improving function, and delaying osteoarthritis progression. While studies indicate enhanced meniscal healing and patient outcomes with the combined approach, further long-term research is required to fully understand the benefits and optimize surgical techniques.

Competing interests

The authors declare that they have no conflicts of interest.

Abbreviations

HTO	high tibial osteotomy
MMPRT	medial meniscus posterior root tear
MMPR	medial meniscus posterior root
MRI	magnetic resonance imaging
LLR	long leg radiographs

Author details

Kyun-Ho Shin[1]* and Seung-Beom Han[2]

1 Department of Orthopedic Surgery, Nanoori Hospital, Incheon, South Korea

2 Department of Orthopedic Surgery, Anam Hospital, Korea University College of Medicine, Seoul, South Korea

*Address all correspondence to: kyunho.shin@gmail.com

References

[1] Allaire R et al. Biomechanical consequences of a tear of the posterior root of the medial meniscus. Similar to total meniscectomy. The Journal of Bone and Joint Surgery. American Volume. 2008;**90**(9):1922-1931

[2] Marzo JM, Gurske-DePerio J. Effects of medial meniscus posterior horn avulsion and repair on tibiofemoral contact area and peak contact pressure with clinical implications. The American Journal of Sports Medicine. 2009;**37**(1):124-129

[3] Kim JH et al. Arthroscopic suture anchor repair versus pullout suture repair in posterior root tear of the medial meniscus: A prospective comparison study. Arthroscopy. 2011;**27**(12):1644-1653

[4] Jiang EX et al. Clinical factors associated with successful meniscal root repairs: A systematic review. The Knee. 2019;**26**(2):285-291

[5] Moon HS et al. Early surgical repair of medial meniscus posterior root tear minimizes the progression of meniscal extrusion: 2-year follow-up of clinical and radiographic parameters after arthroscopic Transtibial pull-out repair. The American Journal of Sports Medicine. 2020;**48**(11):2692-2702

[6] Chung KS et al. Preoperative varus alignment and postoperative meniscus extrusion are the main long-term predictive factors of clinical failure of meniscal root repair. Knee Surgery, Sports Traumatology, Arthroscopy. 2021;**29**(12):4122-4130

[7] Moon HK et al. Prognostic factors of arthroscopic pull-out repair for a posterior root tear of the medial meniscus. The American Journal of Sports Medicine. 2012;**40**(5):1138-1143

[8] Bonasia DE et al. Medial opening wedge high tibial osteotomy for medial compartment overload/arthritis in the varus knee: Prognostic factors. The American Journal of Sports Medicine. 2014;**42**(3):690-698

[9] Ferruzzi A et al. Cartilage repair procedures associated with high tibial osteotomy in varus knees: Clinical results at 11 years' follow-up. The Knee. 2014;**21**(2):445-450

[10] Floerkemeier S et al. Outcome after high tibial open-wedge osteotomy: A retrospective evaluation of 533 patients. Knee Surgery, Sports Traumatology, Arthroscopy. 2013;**21**(1):170-180

[11] Jung WH et al. Second-look arthroscopic assessment of cartilage regeneration after medial opening-wedge high tibial osteotomy. Arthroscopy. 2014;**30**(1):72-79

[12] Jung WH et al. Comparison of results of medial opening-wedge high tibial osteotomy with and without subchondral drilling. Arthroscopy. 2015;**31**(4):673-679

[13] Kim KI et al. Change of chondral lesions and predictive factors after medial open-wedge high tibial osteotomy with a locked plate system. The American Journal of Sports Medicine. 2017;**45**(7):1615-1621

[14] Sterett WI et al. Chondral resurfacing and high tibial osteotomy in the varus knee: Survivorship analysis. The American Journal of Sports Medicine. 2010;**38**(7):1420-1424

[15] Wakabayashi S et al. A comparison of the healing potential of fibrillated cartilage versus eburnated bone in osteoarthritic knees after high tibial osteotomy: An arthroscopic study with 1-year follow-up. Arthroscopy. 2002;**18**(3):272-278

[16] Lee HI, Park D, Cho J. Clinical and radiological results with second-look arthroscopic findings after open wedge high tibial osteotomy without arthroscopic procedures for medial meniscal root tears. Knee Surgery & Related Research. 2018;**30**(1):34-41

[17] Nha KW et al. Second-look arthroscopic findings after open-wedge high tibia osteotomy focusing on the posterior root tears of the medial meniscus. Arthroscopy. 2013;**29**(2):226-231

[18] Seo HS, Lee SC, Jung KA. Second-look arthroscopic findings after repairs of posterior root tears of the medial meniscus. The American Journal of Sports Medicine. 2011;**39**(1):99-107

[19] Kyun-Ho S et al. Effect of concurrent repair of medial meniscal posterior root tears during high tibial osteotomy for medial osteoarthritis during short-term follow-up: A systematic review and meta-analysis. BMC Musculoskeletal Disorders. 2021;**22**(1):623

[20] Wang H et al. The efficacy of medial meniscal posterior root tear repair with or without high tibial osteotomy: A systematic review. BMC Musculoskeletal Disorders. 2023;**24**(1):464

[21] Andrews SH et al. The structural and compositional transition of the meniscal roots into the fibrocartilage of the menisci. Journal of Anatomy. 2015;**226**(2):169-174

[22] Johannsen AM et al. Qualitative and quantitative anatomic analysis of the posterior root attachments of the medial and lateral menisci. The American Journal of Sports Medicine. 2012;**40**(10):2342-2347

[23] Pache S et al. Meniscal root tears: Current concepts review. The Archives of Bone and Joint Surgery. 2018;**6**(4):250-259

[24] Pagnani MJ, Cooper DE, Warren RF. Extrusion of the medial meniscus. Arthroscopy. 1991;**7**(3):297-300

[25] LaPrade CM et al. Meniscal root tears: A classification system based on tear morphology. The American Journal of Sports Medicine. 2015;**43**(2):363-369

[26] Moon HS et al. Early surgical repair of medial meniscus posterior root tear minimizes the progression of meniscal extrusion: Response. The American Journal of Sports Medicine. 2021;**49**(1):NP3-NP5

[27] Bernard CD et al. Medial meniscus posterior root tear treatment: A matched cohort comparison of nonoperative management, partial Meniscectomy, and repair. The American Journal of Sports Medicine. 2020;**48**(1):128-132

[28] Hiranaka T et al. Steep medial tibial slope and prolonged delay to surgery are associated with bilateral medial meniscus posterior root tear. Knee Surgery, Sports Traumatology, Arthroscopy. 2021;**29**(4):1052-1057

[29] Lee JI et al. Analysis of affecting factors of the fate of medial meniscus posterior root tear based on treatment strategies. Journal of Clinical Medicine. 2021;**10**(4):557

[30] Yanagisawa S et al. Association between postoperative meniscal extrusion and clinical outcomes of the pullout fixation technique for medial

meniscus posterior root tear. Asia-Pacific Journal of Sports Medicine, Arthroscopy, Rehabilitation and Technology. 2020;**21**:27-31

[31] Bhatia S et al. Meniscal root tears: Significance, diagnosis, and treatment. The American Journal of Sports Medicine. 2014;**42**(12):3016-3030

[32] Furumatsu T et al. Injury patterns of medial meniscus posterior root tears. Orthopaedics & Traumatology, Surgery & Research. 2019;**105**(1):107-111

[33] Walker PS et al. Function of the medial meniscus in force transmission and stability. Journal of Biomechanics. 2015;**48**(8):1383-1388

[34] Vedi V et al. Meniscal movement. An in-vivo study using dynamic MRI. Journal of Bone and Joint Surgery. British Volume (London). 1999;**81**(1):37-41

[35] Park DY et al. The degeneration of meniscus roots is accompanied by fibrocartilage formation, which may precede meniscus root tears in osteoarthritic knees. The American Journal of Sports Medicine. 2015;**43**(12):3034-3044

[36] Bin SI, Kim JM, Shin SJ. Radial tears of the posterior horn of the medial meniscus. Arthroscopy. 2004;**20**(4):373-378

[37] Habata T et al. Clinical features of the posterior horn tear in the medial meniscus. Archives of Orthopaedic and Trauma Surgery. 2004;**124**(9):642-645

[38] Bae JH et al. Predictive value of painful popping for a posterior root tear of the medial meniscus in middle-aged to older Asian patients. Arthroscopy. 2013;**29**(3):545-549

[39] Brody JM et al. Lateral meniscus root tear and meniscus extrusion with anterior cruciate ligament tear. Radiology. 2006;**239**(3):805-810

[40] Kim YJ et al. Posterior root tear of the medial meniscus in multiple knee ligament injuries. The Knee. 2010;**17**(5):324-328

[41] Kosy JD et al. Meniscal root tears occur frequently in multi-ligament knee injury and can be predicted by associated MRI injury patterns. Knee Surgery, Sports Traumatology, Arthroscopy. 2018;**26**(12):3731-3737

[42] Ra HJ et al. Traumatic posterior root tear of the medial meniscus in patients with severe medial instability of the knee. Knee Surgery, Sports Traumatology, Arthroscopy. 2015;**23**(10):3121-3126

[43] Lee JH et al. Arthroscopic pullout suture repair of posterior root tear of the medial meniscus: Radiographic and clinical results with a 2-year follow-up. Arthroscopy. 2009;**25**(9):951-958

[44] Akmese R et al. A new clinical sign for diagnosing medial meniscus posterior root tear. Orthopaedic Journal of Sports Medicine. 2021;**9**(1):2325967120975511

[45] Lee SY, Jee WH, Kim JM. Radial tear of the medial meniscal root: Reliability and accuracy of MRI for diagnosis. AJR. American Journal of Roentgenology. 2008;**191**(1):81-85

[46] Choi SH et al. The MRI findings of meniscal root tear of the medial meniscus: Emphasis on coronal, sagittal and axial images. Knee Surgery, Sports Traumatology, Arthroscopy. 2012;**20**(10):2098-2103

[47] Harper KW et al. Radial meniscal tears: Significance, incidence, and MR appearance. AJR. American Journal of Roentgenology. 2005;**185**(6):1429-1434

[48] Lee YG et al. Magnetic resonance imaging findings of surgically proven medial meniscus root tear: Tear configuration and associated knee abnormalities. Journal of Computer Assisted Tomography. 2008;**32**(3):452-457

[49] Choi CJ et al. Magnetic resonance imaging evidence of meniscal extrusion in medial meniscus posterior root tear. Arthroscopy. 2010;**26**(12):1602-1606

[50] Costa CR, Morrison WB, Carrino JA. Medial meniscus extrusion on knee MRI: Is extent associated with severity of degeneration or type of tear? AJR. American Journal of Roentgenology. 2004;**183**(1):17-23

[51] Furumatsu T et al. Meniscus extrusion is a predisposing factor for determining arthroscopic treatments in partial medial meniscus posterior root tears. Knee Surgery & Related Research. 2023;**35**(1):8

[52] Javaid MK et al. Pre radiographic MRI findings are associated with onset of knee symptoms: The most study. Osteoarthritis and Cartilage. 2010;**18**(3):323-328

[53] Asawatreratanakul P et al. Screening for or diagnosing medial meniscal root injury using peripheral medial joint space width ratio in plain radiographs. Scientific Reports. 2023;**13**(1):4982

[54] Gale DR et al. Meniscal subluxation: Association with osteoarthritis and joint space narrowing. Osteoarthritis and Cartilage. 1999;7(6):526-532

[55] Kodama Y et al. Preliminary diagnosis of medial meniscus posterior root tears using the Rosenberg radiographic view. Knee Surgery & Related Research. 2019;**31**(1):9

[56] Lee KH et al. Slot-scan digital radiography of the lower extremities: A comparison to computed radiography with respect to image quality and radiation dose. Korean Journal of Radiology. 2009;**10**(1):51-57

[57] Colyn W et al. The lateral joint line opening: A radiographic indicative parameter for high grade varus knees. Journal of Experimental Orthopaedics. 2022;**9**(1):51

[58] Shin KH et al. Preoperative supine radiographs are more accurate than standing radiographs for preoperative planning in medial open-wedge high tibial osteotomy. Arthroscopy. 2020;**36**(6):1655-1664

[59] Feucht MJ et al. Isolated high tibial osteotomy is appropriate in less than two-thirds of varus knees if excessive overcorrection of the medial proximal tibial angle should be avoided. Knee Surgery, Sports Traumatology, Arthroscopy. 2021;**29**(10):3299-3309

[60] Padalecki JR et al. Biomechanical consequences of a complete radial tear adjacent to the medial meniscus posterior root attachment site: in situ pull-out repair restores derangement of joint mechanics. The American Journal of Sports Medicine. 2014;**42**(3):699-707

[61] Seo JH et al. Effect of repair of radial tears at the root of the posterior horn of the medial meniscus with the pullout suture technique: A biomechanical study using porcine knees. Arthroscopy. 2009;**25**(11):1281-1287

[62] Jing L et al. Second-look arthroscopic findings after medial open-wedge high tibial osteotomy combined with all-inside repair of medial meniscus posterior root tears. Journal of Orthopaedic Surgery (Hong Kong). 2020;**28**(1):2309499019888836

[63] Lee OS, Lee SH, Lee YS. Comparison of the radiologic, arthroscopic, and clinical outcomes between repaired versus unrepaired medial meniscus posterior horn root tear during open wedge high tibial osteotomy. The Journal of Knee Surgery. 2021;**34**(1):57-66

[64] Ke X et al. Concurrent arthroscopic meniscal repair during open-wedge high tibial osteotomy is not clinically beneficial for medial meniscus posterior root tears. Knee Surgery, Sports Traumatology, Arthroscopy. 2021;**29**(3):955-965

[65] Lee DW, Lee SH, Kim JG. Outcomes of medial meniscal posterior root repair during proximal tibial osteotomy: Is root repair beneficial? Arthroscopy. 2020;**36**(9):2466-2475

[66] Kim YM et al. Remodified Mason-Allen suture technique concomitant with high tibial osteotomy for medial meniscus posterior root tears improved the healing of the repaired root and suppressed osteoarthritis progression. Knee Surgery, Sports Traumatology, Arthroscopy. 2021;**29**(4):1258-1268

[67] Choi NH, Son KM, Victoroff BN. Arthroscopic all-inside repair for a tear of posterior root of the medial meniscus: A technical note. Knee Surgery, Sports Traumatology, Arthroscopy. 2008;**16**(9):891-893

[68] Jung WH et al. Arthroscopic, suture anchor repair through a novel medial quadriceptal portal for medial meniscal root tear. Knee Surgery, Sports Traumatology, Arthroscopy. 2012;**20**(12):2391-2394

[69] Jung YH et al. All-inside repair for a root tear of the medial meniscus using a suture anchor. The American Journal of Sports Medicine. 2012;**40**(6):1406-1411

[70] Lee SK et al. Medial meniscal root repair using curved guide and soft suture anchor. Clinics in Orthopedic Surgery. 2018;**10**(1):111-115

[71] Cerminara AJ et al. Biomechanical evaluation of a transtibial pull-out meniscal root repair: Challenging the bungee effect. The American Journal of Sports Medicine. 2014;**42**(12):2988-2995

[72] Feucht MJ et al. Biomechanical comparison between suture anchor and transtibial pull-out repair for posterior medial meniscus root tears. The American Journal of Sports Medicine. 2014;**42**(1):187-193

[73] Lee DR et al. Current reviews in musculoskeletal medicine: Current controversies for treatment of meniscus root tears. Current Reviews in Musculoskeletal Medicine. 2022;**15**(4):231-243

[74] Chang PS et al. Midterm outcomes of posterior medial meniscus root tear repair: A systematic review. The American Journal of Sports Medicine. 2022;**50**(2):545-553

[75] Nejima S et al. Risk of interference between the tibial tunnel and locking screws in medial meniscus posterior root repair and open wedge high tibial osteotomy. Journal of Experimental Orthopaedics. 2022;**9**(1):25

[76] Srimongkolpitak S, Chernchujit B. Posterior root medial meniscus tear with medial opening wedge high tibial osteotomy: A step-by-step systematic arthroscopic repair technique. Arthroscopy Techniques. 2022;**11**(9):e1515-e1523

Chapter 4

Optimal Corrective Angle in Recent High Tibial Osteotomies

Masataka Deie and Yuki Yamanashi

Abstract

High tibial osteotomy (HTO) is a traditional surgical procedure for medial-type osteoarthritis of the knee. Recently, the procedure has evolved into a type of knee-preserving surgery. Minor correction HTO aims for a tibial correction angle of ≤15 degrees, a femorotibial angle (FTA) of 171 degrees, a medial tibial plateau angle of ≤90 degrees, and a % medial axis (%MA) of 55%. We have achieved good short-term clinical results by preserving as much cartilage and meniscus as possible. These results show high patient satisfaction and good clinical outcomes. We propose a new HTO concept that combines minor correction with joint preservation to maintain good gait and quality of life (QOL), rather than solely focusing on pain relief through lower limb alignment correction. In Japan, where people are living longer, we suggest this new HTO concept for patients aged 50–60 years with osteoarthritis, followed by conversion to primary total knee arthroplasty (TKA) around age 80.

Keywords: %mechanical axis, minor correction, Fujisawa's point, meniscus treatment, cartilage treatment

1. Introduction

Knee osteoarthritis (KOA) is characterized by a progressive loss of articular cartilage accompanied by new bone formation and often synovial proliferation, which may culminate in pain, loss of joint function, and disability [1]. Symptomatic KOA is characterized by radiographic evidence along with persistent joint pain or stiffness. The most common pattern of symptomatic KOA is articular cartilage degeneration predominantly in the medial compartment [2]. Therefore, high tibial osteotomy (HTO) has been the traditional treatment for this condition.

Recent advances in medical technology are changing the concept of surgery itself, as well as the surgical methods and postoperative treatment of HTO surgery. The key to conventional HTO is the transfer of the medial load in the coronal plane to the lateral load, where the articular cartilage is relatively normal [3, 4]. However, recent arthroscopic procedures have improved the postoperative results of partial meniscectomy and suture, as well as cartilage repair, making it possible to repair damaged medial load-bearing tissues of the knee joint, and postoperative rehabilitation has also shortened [5, 6].

Furthermore, improvements in artificial knee joint implants, the introduction of robotic surgery, have improved the postoperative results of TKA [7]. These advances mean that HTO surgery no longer needs to correct a valgus knee, force an abnormal gait, and aim to end a lifetime with a single osteotomy. Therefore, we hypothesize that a combination of open wedge high tibial osteotomy (OWHTO) and intra-articular procedures that correct to near-normal alignment will result in less pain and a functional knee joint.

Our OWHTO [8, 9] aims to repair as much intra-articular tissue as possible in patients aged 30 to 65 with medial-type osteoarthritis of the knee. We strive to correct the alignment to near-normal lower extremity alignment, facilitating easier future conversion to TKA.

The surgical concept for our OWHTO is to perform intra-articular procedures whenever possible, i.e., to induce repair of the injured tissue and to remove pain factors. Correction of coronal alignment should be planned preoperatively to achieve FTA of 171 degrees, medial angle tibial plateau (MPTA) of less than 90 degrees, and %medial axis (%MA) of 55%.

If the correcting angle is more than 15 degrees, double-level osteotomy or other methods should be considered. If the MPTA is greater than 90 degrees, double-level osteotomy or other methods should be considered.

Based on the above concept, the purpose of this article is to review cases in which OWHTO Japanese patients were performed and more than 2 years had passed since the surgery.

This study was approved by the Ethics Review Committee of Aichi Medical University in Japan.

2. Materials and methods

2.1 Patients and evaluations

From April 2018 to March 2022, 75 patients underwent knee osteotomy. We included 63 OWHTO cases, excluding those with double-level osteotomy, anterior cruciate ligament reconstruction, and closed wedge HTO. Seventy-two patients (97%) underwent a second look and plate removal one year after surgery, and 55 patients (87%) were followed up for more than two years.

We recorded patients' characteristics, including age at surgery, sex, body mass index (BMI), Japanese Orthopedic Association (JOA) score, knee injury and osteoarthritis outcome score (KOOS), and any concomitant meniscus or cartilage surgery (meniscectomy, repair, abrasion, drilling, microfracture, and mosaicplasty). Within one month before HTO surgery, patients were examined for range of motion (ROM), visual analog scale (VAS), and functional tests such as the 10 m walk and timed up and go (TUG). Radiographic data, including preoperative KL grades, pre- and postoperative FTA, mechanical axis (as percentages of the medial axis, %MA), and medial proximal tibial angle (MPTA), were reviewed on anteroposterior long leg double standing radiographs. One year after surgery, functional tests such as the 10 m walk and TUG were recorded. Patients also underwent a second look arthroscopy and plate removal at the tibia, during which intraarticular evaluations were performed.

2.2 Surgical procedure and rehabilitation

Two surgeons performed all surgeries under general or lumbar anesthesia. Initially, arthroscopy was conducted to confirm the following:

1. The ACL was functional.
2. The lateral articular cartilage was relatively well maintained (Grade 2 or less of ICRS).
3. The lateral meniscus was normal or had been repaired using the all-inside technique.
4. Patellofemoral joint debridement was indicated for injuries up to Grade 3 of the ICRS.

For the medial tibiofemoral joint, the following treatments were performed:

1. For the medial meniscus, radial tears were repaired, but partial resection was performed for degenerative flap or horizontal tears.
2. For tibial cartilage injuries, drilling and abrasion arthroplasty were performed.
3. For the medial femoral condyle, debridement and bone marrow stimulation were performed. Osteochondral grafting was done for osteochondral defects. Intraoperatively, the surgeon attempted to eliminate as much as possible the source of the medial joint pain.

2.2.1 Tibial osteotomy

2.2.1.1 Incision and initial steps

A transverse incision of approximately 5–7 cm was made in the medial part of the tibia, slightly proximal to the pes anserinus, avoiding subcutaneous tissue and the saphenous nerve. The pes anserinus, including hamstring tendons, was detached from the insertion, and the semitendinosus and gracilis tendons were sutured with threads for marking.

2.2.1.2 Ligament and posterior tibia release

The superficial to deep layers of the medial collateral ligament (MCL) were released from the joint line under the periosteum along the medial side of the patellar tendon. The deeper layers are detached until joint fluid leakage was confirmed, resulting in partial detachment of the capsule. The tibial attachment of the MCL was preserved. The posterior aspect of the tibia was released under the periosteum as much as possible to allow insertion of the retractor toward the posterior aspect of the tibia, without releasing the MCL attachment.

2.2.1.3 Osteotomy procedure

Following the Olympus HTO guide system (Olympus Terumo Biomaterials Corp., Tokyo, Japan), the osteotomy entry point was approximately 4 cm distal to the medial joint crease. A 2.4 mm K-wire was inserted from the anteromedial portion of the tibial tuberosity toward the lateral aspect of the tibia, targeting the fibular head. Fluoroscopy confirmed that the K-wire was inserted approximately 1 cm in front of the lateral border of the tibia. Another K-wire was inserted parallel to the first, approximately 2 cm posterior to the tibia. For the anterior tibia cut, an acceding cut was made at the tibial tuberosity with a thickness 5–7 mm, and a medial open osteotomy was performed. The medial tibia was opened with a spreader, and optimal alignment was checked with fluoroscopy. After confirming the optimal corrective angle, a wedge-shaped hydroxyapatite artificial bone (Neobone; AI medic, Tokyo Japan) was placed into the open gap, depending on size. The detached semitendinosus and gracilis tendons were then reattached. Plate fixation (Tris plate; Olympus Terumo, Biomaterials Corp., Tokyo, Japan) was used to fix the tibia.

2.2.2 Postoperative rehabilitation

The knee was immobilized with the knee brace in the extended position, and muscle strength training was started the next day. From 1 week postoperatively, joint range of motion training and crutch walking training were performed. The patient was allowed to walk with full weight bearing at 4–6 weeks postoperatively and engage in light exercise at 3–4 months postoperatively. At 5–6 months postoperatively, activities such as golf, jogging, and other physical activities were permitted.

3. Statistical analysis

Preoperative and postoperative data were analyzed using a paired t-test, with a p-value of 0.05 or less considered significant.

4. Results

All patients were diagnosed with medial-type osteoarthritis of the knee.

There were 46 male and 22 female patients. Their age was from 45 to 71 years (mean 61.1 ± 5.5 years). Patients' BMI at surgery ranged from 22.3 to 34.2 (mean 26.8 ± 3.4). The KL classification of the medial knee joint was grade I in 4 patients, grade 2 in 28, grade 3 in 30, and grade 4 in 6. The corrected angles were from 6 to 15 degrees (average 11.7 ± 2.0 degrees) (**Table 1**).

4.1 Arthroscopic surgery

Arthroscopic procedures performed at the time of initial surgery included partial resection of the medial meniscus in 45 of the 68 patients and suturing in 4 cases. Four sutures were performed for lateral meniscus injuries. For medial femoral condylar

Sex: Man/female	46/22
Age	45–71 years (average 61.1 ± 5.5 years old)
BMI at the surgery	22.3–34.2 (average 26.8 ± 3.4)
OA grade I/II/III/IV	4/28/30/6
Correcting angle	6 to 15 degrees. (average 11.7 ± 2.0 degrees)

Table 1.
Patients profile at HTO surgery.

cartilage injuries, osteochondral grafting was performed in 3 cases, and drilling was performed in 20 cases for medial femoral condylar cartilage injuries and in 15 cases for tibial cartilage injuries.

4.2 Clinical evaluations

Preoperative joint ROM was −3.3 ± 10.7 degrees at knee extension and 134.2 ± 21.8 degrees at knee flexion. At final follow-up, ROM was-5.3 ± 6.7 degrees at knee extension and 138.0 ± 10.6 degrees at knee flexion. There were no significant differences in ROM between before and after surgery.

Vas score decreased from 52.1 ± 29.1 mm preoperatively to 14.6 ± 16.8 mm postoperatively. Motor function tests showed significant improvement: the 10 m gait from 7.2 ± 2.9 seconds preoperatively to 6.0 ± 1.7 seconds postoperatively, and in the TUG test from 8.4 ± 3.3 seconds preoperatively to 7.2 ± 2.7 postoperatively. Postoperative VAS and motor function tests were significantly improved compared to preoperative values.

The JOA score improved from 71.8 ± 13.1 preoperatively to 88.0 ± 10.1 postoperatively. KOOS scores improved from 59.4 ± 17.0 preoperatively to 83.3 ± 11.2 postoperatively in Total, from 62.9 ± 18.0 preoperatively to 81.3 ± 13.2 postoperatively in Symptom, from 57.8 ± 18.0 preoperatively to 82.9 ± 14.3 postoperatively in Pain, from 71.7 ± 16.7 preoperatively to 90.8 ± 8.5 postoperatively in ADL, and from 59.4 ± 17.0 preoperatively to 83.3 ± 11.2 postoperatively in Sport. The ADL improved from 71.7 ± 16.7 preoperatively to 90.8 ± 8.5 postoperatively, the Sport from 40.1 ± 23.0 preoperatively to 69.1 ± 22.1 postoperatively, and the QOL from 38.0 ± 21.1 preoperatively to 70.9 ± 17.7 postoperatively (**Table 2**). Postoperative JOA and KOOS scores were statistically significantly improved compared to preoperative values.

4.3 X-ray evaluations

X-ray evaluation at the final follow-up showed that the FTA was corrected from 176 to 188 degrees (average 179.8 degrees ±3.1 degrees) preoperatively to 168 to 180 degrees (average 173.6 ± 3.3 degrees) postoperatively. The %MA shifted from −20 to 43.4% (average 21.5% ± 11.3%) preoperatively to 33 to 66% (average 51.4 ± 9.7%) postoperatively. Additionally, MTPA was corrected from 78 to 89 degrees (average

	Preoperative score	Postoperative score	*P* Value
JOA	71.8 ± 13.1	88.0 ± 10.1	< 0.01*
KOOS Total	59.4 ± 17.0	83.3 ± 11.2	< 0.01*
symptom	62.9 ± 18.0	81.3 ± 13.2	< 0.01*
pain	57.8 ± 18.0	82.9 ± 14.3	< 0.01*
ADL	71.7 ± 16.7	90.9 ± 10.2	< 0.01*
sports	40.1 ± 23.0	69.1 ± 22.1	< 0.01*
QOL	38.0 ± 21.1	71.0 ± 17.7	< 0.01*

Date are presented as mean ± SD.
JOA: Japanese orthopedic association, KOOS: knee injury and osteoarthritis outcome score.
**Achieved statistical significance.*

Table 2.
Clinical outcomes.

	Pre operation	Post operation	*P* Value
ROM			
Extension (°)	−3.3 ± 10.7	−5.3 ± 6.7	0.20
Flexion (°)	134.2 ± 21.8	138.0 ± 10.6	0.43
VAS (mm)	52.1 ± 29.1	14.6 ± 16.8	< 0.01*
10 m gait (second)	7.2 ± 2.9	6.0 ± 1.7	< 0.01*
TUG (second)	8.4 ± 3.3	7.2 ± 2.7	< 0.01*
Radiological data			
FTA (°)	179.8 ± 3.1	173.6 ± 3.3	< 0.01*
%MA (%)	21.5 ± 11.3	51.4 ± 9.7	< 0.01*
MTPA (°)	83.2 ± 2.3	89.3 ± 2.7	< 0.01*

Date are presented as mean ± SD.
ROM: range of motion, VAS: visual analogue scale, TUG: time up and go test, FTA: femorotibial angle, MA: mechanical axis.
**Achieved statistical significance.*

Table 3.
Subject characteristics.

83.2 ± 2.3 degrees) preoperatively to 87.9 to 90.5 degrees (average 89.3 ± 2.7 degrees) postoperatively. These data showed significant differences between preoperative and postoperative values (**Table 3**).

4.4 Arthroscopic evaluations

At the second look evaluation during plate removal one year postoperatively, all 4 knees that underwent medial meniscus suturing were healed. Three of the 45 knees that underwent partial resection required additional resection. One of the 4 knees with lateral meniscus sutures had suture failure, necessitating additional partial resection, while the other 3 knees were healed. For cartilage injuries, no additional procedures were performed. The articular cartilage at each site was evaluated as follows.

4.4.1 IKDC cartilage evaluation

- Medial femoral condyle: 3.2 ± 0.09 at 1st surgery to 2.9 ± 0.9 at 2nd look
- Medial tibial plateau: 3.2 ± 0.8 at 1st surgery to 2.9 ± 0.9 at 2nd look
- Lateral femoral condyle: 0.9 ± 0.6 at 1st surgery to 1.1 ± 0.6 at 2nd look
- Lateral tibial plateau: 1.4 ± 0.7 at 1st surgery to 1.6 ± 0.7 at 2nd look
- Femoral groove: 2.2 ± 0.9 at 1st surgery to 2.3 ± 0.8 at 2nd look
- Patella cartilage: 1.4 ± 0.7 at 1st surgery to 1.6 ± 0.8 at 2nd look

None of these differences were significant.

Among the patients in this study, one knee required conversion to TKA at 3 years postoperatively.

5. Representative case

A 64- year- old male with a JOA score of 65 points presented with his right knee pain. His chief complaint was right pain, and he wanted to play tennis and golf. He had been treated with conservative therapies for six months. ROM was −5 to 125 degrees with terminal pain.

KOOS scores were as follows: Symptom 57.1, Pain 30.6, ADL 97.1, Sports 70.0, QOL 62.5, and Total 70.8.

X-rays showed FTA of 180 degrees, MTPA of 85 degrees, and %MA of 45% (**Figure 1**).

These x-rays showed narrowing of the medial joint space and medial osteopathic changes.

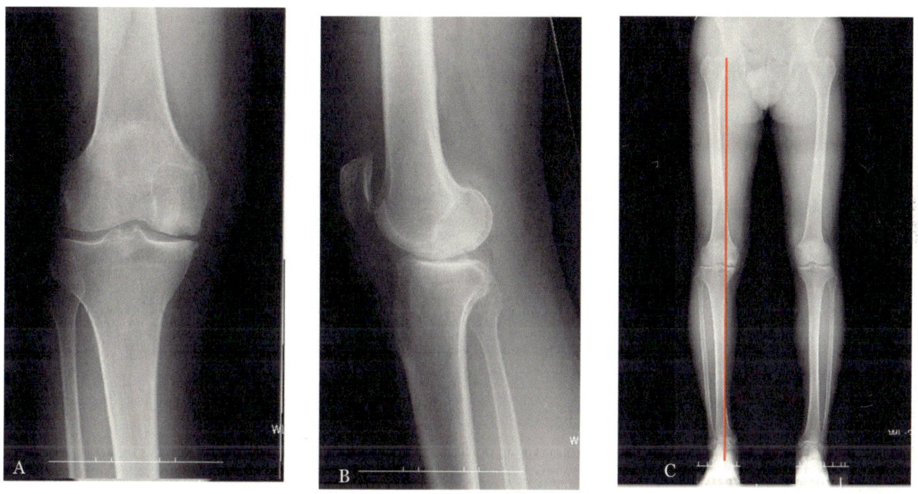

Figure 1.
Preoperative x-rays, (A): Anteroposterior view, (B): Lateral view, and (C): Standing both legs view. The red line indicated the mechanical axis.

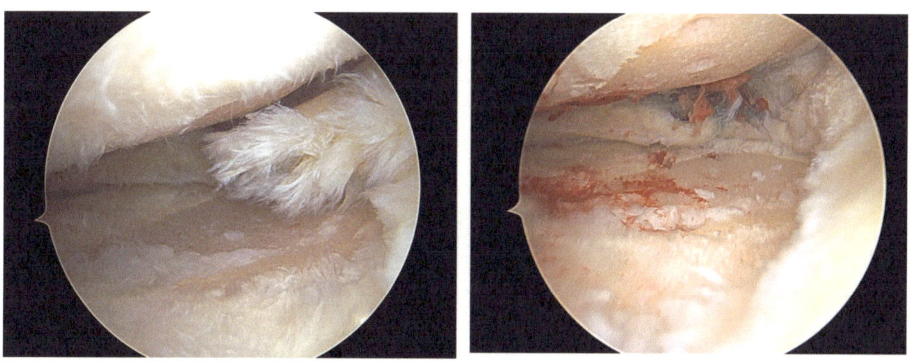

Figure 2.
Arthroscopic views at initial surgery, (A): ICRS grade 4 damage to the medial femoral condyle and medial tibial articular cartilage, and degenerative tear in medial meniscus, and (B): abrasion and drilling were performed, and meniscal sutures and wrapped fibrin clots [10] were added to the remaining portion of the medial meniscus.

Arthroscopic and HTO surgery were performed. The tibia correcting angles was 10 degrees. Medial meniscus sutures, abrasion and drilling with 1.5 mm K-wire at the medial femoral and tibia cartilage lesions (**Figure 2**).

At 7 months post-surgery, he returned to playing golf. At 1 year after HTO, ROM was −3 to 135. The JOA score was 85, KOOS score were as follows: Symptom 64.3, Pain 63.9, ADL 98.5, Sports 75, QOL 43.8, Total 76,2. X-ray showed FTA of 173 degrees, MTPA of 90, and %MA of 52% (**Figure 3**).

At the second look arthroscopy (**Figure 4**), the meniscus was repaired, and the articular surface of the tibiofemoral joint was covered with cartilage-like tissue. The plate and screws were removed. He has returned society and sport activity satisfactorily.

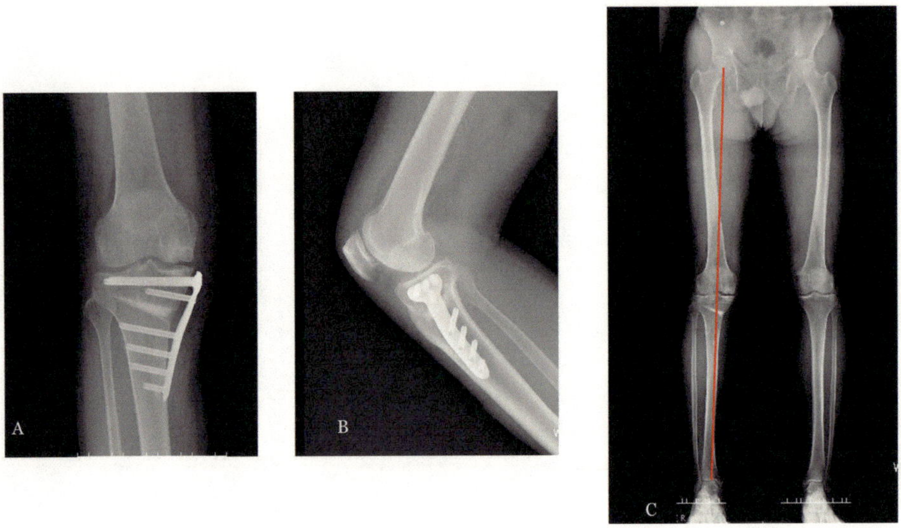

Figure 3.
Postoperative X-rays, (A): Anteroposterior view, (B): Lateral view, x-rays in A and B are before the 2nd look, bone fusion has been achieved, and the joint gap is more open than before surgery, and (C): Standing both legs view: X-rays after plate removal. The red line indicated the mechanical axis.

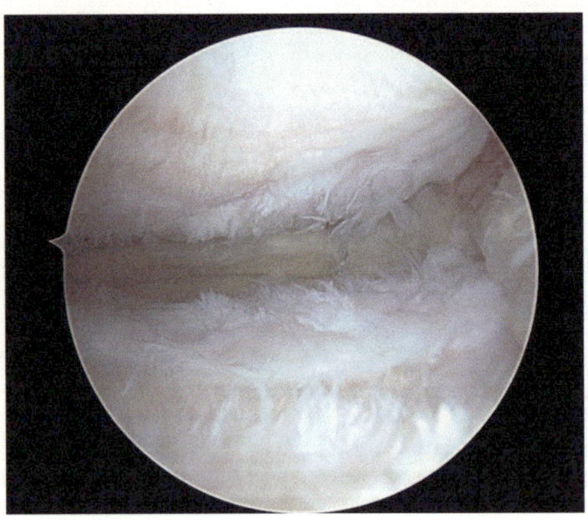

Figure 4.
2nd look arthroscopic view.

6. Discussions

In this study, we have performed OWHTO with a correction of less than 15 degrees, incorporating a firm intra-articular procedure, the FTA of 173 degrees, MTPA of 89 degrees, and %MA of 53%, following the new concept of HTO. The results indicate that patients are satisfied both functionally and clinically. Although long-term results have not yet been studied, we found that the new concept HTO can achieve satisfactory clinical results if the meniscus and cartilage are treated as much as possible by arthroscopic surgery in addition to minor correction.

The problems with conventional HTO surgery include a long postoperative immobilization period, delaying return to society, and overcorrection to prevent recurrence of varus deformity, sometimes resulting in a cosmetically problematic gait due to excessive valgus deformity. Additionally, the conventional surgical concept of HTO focused mainly on eliminating pain by correcting alignment rather than intra-articular procedures, necessitating a significant change in the axis of loading [2–4].

Under these views, minor correction HTO was not recommended for fear of recurrence of internal rotation and recurrence of pain. However, our investigation found that minor correction is sufficient not only to correct the alignment, but also to achieve satisfactory results with partial meniscectomy, suture, and cartilage repair. It is well known that pain relief cannot be achieved solely with debridement such as partial meniscectomy, and the cartilage in the injured area is not fully repaired [11].

The second look findings at 1 year postoperatively revealed that in cases where the meniscus was repairable, it remained so, and articular cartilage damage had not progressed. There was no progression of patellofemoral osteoarthritis, a known problem with OWHTO. These results suggest that these surgical procedures alone do not provide satisfactory results, but that minor correction HTO in addition to these intra-articular treatments provides satisfactory surgical outcomes. In the long term, we are also concerned about the progression of OA, such as recurrence of varus deformity and pain, but because the correction angle of HTO is small, we believe that conversion to TKA is relatively easy.

Fujisawa et al. recommended aligning the weight-bearing line of HTO through the 65–70% coordinate of the width of the tibial plateau, recently refined to 62.5% (62–66%) [4]. This concept was widely accepted in the era of 60–70 years of life expectancy. Today, the average life expectancy is over 70 years globally, and in Japan, it is over 85 years for women and 80 years for men, making the era of a 100-year life expectancy [12].

However, when TKA is performed on patients with medial OA at the age of 50–60 years who have developed knee joint disorders, there is a risk of revision TKA. Additionally, if a revision TKA is performed, a decline in joint function is unavoidable.

If patients suffer from knee OA in their 50s, they should undergo HTO to preserve the joints and exercise with their own joints until the age of 70–80. As OA progresses, the patient should undergo primary TKA to maintain as much activity as possible until the end of life. Therefore, we recommend minor correction HTO to enable smooth conversion from HTO to TKA.

7. Conclusions

The new concept of OWHTO that we have proposed has achieved good postoperative results in the short term. With advances in surgical techniques, implants, and rehabilitation, as well as the extension of life expectancy, we recommend the minor correction OWHTO, which is different from the conventional concept, as an alternative to knee around surgery.

Acknowledgements

We are deeply grateful to Dr. Machiko Akao, Dr. Takuya Takada, and Dr. Kyosuke Kobayakawa of the Department of Orthopedic Surgery, Aichi Medical University, for their invaluable assistance with the surgeries and data analysis. We are also extend my sincere thanks to Dr. Syungo Sasamine of Hiroshima Citizen Hospital for his help in image analysis.

Conflict of interest

The authors declare no conflict of interest.

Author details

Masataka Deie[1*] and Yuki Yamanashi[2]

1 Hiroshima Citizen Hospital, Hiroshima, Japan

2 Aichi Medical University, Nagakute, Japan

*Address all correspondence to: masatakadeie@yahoo.co.jp

References

[1] Abramson SB, Attur M. Developments in the scientific understanding of osteoarthritis. Arthritis Research and Therapy. 2009;**11**:227

[2] Mina C, Garrett WE Jr, Pietrobon R, Glisson R, Higgins L. High tibial osteotomy for unloading osteochondral defects in the medial compartment of the knee. The American Journal of Sports Medicine. 2008;**36**:949-955

[3] Coventry MB, Ilstrup DM, Wallrichs SL. Proximal tibial osteotomy a critical long-term study of eighty-seven cases. The Journal of Bone and Joint Surgery. American Volume. 1993;**75**:196-201

[4] Fujisawa Y, Masuhara K, Shiomi S. The effect of high tibial osteotomy on osteoarthritis of the knee. An arthroscopic study of 54knee joints. Clinical in Orthopedic Clinic of North. America. 1979;**10**:585-608

[5] Dawson M, Elson D, Claes S, Predescu V, Khakha R, Espejo-Reina A, et al. Osteotomy around the painful degenerative varus knee has broader indications than conventionally described but must follow a strict planning process: ESSKA formal consensus part I. Knee Surgery, Sports Traumatology, Arthroscopy. 2024;**32**(7):1891-1901

[6] Ollivier M, Claes S, Mabrouk A, Elson D, Espejo-Reina A, Predescu V, et al. Surgical strategy and complication management of osteotomy around the painful degenerative varus knee: ESSKA formal consensus part II. Knee Surgery, Sports Traumatology, Arthroscopy. 2024;**32**(8):2194-2205

[7] Pagan CA, Karasavvidis T, Cohen-Rosenblum AR, Hannon CP, Lombardi AV Jr, Vigdorchik JM. Technology in Total Knee Arthroplasty in 2023. The Journal of Arthroplasty. 2024;**39**:S54-S59

[8] Tsukada S, Wakui M. Is overcorrection preferable for repair of degenerated articular cartilage after open-wedge high tibial osteotomy? Knee Surgery, Sports Traumatology, Arthroscopy. 2017;**25**:785-792

[9] Deie M, Hoso T, Shimada N, Iwaki D, Nakamae A, Ochi M. Differences between opening versus closing high tibial osteotomy on clinical outcome and gait analysis. The Knee. 2015;**21**:1046-1051

[10] Yamanashi Y, Kato T, Akao M, Takata T, Kobayakawa K, Deie M. Meniscal repair using fibrin clots made from bone marrow blood wrapped in a Polyglycolic acid sheet. Arthroscopy Techniques. 2021;**23**:e2541-e2546

[11] Moseley JB, O'Malley K, Petersen NJ, Menke TJ, Brody BA, Kuykendall DH, et al. A controlled trial of arthroscopic surgery for osteoarthritis of the knee. The New England Journal of Medicine. 2002;**347**(2):81-88

[12] Ministry of health. Labor and Welfare. Japan: World Health Statistics; 2024. Available from: https://www.mhlw.go.jp/toukei/saikin/hw/life/life10/01.html

Chapter 5

Design and 3D Printing of Customized Osteosynthesis Instruments for Osteotomies

Mikel Sánchez, Alexis Fernández, Leonor López de Dicastillo, Jaime Oraa, Xabier Sánchez, Jorge Guadilla, Nicolás Fiz and Diego Delgado

Abstract

In recent years, the use of 3D technology in the medical field, especially in orthopedic surgery, has increased considerably. This valuable tool can be used both in preoperative planning and during the surgical procedure itself. The application of this technology may be of particular interest in osteotomy surgeries, both to correct rotational malalignment and to treat degenerative joint diseases. Achieving an ideal osteosynthesis that fits perfectly after correction of the bone deformity is very difficult, in spite of the advantage of customized guides. This is due to the deformity of the bone caused by the fracture callus. The use of technology and 3D printing makes it possible to plan the surgery with great precision as well as to design and manufacture personalized surgical material that fits the patient optimally, favoring implantation.

Keywords: 3D printing, 3D technology, derotation osteotomy, malrotation, osteosynthesis

1. Introduction

Orthopedic surgeons are very familiar with the visualization of clinical images for diagnostic use, to appreciate the relationships between anatomical structures and to plan surgical interventions. Images are used to communicate findings to other colleagues and to convey details of a surgical technique.

Although 3D printers have been successfully employed in several specialties, such as plastic surgery, dental and maxillofacial surgery, and urology, their use in orthopedic surgery is still in its infancy and little known to many specialists, although it offers huge advantages and benefits [1].

3D printed models provide us with tangible depth information about the anatomical and pathological conditions of different structures. It has the advantage of improving the planning of the surgical technique with patient-specific models, increasing diagnostic quality, and decreasing exposure time and general anesthesia. These models also improve communication between medical teams and facilitate information for the patient as well as for other doctors in training [2–6].

2. From image to 3D model

Making a 3D printed model of an anatomical structure from imaging tests involves converting data stored in image format to a 3D printing format. The need for a 3D printed model arises in difficult or complex cases or patients with multiple treatment variables where a definitive solution is not clear. It is necessary to clearly define what the purpose of the model is, to decide which structures should be included in the print if it will be necessary to manipulate and/or cut it easily, and if the model is to be introduced in the surgical field and therefore sterilized (**Figure 1**).

The imaging study must be tailored to acquire high-quality images of the anatomical structure to be printed. Computed tomography (CT) is the most commonly used imaging model, although models can be obtained from magnetic resonance imaging (MRI), recommended in pediatric patients to avoid radiation. In cases where it is important to visualize surrounding vascular structures, cartilage or ligaments in addition to bone, a combined acquisition of CT with the addition of contrast and MRI sequences could be obtained. CT images are considered to be two and a half dimensional as they show cross-sectional slices with known distances between them. In this way, these slices can be oriented in space.

Acquired images should have a slice thickness of 1–2 mm in both CT and MRI to create 3D models, and gaps between slices should be avoided. Adjustments in the image acquisition should be aimed at decreasing noise to improve the quality of the final 3D model print. Artifacts in the acquired image datasets will also be represented in the printed model. This is a frequent problem in calcifications, heterotopic bone or in the presence of metallic implants. The application of a metallic artifact reduction algorithm available on some modern CT machines helps to improve the image quality obtained. Without adequate images of an anatomical structure, it is impossible to isolate it accurately in order to produce a precisely printed model. Therefore, communication between surgeons, radiologists, and engineers is key [7].

An important step in creating a 3D model is image segmentation. This refers to the process of isolating the structure of interest from the other anatomical structures present and precisely defining the boundaries between the different structures to create patient-specific models. Segmentation methods are based on pixel density

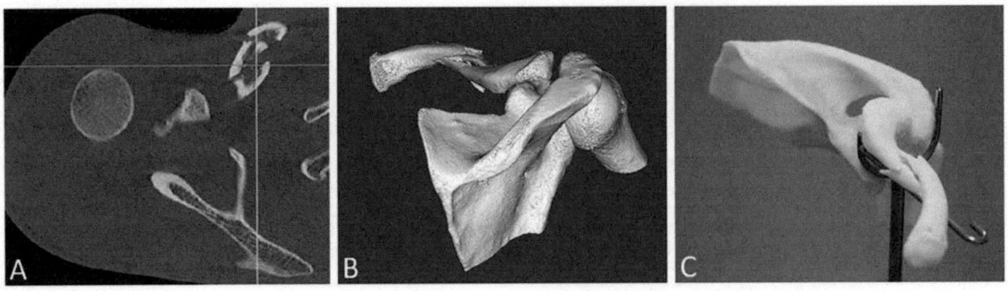

Figure 1.
Design and 3D printing process. From the images (A) obtained of the patient, a 3D design (B) is generated and then printed (C).

differences in CT or signal intensity in MRI. The segmented anatomy is converted to a 3D object that represents its geometry with a series of connected polygons. It is referred to as a 3D mesh because the model is not solid, but has the appearance of a net or mesh [8, 9]. Several 3D printing models work according to the principles of either additive or subtractive manufacturing. In the additive manufacturing model, the material is added line by line until the model is complete. In the subtractive model, the printer removes the excess material from a compact block.

At the time of printing, there is a wide variety of materials used to make 3D models, such as printable acrylonitrile butadiene styrene (ABS) polymers, plastics (polylactic acid (PLA), resins, and nylon) and metals (aluminum, bronze, copper, gold, and titanium). Apart from the different materials and technologies, 3D printers also differ in resolution. The higher the resolution, the better the quality of the final product, and this depends on the material dots per inch (dpi) they are able to work with. There are printers with a minimum of 250 dpi up to a maximum of 1600 dpi [10, 11].

3. Applications in orthopedic surgery

Since its emergence in the 1980s by Chuck Hull, 3D printing has been used in surgery to make pre-surgical anatomical models, guides for total arthroplasty, guides for fixation and corrective osteotomies, or implants adapted to the patient.

Anatomical models are commonly used to visualize a complex fracture or deformity, a large bone-invasive injury that may involve important surrounding anatomical structures, or a congenital defect requiring reconstructive surgery. These models allow: (1) pre-surgical visualization of the patient's anatomy, which improves spatial perception and helps the surgeon to prepare for surgery, (2) Simulate the surgery or osteotomy as it is a 1:1 scale model improving the efficiency of the surgery, (3) Choose and pre-mold the fixation/osteosynthesis system, which can save time during surgery which is beneficial for the patient, (4) Choose a total arthroplasty system prior to surgery, and (5) Have intraoperative references if the model is made in sterilizable materials.

3D printing also creates patient-specific instruments and cutting blocks for the femoral and tibial components, adapting them to the patient's anatomy according to preset cutting references [12]. Many manufacturers currently offer these solutions for total knee, shoulder, and hip arthroplasty [13–15].

When it comes to osteotomies, the guides resulting from a planned surgery may include a fixation plate that can be prefabricated or customized as an important part of the surgical guide. There are several ways to achieve a customized fixation plate. The simplest manner is to have a 3D model of the desired correction result and to manually design the plate on the model. It is then sterilized and used during surgery. Another way is the direct 3D printing of a metal part. This technique has been successfully applied in acetabular osteotomies, tibial osteotomies, distal radial osteotomies, hip dysplasia corrective osteotomies, and long bone axis corrective osteotomies [16–24].

Finally, those patients with specific needs, who are out of standard in size or shape, can get a reconstruction system tailored to their individual needs.

The following details techniques and cases related to the use of personalized 3D printing for use in osteotomies, as it is one of the most widespread applications that can help the surgeon the most.

4. Application of 3D technology in osteotomies to correct rotational malalignment

As said before, in recent years there has been a significant increase in the use of 3D technology in orthopedic surgery [25]. Currently, surgical interventions to correct malrotation depend on intraoperative clinical and radiological data, which are collected by an observer. Thus, the current aim is to achieve better accuracy of malalignment correction through the development of new surgical guides.

The use of this tool both for preoperative surgical planning of different situations (for instance, malrotation of femur and tibia and dealignment in the coronal plane of these two long bones) and for the surgical procedure itself has been spread out [25]. Most published articles present innovative techniques in the use of 3D-printed guides for different types of surgical interventions [26–28]. The implementation of 3D technology has made it possible to develop customized and personalized cutting guides for specific patients, as well as to manufacture customized titanium osteosynthesis plates to achieve osteotomy stabilization [25]. Thus, depending on the site of osteotomy, the presence of fracture, the size of the callus or even the preference of the surgeon, conventional nails, plates, and external fixators or personalized plates can be used to achieve the fixation while the osteotomy heals.

CT images of the affected limb are treated with 3D reconstruction software, obtaining a 3D composition of the affected bone. The bone rotational malalignment is measured by the software according to the natural position using the contralateral limb as a reference. After correcting the malrotation, the bone models and the surgical material required for the surgery are designed and printed.

4.1 Primary or constitutional malrotations

A common reason for pain in the hip, knee, and ankle is the constitutional or non-posttraumatic rotational malalignment of the lower limbs. Knowing the usual signs and results from an initial examination is the initial step toward a correct diagnosis. Advanced imaging tests and procedures can help with diagnosis and planning for surgery. Surgical treatment of these deformities is unusual, but it could help patients with painful and dysfunctional deformities who have been correctly screened [29].

Pathological rotational abnormalities of the femur and tibia can cause pain and patellofemoral instability and can lead to other pathologies such as ischiofemoral impingement (IFI), femoroacetabular impingement (FAI), and joint degeneration (**Figure 2**) [29–32].

Clinical evaluation must be meticulous since many benign rotational variations may be present in children and adults, and it is important to differentiate normal variability from pathological scenarios. A detailed physical examination is mandatory, starting with the general appearance (height, posture, and signs of asymmetry of the limb or spine that may also be present in syndromic conditions) and followed by an assessment of the rotational profile of both the femur and tibia. Finally, functional assessment of the limb during gait should be checked for asymmetries and deviations from normal.

As described above, digital analysis and preoperative planning are performed in those cases that have a symptomatic hip or knee due to the malrotation and have not a normalized quality of life. After virtual surgical correction, a 3D model reconstruction from CT images is generated, and an adapted guide to the bone surface is designed. It helps in performing the osteotomy (**Figure 3**), achieving the required rotational correction as described in the later clinical case [27].

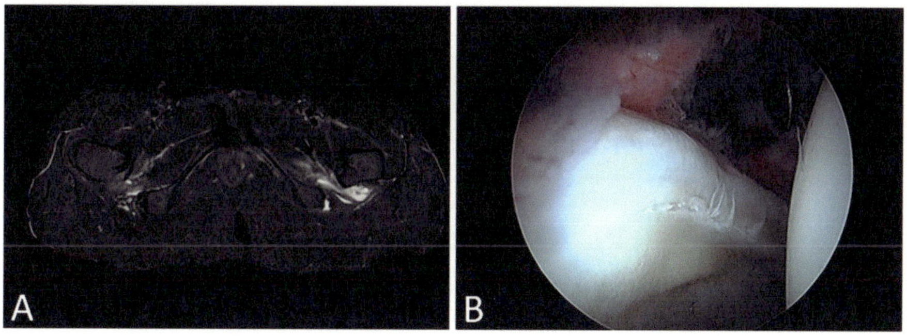

Figure 2.
Constitutional rotational malalignment of the lower extremities. Excessive anteversion of the proximal femur causes impingement between the ischium and lesser trochanter, and this leads to quadratus femoris muscle irritation and buttock pain (ischiofemoral impingement) (A). Both excessive antetorsion and retrotorsion can cause acetabular labral and cartilage injury (B).

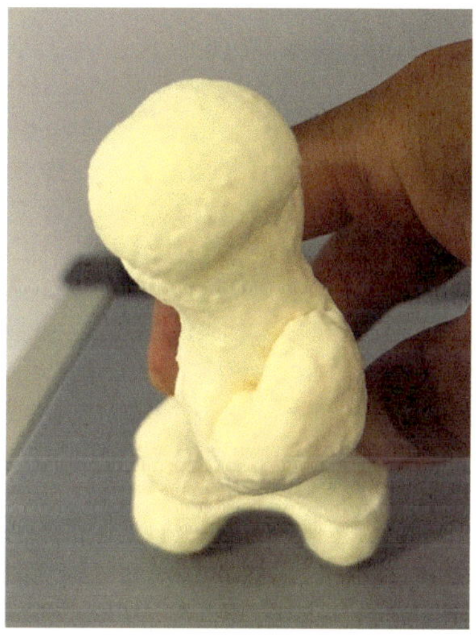

Figure 3.
3D printed model of a case of excessive anteversion in a 12-year-old girl.

Once both the result of the correction planning and the design of the guide are satisfactory, the part is printed on a 3D printer and sterilized for use during surgery. Intramedullary nailing is usually the first choice for osteotomy fixation (**Figure 4**), both in the femur and tibia, aiming for a faster postoperative protocol, although plate fixation may also be a feasible option. The point of approach is conditioned by the site where the osteotomy is planned. As we need to expose the cortical bone to fit the guide, we perform the osteotomy with a conventional orthopedic saw. The detailed surgical technique is the same as the one detailed in the clinical case of the next section.

4.2 Malrotations resulting from fractures

3D technology can be used to treat some bone deformities resulting from fractures. Femoral diaphyseal fractures are frequent in our practice, with traffic accidents being the most common cause [1, 2]. The gold standard in the treatment of these

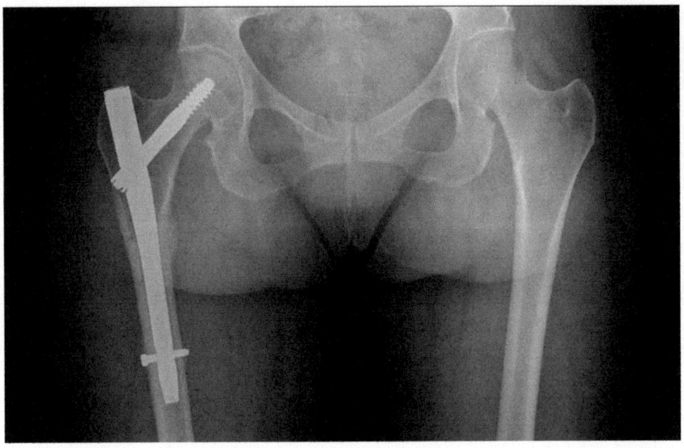

Figure 4.
Case of A twenty-five-year-old woman with buttock and groin pain due to an antetorsion of 45° degrees (same case as **Figure 2A***). A hip arthroscopy and a subtrochanteric osteotomy were performed.*

fractures is intramedullary nailing, which offers good results in terms of consolidation and functional recovery. It is performed percutaneously without the need to open the fracture focus [3, 4]. Nevertheless, rotational misalignment is a recognized medical issue after this technique. A rotational difference of more than 15° with respect to the non-injured side may be associated with functional difficulties. [5, 6].

Malrotation of the femur is determined by calculating the femoral version, which is established according to the procedure reported by Jeanmart et al. [33]. It defines the angle between a line traced through the axis of the femoral neck and a line tangent to the dorsal contours of the femoral condyles [34].

Exceedance on both sides of mean values of the anteversion of the femur ranging from 10° to 15° may result in pathological conditions [35]. In patients with ischio-femoral impingement, concomitant femoroacetabular impingement and posterior extra-articular hip impingement, excessive femoral anteversion can cause anterior knee pain and instability as well as anterior hip pain and labral tears. It can also lead to internal rotation during walking, causing difficulties when walking, running, and playing sports. Conversely, poor femoral anteversion (or femoral retroversion) can lead to labral and articular cartilage damage of the hip, joint degeneration, and gait with external rotation [6, 10–13].

When a patient presents a history of femoral diaphyseal, a detailed physical examination is the first step. It is important to explore hip mobility and compare it with the contralateral side. A significant difference in internal and external rotation between healthy and pathological hips should raise suspicion of malrotation. It is also important to observe the patient's gait, with the possibility of in-toe or out-toe gait. If malrotation is suspected, a complete set of X-rays and telemetry should be requested. If any pathological finding is presented in these tests, a CT scan must be conducted. The CT scan makes it possible to assess fracture consolidation and also calculate malrotation of the limb, evaluating the healthy side as a reference. The CT scan can accurately determine the degrees of malrotation, allowing to design of a specific and personalized surgical guide [26, 27].

4.2.1 Clinical case

The patient was a 40-year-old man with a history of left femur diaphyseal fracture after a traffic accident 2 years ago. He had previously undergone surgery at another orthopedic center and underwent intramedullary nailing with locking screws. Due to the delay of union, they decided to dynamize fracture focus by removing the nail distal locking screw, resulting in malrotation of the fracture site. The CT scan performed showed an external rotation of the distal fragment of 43° concerning the contralateral femur. A surgical plan was designed for the nail removal and new intramedullary nailing, calculating the rotation to correct. Personalized guides were designed and 3D printed for correction.

The osteotomy guides were designed to be tailored to the bone surface of the femur and to manage the bone fragments rotation (Materialize Magics, Materialize, Leuven, Belgium) (NX Unigraphics, Siemens, TX, USA). A set of three surgical pieces was designed, including a first piece for the proximal bone fragment, a second piece for the distal bone fragment, and a third one acting as a bridge between the first two pieces to provide the necessary degree of rotation.

A postero-lateral approach was conducted between the lateral intermuscular septum and the vastus lateralis to reach the diaphysis of the femur. Two monocortical Kirschner wires and two monocortical screws were used to fix each of the first two surgical guides to the bone surface. Correct rotational positioning and placement was ensured by the precise adaptation of the 3D printed guides to the fracture lips and osteophytes. The osteosynthesis material used in the previous surgery (T2 femoral nail) was then removed. Femoral osteotomy was performed along the anterior fracture site, and then, the external femoral rotation was corrected by rotating the distal femoral fragment. The third 3D printed guide was then used to connect the other two and provided the correct degree of femoral rotation. The first two guides were then connected using the third 3D printed guide, achieving the desired degree of rotation. Lastly, a new T2 femoral nail (Stryker) with proximal and distal locking was inserted. It was not necessary to remove the guides to place the nail as the screws were monocortical, maintaining the correction and stability of the osteotomy. When the nail was in place, the surgical guides were removed, and the final result was assessed under fluoroscopy (**Figure 5**).

The patient showed favorable evolution. Serial radiographs were performed to assess the correct consolidation of the osteotomy. In the sixth month, a control CT scan was requested, which showed complete consolidation in the preoperatively

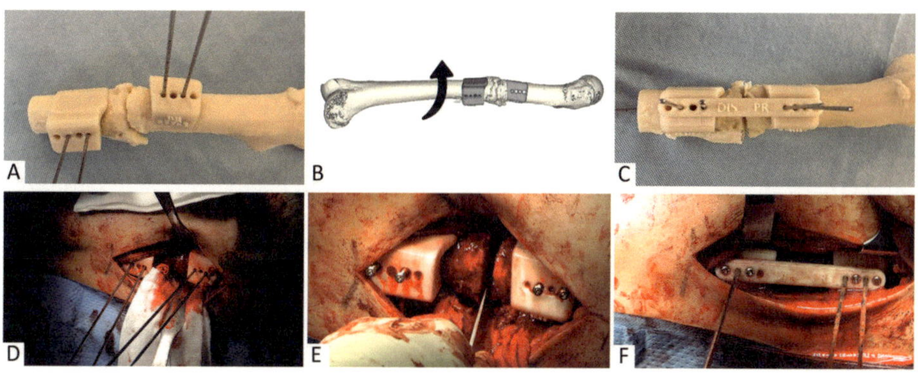

Figure 5.
Surgical procedure. After exposing the femoral diaphysis, guides are fixed to correctly adapt them to the bone (A, D), and then the rotation of the distal femoral fragment is performed (B, E.). Once the wires are aligned, the third 3D- printed guide is used to connect the other two, providing the correct femoral rotation degree (C, F). Modified from Oraa et al. [27].

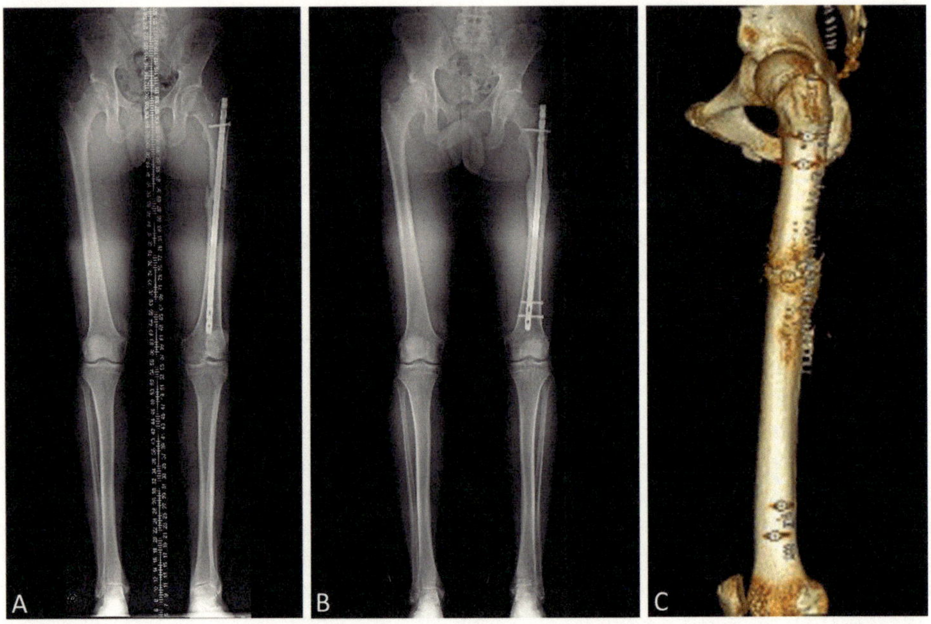

Figure 6.
Imaging study before and after surgery. Teleradiographs were taken to assess rotation before (A) and after osteotomy (B). CT scan indicated whether the alignment of the femur was correct after surgery (C). Modified from Oraa et al. [27].

planned position, achieving a physiological angle femoral anteversion angle of 10°, similar to that of the contralateral hip (**Figure 6**).

5. Application of 3D technology for osteotomies in degenerative knee joint disease

Osteotomies are a growing alternative in the treatment of knee osteoarthritis in adult patients with alterations of the biomechanical axes. This technique is intended to relieve pain, delay knee prosthetic surgery, or prevent early degenerative pathology when meniscectomy is performed or when local chondral lesions are present in a compartment in young people [15, 16]. These treatments are becoming more and more precise thanks to new technological advances such as customized 3D guides that shorten surgical times and allow patients to recover quickly [36]. Tibial knee osteotomy is used in the management of medial compartment osteoarthritis in patients with varus malalignment [18, 19]. Effective tibial knee osteotomy begins with proper patient selection. Although there is never a perfect case, it is preferable that the patient be relatively young, with unicompartmental chondropathy, without associated bone pathologies that could complicate the consolidation of the osteotomy, and that the patient be cooperative and involved in the post-surgical process involved in this type of intervention.

The physical examination is equally important to assess joint balance, ligament stability, patellofemoral compartment, and axial evaluation and to discard associated pathologies such as hip pathologies. The planning of the surgery is very important using weight-bearing X-ray to assess the state of the joint, severity, patella height, and patellar tracking and to discard possible degenerative pathology. Telemetry allows the measurement of axes and the assessment of the limb as a whole and ruling out associated biomechanical pathologies. MRI provides information on the degenerative state of these compartments in terms of cartilage, meniscus, and ligaments.

Finally, until the advent of 3D CT, planning was carried out in 2D, which did not provide such precise information and did not allow corrections to be made in the axial plane. However, 3D CT provides three-dimensional information about the entire limb, which allows for more precise surgical planning, as well as anticipating possible unforeseen events. With this type of imaging study, it is also possible to correct possible errors in X-rays and telemetry. Finally, 3D CT allows the design and printing of a 3D model of the limb and the customization of the guides with great precision [27]. With better planning, patients will undergo customized surgeries with fewer errors, shorter surgical times, and better recoveries.

5.1 Clinical case

The patient was a 57-year-old male with a history of internal meniscopathy with an associated chondral lesion in the internal femoral condyle, which did not respond to conservative treatment. After a complete imaging study (**Figure 7**), telemetry showed an internal biomechanical axis, with a varus axis of 6°. The X-ray images revealed an impingement of the internal articular compartment, without medial osteophytes, correct patellar height, no apparent joint degeneration, and adequate patellar tracking. The MRI showed a complex tear of the internal meniscus with a chondral lesion of the internal femoral condyle and reactive edema. The information

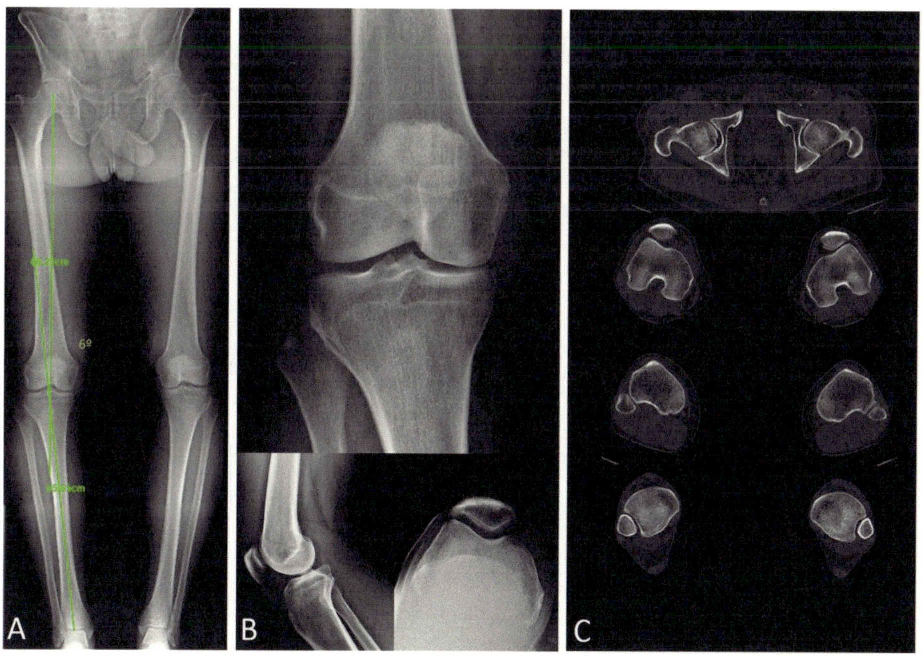

Figure 7.
Imaging studies. By analyzing the axis with telemetry (A), the state of the joint with X-rays (B), and the knee in all planes on CT (C), appropriate surgical planning can be performed.

provided by the pre-surgical CT scan made it possible to study the joint in all its planes, to assess associated pathologies or possible malrotations of the limb and evaluate the patient's bone surfaces to design personalized osteotomy guides.

Once the image studies were analyzed, the 3D model of the tibia was made and the surgery was planned virtually, calculating aspects such as the tibial cut and the place where to perform the fibula osteotomy. Based on this planning, all the surgical material necessary for the osteotomy was designed. Subsequently, the anatomical model, the cutting guides, the osteosynthesis plate, and the final result were 3D printed (**Figure 8**).

During the surgery, an arthroscopic examination revealed the absence of pathology in the external and patellofemoral compartment, which allowed the osteotomy to proceed. After cleaning the internal compartment, a meniscectomy was conducted due to the complex meniscal tear, and the spongolisation of the internal femoral condyle was performed due to the chondral lesion. In a second step, an anterior lateral approach to the knee was carried out to access the proximal tibia and fibula. An oblique incision was made in front of the lateral collateral

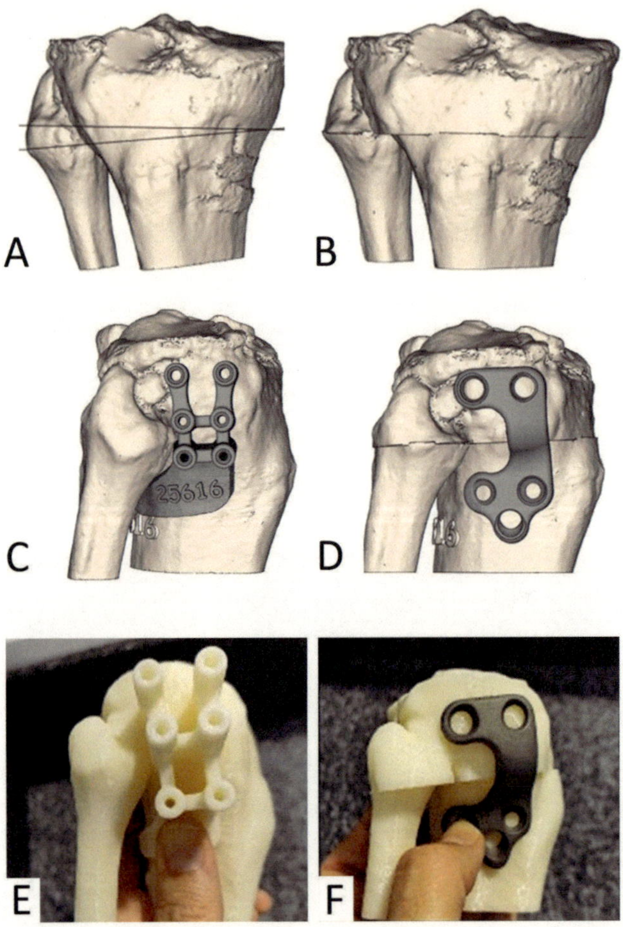

Figure 8.
Surgical planning. Based on the 3D design, the cutting planes were calculated (A) and the final result was evaluated (B). Subsequently, both the cutting guides (C) and the osteosynthesis plate (D) were designed, and they were printed in 3D for their use during the surgery (E-F).

ligament, and a flap from the extensor and tibialis anterior muscles was detached, allowing anterior visualization of the tibia and fibula while respecting the lateral collateral ligament.

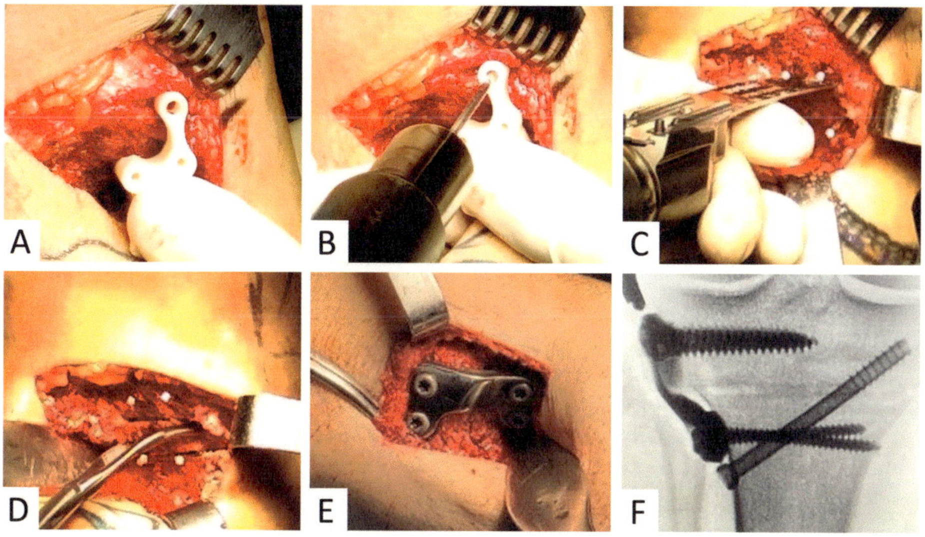

Figure 9.
Surgical procedure. After the placement of the cutting guide (A) and its fixation to the bone (B), the tibial cut was performed (C). Once the bone wedge was removed (D), the osteosynthesis plate was placed (E), and its positioning was checked by radiological control (F).

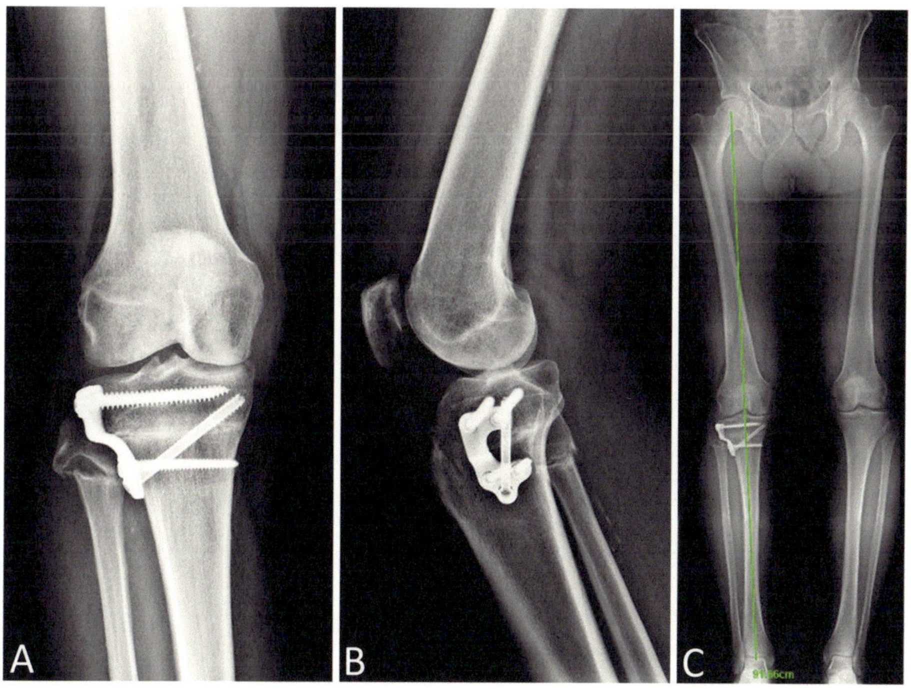

Figure 10.
Post-surgical imaging study. Post-surgical anteroposterior (A) and lateral (B) radiographs showed a good result of the surgery. Post-surgical telemetry (C) also showed correction of the biomechanical axes.

The planned fibula osteotomy was then performed according to the pre-surgical planning. For the tibial osteotomy, the guide designed to adapt to the patient's bony anatomy, and its fixation with needles was placed. After radiological examination, the guide was removed, and the anterior osteotomy of the anterior tibial tuberosity was performed so as not to influence the patella height, and then, the tibial cut was made. The bone wedge was then removed, and the anatomical osteosynthesis plate was placed, also achieved thanks to the 3D design (**Figure 9**).

X-rays showed that the osteotomy was adequately closed. These guides also facilitate the guided placement of an oblique partial thread screw, which allows greater bone contact and helps to achieve a good consolidation of the osteotomy. Post-surgical telemetry showed the correction of the biomechanical axes required during planning (**Figure 10**).

6. Conclusion

The use of 3D technology in orthopedic surgery includes both the design and printing of anatomical models and surgical materials. The introduction of this technology in this field allows the surgeon to plan the surgery with greater precision as well as to design personalized material suitable for each patient. All this means an optimization in surgical intervention that has a positive impact on the clinical outcome of the patient.

Author details

Mikel Sánchez[1,2]*, Alexis Fernández[1], Leonor López de Dicastillo[1], Jaime Oraa[1], Xabier Sánchez[3], Jorge Guadilla[1], Nicolás Fiz[1] and Diego Delgado[2]

1 Arthroscopic Surgery Unit, Hospital Vithas Vitoria, Vitoria-Gasteiz, Spain

2 Advanced Biological Therapy Unit, Hospital Vithas Vitoria, Vitoria-Gasteiz, Spain

3 Osteomodel, San Sebastián, Spain

*Address all correspondence to: mikel.sanchez@ucatrauma.com

References

[1] O'Connor O, Patel R, Thahir A, Sy J, Jou E. The use of three-dimensional printing in orthopaedics: a systematic review and meta-analysis. Archives of Bone and Joint Surgery. 2024;**12**(7):441-456

[2] Karlin L, Weinstock P, Hedequist D, Prabhu SP. The surgical treatment of spinal deformity in children with myelomeningocele: The role of personalized three-dimensional printed models. Journal of Pediatric Orthopaedics. Part B. 2017;**26**(4):375-382

[3] Webb PA. A review of rapid prototyping (RP) techniques in the medical and biomedical sector. Journal of Medical Engineering & Technology. 2000;**24**(4):149-153

[4] Matsumoto JS, Morris JM, Foley TA, Williamson EE, Leng S, McGee KP, et al. Three-dimensional physical modeling: Applications and experience at Mayo Clinic. Radiographics. 2015;**35**(7):1989-2006

[5] Bücking TM, Hill ER, Robertson JL, Maneas E, Plumb AA, Nikitichev DI. From medical imaging data to 3D printed anatomical models. PLoS One. 2017;**12**(5):e0178540

[6] Rengier F, Mehndiratta A, von Tengg-Kobligk H, Zechmann CM, Unterhinninghofen R, Kauczor HU, et al. 3D printing based on imaging data: Review of medical applications. International Journal of Computer Assisted Radiology and Surgery. 2010;**5**(4):335-341

[7] Mitsouras D, Liacouras P, Imanzadeh A, Giannopoulos AA, Cai T, Kumamaru KK, et al. Medical 3D printing for the radiologist. Radiographics. 2015;**35**(7):1965-1988

[8] Heller M, Bauer HK, Goetze E, Gielisch M, Roth KE, Drees P, et al. Applications of patient-specific 3D printing in medicine. International Journal of Computerized Dentistry. 2016;**19**(4):323-339

[9] Shui W, Zhou M, Chen S, Pan Z, Deng Q, Yao Y, et al. The production of digital and printed resources from multiple modalities using visualization and three-dimensional printing techniques. International Journal of Computer Assisted Radiology and Surgery. 2017;**12**(1):13-23

[10] Ventola CL. Medical applications for 3D printing: Current and projected uses. Pharmacy and Therapeutics. 2014;**39**(10):704-711

[11] Zambouri A. Preoperative evaluation and preparation for anesthesia and surgery. Hippokratia. 2007;**11**(1):13-21

[12] Howell SM, Kuznik K, Hull ML, Siston RA. Results of an initial experience with custom-fit positioning total knee arthroplasty in a series of 48 patients. Orthopedics. 2008;**31**(9):857-863

[13] Slamin J, Parsley B. Evolution of customization design for total knee arthroplasty. Current Reviews in Musculoskeletal Medicine. 2012;**5**(4):290-295

[14] McLawhorn AS, Carroll KM, Blevins JL, DeNegre ST, Mayman DJ, Jerabek SA. Template-directed instrumentation reduces cost and improves efficiency for Total knee arthroplasty: An economic decision

analysis and pilot study. The Journal of Arthroplasty. 2015;**30**(10):1699-1704

[15] Gauci MO, Boileau P, Baba M, Chaoui J, Walch G. Patient-specific glenoid guides provide accuracy and reproducibility in total shoulder arthroplasty. Bone Joint Journal. 2016;**98-B**(8):1080-1085

[16] Chen X, Chen X, Zhang G, Lin H, Yu Z, Wu C, et al. Accurate fixation of plates and screws for the treatment of acetabular fractures using 3D-printed guiding templates: An experimental study. Injury. 2017;**48**(6):1147-1154

[17] Du H, Tian XX, Li TS, Yang JS, Li KH, Pei GX, et al. Use of patient-specific templates in hip resurfacing arthroplasty: Experience from sixteen cases. International Orthopaedics. 2013;**37**(5):777-782

[18] Otsuki B, Takemoto M, Kawanabe K, Awa Y, Akiyama H, Fujibayashi S, et al. Developing a novel custom cutting guide for curved peri-acetabular osteotomy. International Orthopaedics. 2013;**37**(6):1033-1038

[19] Cartiaux O, Paul L, Francq BG, Banse X, Docquier PL. Improved accuracy with 3D planning and patient-specific instruments during simulated pelvic bone tumor surgery. Annals of Biomedical Engineering. 2014;**42**(1):205-213

[20] Cernat E, Docquier PL, Paul L, Banse X, Codorean IB. Patient specific instruments for complex tumor resection-reconstruction surgery within the pelvis: A series of 4 cases. Chirurgia (Bucur). 2016;**111**(5):439-444

[21] Chung KJ, Huang B, Choi CH, Park YW, Kim HN. Utility of 3D printing for complex distal Tibial fractures and malleolar avulsion fractures: Technical tip. Foot and Ankle International. 2015;**36**(12):1504-1510

[22] de Muinck Keizer RJO, Lechner KM, Mulders M, a. M, Schep NWL, Eygendaal D, Goslings JC. Three-dimensional virtual planning of corrective osteotomies of distal radius malunions: a systematic review and meta-analysis. Strategies in Trauma and Limb Reconstruction. 2017;**12**(2):77-89

[23] Honigmann P, Thieringer F, Steiger R, Haefeli M, Schumacher R, Henning J. A simple 3-dimensional printed aid for a corrective palmar opening wedge osteotomy of the distal radius. The Journal of Hand Surgery. 2016;**41**(3):464-469

[24] Schweizer A, Fürnstahl P, Nagy L. Three-dimensional correction of distal radius intra-articular malunions using patient-specific drill guides. The Journal of Hand Surgery. 2013;**38**(12):2339-2347

[25] Oraa J, Fiz N, González S, Beitia M, Sánchez X, Delgado D, et al. Derotation tibial osteotomy with custom cutting guides and custom osteosynthesis plate printed with 3D technology: Case and technical note. Annals of 3D Printed Medicine. 2023;**9**:100093

[26] Fiz N, Delgado D, Sánchez X, Sánchez P, Bilbao AM, Oraa J, et al. Application of 3D technology and printing for femoral derotation osteotomy: Case and technical report. The Annals of Translational Medicine. 2017;**5**(20):400

[27] Oraa J, Beitia M, Fiz N, González S, Sánchez X, Delgado D, et al. Custom 3D-printed cutting guides for femoral osteotomy in rotational malalignment due to Diaphyseal fractures: Surgical technique and case series. Journal of Clinical Medicine. 2021;**10**(15):3366

[28] Victor J, Premanathan A. Virtual 3D planning and patient specific surgical guides for osteotomies around the knee: a feasibility and proof-of-concept study. Bone Joint Journal. 2013;**95-B**(11 Suppl A):153-158

[29] Gruskay JA, Fragomen AT, Rozbruch SR. Idiopathic rotational abnormalities of the lower extremities in children and adults. Journal of Bone and Joint Surgery Reviews. 2019;**7**(1):e3

[30] Boschung A, Antioco T, Steppacher SD, Tannast M, Novais EN, Kim YJ, et al. Limited external rotation and hip extension due to posterior extra-articular Ischiofemoral hip impingement in female patients with increased femoral Anteversion: Implications for sports, sexual, and daily activities. The American Journal of Sports Medicine. 2023;**51**(4):1015-1023

[31] Dablan A, Oktay C, Çevikol C. Ischiofemoral impingement syndrome: Effect of morphological variations on the diagnosis. Current Medical Imaging. 2021;**17**(5):595-601

[32] Gómez-Hoyos J, Schröder R, Reddy M, Palmer IJ, Martin HD. Femoral neck Anteversion and lesser trochanteric retroversion in patients with Ischiofemoral impingement: A case-control magnetic resonance imaging study. Arthroscopy. 2016;**32**(1):13-18

[33] Jeanmart L, Baert AL, Wackenheim A. Atlas of Pathological Computer Tomography: Volume 3: Computer Tomography of Neck, Chest, Spine and Limbs [Internet]. Berlin Heidelberg: Springer-Verlag; 1983. Available from: https://www.springer.com/gp/book/9783642685385 [Accessed: June 24, 2020]

[34] Wissing H, Buddenbrock B. Determining rotational errors of the femur by axial computerized tomography in comparison with clinical and conventional radiologic determination. Unfallchirurgie. 1993;**19**(3):145-157

[35] Fabry G, MacEwen GD, Shands AR. Torsion of the femur. A follow-up study in normal and abnormal conditions. The Journal of Bone and Joint Surgery. American Volume. 1973;**55**(8):1726-1738

[36] Zaffagnini S, Dal Fabbro G, Belvedere C, Leardini A, Caravelli S, Lucidi GA, et al. Custom-made devices represent a promising tool to increase correction accuracy of high Tibial osteotomy: A systematic review of the literature and presentation of pilot cases with a new 3D-printed system. Journal of Clinical Medicine. 2022;**11**(19):5717

Chapter 6

Infection Control

Munehiro Ogawa and Yasuhito Tanaka

Abstract

Knee osteoarthritis (KOA) is a degenerative disease that often results in joint deformity and dysfunction. Among treatment options, high tibial osteotomy (HTO), a joint-sparing surgical technique, effectively treats medial compartment KOA by redistributing load and improving joint alignment. Despite advancements in surgical technique and infection prevention, surgical site infection (SSI) remains a significant complication. This review examines the incidence, risk factors, and management strategies for SSIs following around-knee osteotomy, particularly HTO. While deep SSIs are rare, they pose significant risks such as revision surgery, loss of corrected alignment, and nonunion. Potential risk factors include smoking, diabetes, advanced age, male sex, and use of artificial bone grafts. First-line management typically involves debridement, antibiotics, and implant retention, with additional multifaceted measures for infection control and bone or soft tissue reconstruction in the event of severe complications such as osteomyelitis or infected nonunion. Promising techniques, including negative pressure wound therapy, continuous local antibiotic perfusion, Masquelet technique, and antibiotic-impregnated calcium phosphate cement, have shown success in managing post-traumatic osteomyelitis and periprosthetic joint infections and may benefit osteotomy-related infection. However, the rarity and heterogeneity of SSI hinder standardized treatment protocols. Therefore, large multicenter studies are needed to enhance prevention strategies and improve patient outcomes.

Keywords: around-knee osteotomy, high tibial osteotomy, surgical site infection, infection control, infected nonunion

1. Introduction

Knee osteoarthritis (KOA) is a degenerative condition characterized by the deterioration of cartilage in the knee joint, which leads to a reduction in joint function and is often associated with lower limb deformities [1]. High tibial osteotomy (HTO) is a widely used knee-joint-preserving surgical procedure for the treatment of KOA. This procedure improves alignment and redistributes load stresses in patients with unilateral KOA and associated deformities, thereby alleviating symptoms and slowing the disease progression [2–5]. The surgical technique has evolved from closed-wedge high tibial osteotomy (CWHTO), which was first described by Coventry in 1965 [6]. Since then, various techniques have been developed, collectively referred to as around-knee

IntechOpen

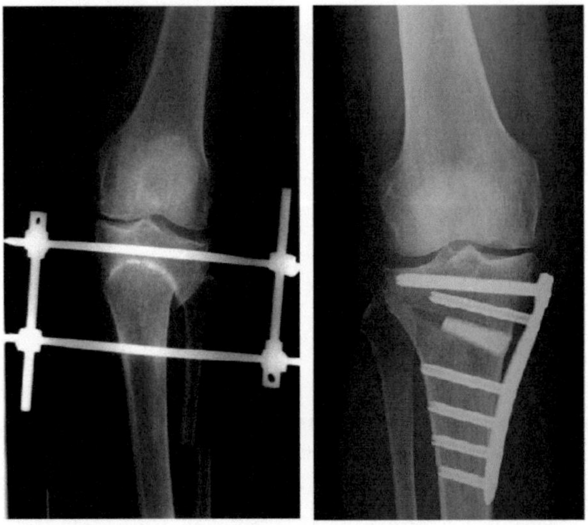

Figure 1.
Barrel vault osteotomy and modern MOWHTO with locking plate and artificial bone (β-tricalcium phosphate) improved osteotomy stability and allowed early weight bearing, contributing to the widespread use of HTO.

osteotomy (AKO) [7–9]. Among these techniques, the development of medial wedge open-wedge high tibial osteotomy (MOWHTO) utilizing a locking plate improved osteotomy stability and allowed early weight bearing, which has contributed to the widespread adoption of this technique (**Figure 1**) [10, 11]. This innovation has led to increased demand, particularly in response to an aging population and greater sports participation [12].

HTO is often recommended for young, active patients with medial compartment osteoarthritis, as it redistributes load away from the medial compartment by slightly realigning the mechanical axis toward the lateral compartment [13–17]. Recently, combining MOWHTO with arthroscopic knee surgery for cartilage and meniscus repair has gained popularity, as this approach enhances the healing process [18–20]. Although HTO generally produces favorable short- and long-term outcomes [21–23], complications can occur, such as superficial and deep surgical site infections (SSI), delayed union, nonunion, hardware failure, hematoma formation, neurovascular disorder, and hinge fractures. Despite advancements in infection prevention and surgical techniques, postoperative infection remains a significant complication, potentially leading to frequent reoperation, loss of correction, and nonunion [13, 24]. While surgical techniques and rehabilitation have advanced, evidence-based treatment strategies for managing infection following AKO remain controversial owing to the rarity and heterogeneity of such cases, as well as the limited available research on infection control following osteotomy. This chapter provides a comprehensive overview of infection control after osteotomy, with a focus on the incidence, risk factors, and treatment strategies in this specialized field.

2. Incidence

SSIs following AKO are relatively uncommon but can lead to significant complications, including repeated surgeries and adverse clinical and radiological results

[11, 13, 14, 24–26]. Despite several studies on SSIs following osteotomy, comprehensive data remain limited, mostly consisting of small case series from single-center studies, particularly those focusing on HTO [13, 27, 28]. Furthermore, these studies often lack clear definitions of infection, and variations in surgical methods, fixation techniques, study designs, patient demographics, implant types, and other variables hinder direct comparisons between studies [13, 26, 29]. According to the Centers for Disease Control and Prevention, superficial SSIs are usually treated with systemic antibiotics based on visible symptoms such as redness and swelling around the surgery site. In contrast, deep SSIs present with abscesses, purulent drainage, fever, and significantly elevated inflammatory markers and require surgical intervention [30, 31].

A systematic review by Anagnostakos et al. (2013) reported an incidence of superficial SSIs ranging from 1 to 9%, with deep SSIs occurring between 0.5 and 4.7% [13]. This review analyzed 26 studies involving 2026 patients and 2210 knees undergoing MOWHTO and CWHTO. Advancements in surgical techniques, particularly the use of locking plates and allograft bone wedges, have contributed to the widespread use of MOWHTO. However, factors such as hematomas at the osteotomy site, improper plate placement in areas with thin subcutaneous tissue, and the creation of dead spaces exposing the bone marrow have been associated with higher postoperative infection rates [32, 33]. Recent studies on OWHTO using locking plates have reported deep infection rates of 2% by Sidhu R et al. [34] and 4.9% by Liu TW et al. [26], respectively. Given the rarity of infection-related complications after HTO, large-scale, multicenter studies are essential for better understanding and prevention [13, 14, 27, 35, 36]. A national database study by Kawata et al., involving 12,853 patients, identified a 1.52% incidence of superficial SSIs and 0.39% incidence of deep SSIs [14]. However, the study's median follow-up of 34 days (limited to the postoperative hospital stay) suggests these rates may underestimate the actual SSI rates. Nonetheless, infection was identified as the most frequent early complication after HTO in this large national study. In a study by Hancock et al., which included 755 patients (822 osteotomies) from a high-volume AKO center with a mean follow-up of 6.3 years, deep SSI rates were reported to be 1.2% across all knee osteotomies and 1.6% for HTO alone [37]. Although recent surgical advancements have likely contributed to reducing infection rates, SSIs remain a significant concern during the early postoperative phase [14, 27, 37]. As surgical techniques continue to improve and the demand for osteotomies increases among young, more active patients, understanding the risk factors for SSIs and implementing effective preventive strategies will be essential for reducing complications and improving long-term clinical outcomes.

3. Risk factors

Recognizing the factors that increase the likelihood of postsurgical infections in AKO is crucial for reducing severe complications and improving patient outcomes. Identifying these risk factors helps prevent infections and make informed decisions about selecting the appropriate candidates for surgery. Similar to the incidence of SSI, many studies examining risk factors rely on single-center data with small sample sizes, which may introduce bias [13]. To achieve more accurate results, large-scale, multicenter studies are needed to better understand these factors, leading to more reliable findings. Such studies will also enhance patient education regarding potential complications and help refine the selection process. A variety of risk factors have been identified in previous reports as possible risk factors, including patient-related factors such as smoking, diabetes, sex, and age, as well as surgical factors such as the use of artificial bones [14, 26, 27, 29, 37]. These factors are discussed in more detail in the subsequent section.

3.1 Smoking

Smoking is widely recognized as a significant risk factor for complications following orthopedic procedures, including AKO [11, 13, 38–49]. Patients who smoke and undergo MOWHTO are at an increased risk of SSI and nonunion due to the detrimental impact of smoking on the immune system and wound healing. Smoking suppresses immune functions, including immunoglobulin levels, immune cell ratios, and phagocyte activity, all of which contribute to the risk of infection [50, 51]. Furthermore, smoking disrupts endothelial function and directly impairs the healing process *via* substances such as nicotine, nitric oxide, and carbon monoxide [14, 50–52]. These substances hinder oxygen distribution to tissues, impair tissue regeneration, and thus contribute to higher rates of SSI among smokers [53–55]. Although the precise impact of smoking on postoperative infections following HTO remains unclear, smoking cessation programs have proven to be effective in reducing complications in orthopedic surgeries. Therefore, patients should be strongly encouraged to quit smoking before undergoing elective procedures such as MOWHTO, as smoking increases the likelihood of osteotomy failure and nonunion [46, 48, 49]. Further research is required to determine the optimal timing and duration of smoking cessation to mitigate these risks [14].

3.2 Diabetes mellitus

Diabetes is a well-established risk factor for postoperative complications, including SSI after AKO [25, 26] and periprosthetic joint infections (PJI) following procedures such as total knee arthroplasty (TKA) [56–61]. Studies have shown that diabetes increases the risk of infection by impairing immune function, especially leukocyte activity, which reduces the body's ability to combat infections [62, 63]. Additionally, hyperglycemia impairs wound healing by causing microangiopathy, leading to ischemia, and reducing the effectiveness of antibiotics [64, 65]. Research indicates that patients with diabetes experience higher rates of deep infections post-surgery, with those with poor glycemic control at an even greater risk. Effective management of blood glucose levels during the perioperative period can help reduce the risk of infection [56, 59, 66]. Furthermore, other factors such as the duration of surgery also play a role in influencing infection rates [14, 61].

3.3 Age

Age significantly influences the risk of SSI after orthopedic procedures, including AKO [26, 67–69]. For TKA, younger patients show a higher incidence of SSI compared to older patients, possibly due to factors such as higher activity levels or other reasons that are not fully understood [70–73]. However, younger age is generally considered a protective factor against infections following surgeries, such as HTO, likely due to better tissue oxygenation and a higher capacity for tissue recovery and resistance to infection [74–77]. On the other hand, older age is typically associated with an increased risk of infection after orthopedic surgery. For example, a study by Kaye et al. reported a 1.1% annual increase in SSI risk between the ages of 17 and 65 years, but after the age of 65, the risk appeared to decrease by 1.2% annually [78]. Notably, the majority of patients undergoing HTO are under 65 years of age, suggesting that age-related risks may vary depending on the procedure and patient characteristics.

3.4 Sex

Male sex has been identified as a significant risk factor for SSI, including AKO [14, 79]. Similarly, men face a higher risk of PJIs after total knee and hip arthroplasty [42, 71, 80, 81] and other orthopedic procedures, such as anterior cruciate ligament reconstruction [82, 83]. This increased risk is partially attributed to the biological differences between men and women; for example, men often engage in higher levels of activity, which may increase their exposure to factors that elevate the likelihood of infection [79]. Additionally, studies of biological differences suggest that estrogen plays a positive role in wound healing by regulating genes involved in tissue regeneration and matrix production, whereas androgens may have a negative impact on the healing process [25].

3.5 Bone grafting in OWHTO

In OWHTO, several options are available for filling the osteotomy gap. These include natural bone grafts (e.g., iliac crest), artificial bone graft substitutes such as beta-tricalcium phosphate and hydroxyapatite, or leaving the gap unfilled. Each approach has its own set of advantages and disadvantages [26]. Bone grafting promotes bone union and stabilizes the osteotomy gap, particularly in cases where the gap is large (≥10 mm) [84, 85]. However, different types of grafts come with potential drawbacks. For example, the use of allografts or artificial bone grafts may increase the risk of complications, such as weak antibacterial properties, biocompatibility, and potential immunological rejection [86]. While autogenous bone grafting is highly effective, it is associated with certain risks. These include increased surgical trauma, longer operation times, and donor-site morbidity. Artificial bone graft substitutes, on the other hand, eliminate these donor-site morbidity and reduce the risk of disease transmission or immune-related complications [87]. Despite their benefit, surgeons must carefully assess the advantages and disadvantages of each option according to the patient's specific needs. Studies have shown that artificial bone grafts can be safely used [88–90]; however, the potential risk of SSI following HTO must be considered [14, 33].

4. Management strategies for deep SSI following AKO

The management of deep SSIs following AKO remains a challenge, as most available evidence are derived from small-scale, single-center studies. These infections are typically managed through various approaches, including retaining or removing of internal fixation devices, using surgical drains or vacuum-assisted dressings, administering antibiotics both locally and systemically, and performing additional procedures for bone and soft tissue reconstruction [37]. Due to the variability in reported methods, no universally accepted treatment guidelines have been establish. Typically, the initial management involves debridement, antibiotics, and implant retention (DAIR) (**Figure 2**). In some cases, the removal of foreign materials is required for

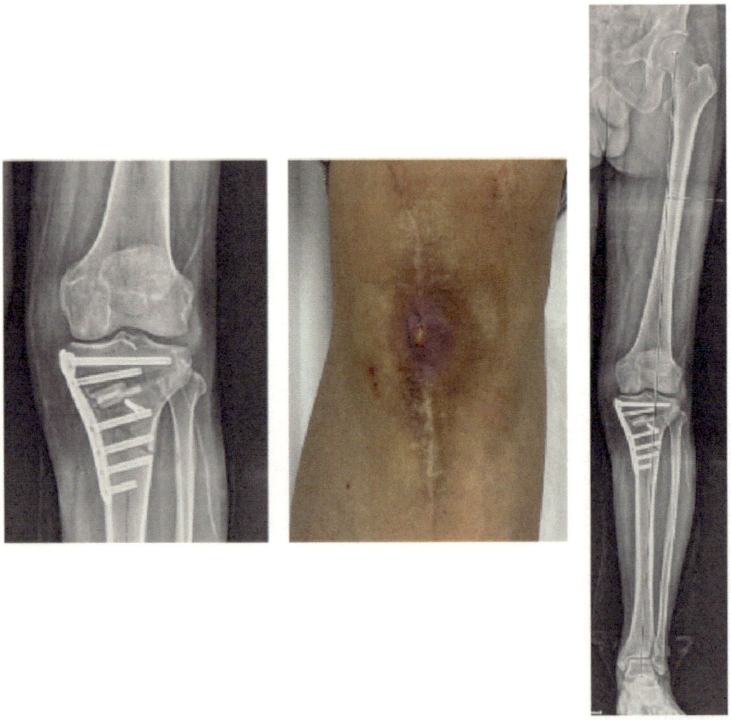

Figure 2.
Infection after medial open-wedge distal tibial osteotomy (MOWDTO), fistula in the wound, DAIR could control infection without corrective loss of alignment.

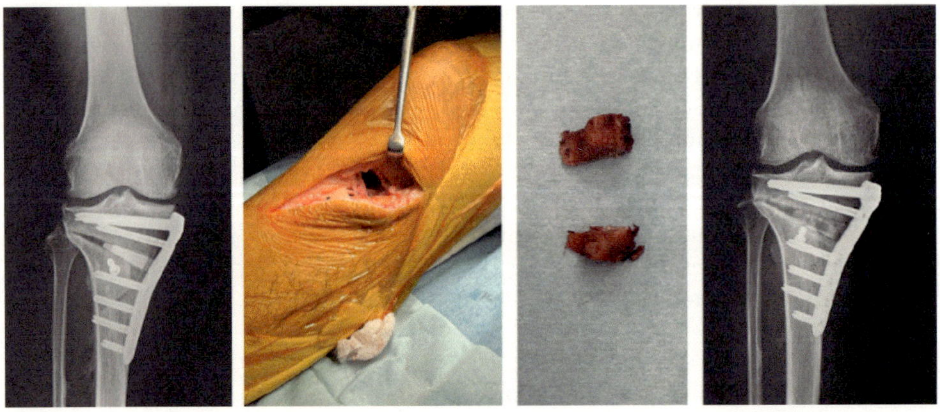

Figure 3.
Infection after medial open-wedge distal tibial osteotomy (MOWDTO), with deep abscess, debridement including artificial bone, and reoperation with bone graft from iliac bone after confirmation of infection control.

infection control (**Figure 3**). However, during the early postoperative period, when bone union is not yet achieved, implant removal poses a risk of losing the corrected alignment. Therefore, the decision to remove implants after HTO must be carefully considered [13, 24, 91].

4.1 Debridement, antibiotics, and implant retention (DAIR)

The European Society of Sports Traumatology, Knee Surgery, and Arthroscopy (ESSKA) provides consensus recommendations for the management of painful degenerative knee osteotomies (**Figure 4**) [92]. They advocate debridement, antibiotics, and implant retention (DAIR) as the first-line treatment for patients presenting with purulent discharge, abscesses, and elevated inflammatory markers. If infection

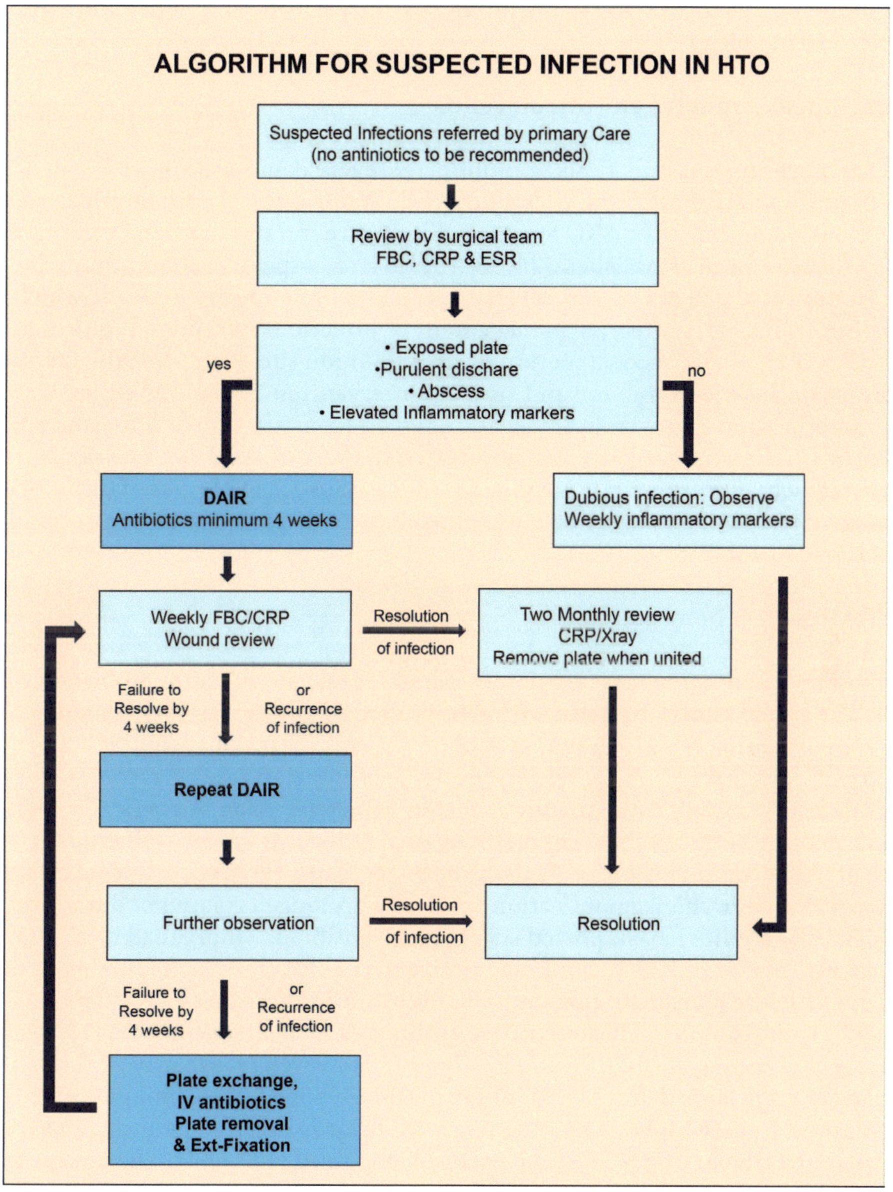

Figure 4.
ESSKA consensus document algorithm for treatment of osteotomy infection. ESR: erythrocyte sedimentation rate; FBC: full blood count.

persists, external fixation or plate removal should be considered. While the consensus emphasizes the need for further research to enhance the evidence on infection control after knee osteotomy, Hancock et al. reported favorable outcomes [37]. In a study involving 822 osteotomy cases with 755 patients, deep infections occurred in only nine cases (1.2%). Notably, none of these patients required external fixation, reoperation, or infectious nonunion when managed according to the DAIR principles. Early detection and the application of DAIR principles significantly increase the likelihood of treating infection without additional procedures or external fixation. The findings of this study support the ESSKA algorithm as an effective method for infection control in knee osteotomies.

4.2 Infectious nonunion and osteomyelitis

Osteomyelitis and infectious nonunion are severe complications that can occur due to postoperative infection following AKO. While cases of osteomyelitis and infectious nonunion after AKO are exceedingly rare, no standardized treatment protocols have been established [24, 93–95]. In a retrospective cohort study by van Houten et al., 19 out of 280 HTO cases resulted in nonunion, two of which were infectious [49]. Effective management of infectious nonunion requires both infection control and reconstruction of the nonunion site. This typically involves appropriate antibiotic therapy and surgical intervention, including lesion curettage, stabilization of unstable areas, and staged reconstruction of bone and soft tissue [96]. The primary pathogen implicated in these cases is *Staphylococcus aureus*, which may necessitate localized treatments, such as the use of antibiotic-impregnated PMMA beads or calcium phosphate bone paste to achieve optimal infection control [24].

4.3 Treatment of bone defects

Biofilm formation in infected tissues is highly resistant to antimicrobial agents [97]. The eradication of bacteria within bone canals is particularly challenging as intravenous antibiotics alone cannot achieve the concentrations required locally for infection control [96]. Therefore, curettage of infected areas is recommended. Bone defects resulting from infection-related bone resorption or surgical curettage can be managed effectively using methods such as Ilizarov external fixation or bone grafting combined with soft tissue coverage flaps. However, external fixation is associated with a high complication rate and a prolonged treatment duration [98]. Several studies have reported success with antibiotic-impregnated calcium phosphate cement (AICPC) combined with external fixation for stabilizing bone defects. Calcium phosphate cement (CPC) is biocompatible, osteoconductive [24, 99], compatible with heat-sensitive antibiotics such as vancomycin [100], and capable of retaining antibiotics effectively [99]. However, its use may be limited in cases of large bone defects [101]. For critical-size bone loss, techniques such as the Masquelet method, bone lengthening with Ilizarov external fixation, and free vascularized fibular graft (FVFG) have been employed [102–104]. The Masquelet technique, which involves using an induced membrane for bone reconstruction, shows high infection control and bone union rates, making it a promising option for AKO-related infectious nonunion. Compared to the Ilizarov method, the Masquelet technique is simpler to perform and is more suitable for elderly patients [105]. In cases of infected pseudoarthrosis or severe joint degeneration, staged TKA following debridement and inflammation control is another viable treatment option [93, 94, 106, 107].

4.4 Soft tissue reconstruction

Negative Pressure Wound Therapy (NPWT), also known as vacuum-assisted closure, promotes wound healing by removing excess exudate and stimulating angiogenesis. Since its introduction in 1997, NPWT has been widely used as an adjunct in trauma treatment. It aids in the removal of necrotic tissue, enhances tissue oxygenation, promotes granulation tissue formations, and reduces infection rates [108]. Flap transplantation is another common method for repairing soft tissue defects in the lower limbs. Recent advancements in microsurgical techniques have allowed continuous refinement of flap designs. The key to successful treatment lies in selecting the appropriate flap technique based on the location, extent, and nature of the defect to ensure proper wound coverage and healing (**Figure 5**) [109].

4.5 Local therapy and reconstruction techniques

Continuous Local Antibiotic Perfusion (CLAP) involves the continuous infusion of antibiotics into the infected area while applying negative pressure to circulate the medication. This method enables the targeted delivery of high concentrations of antibiotic over an extended duration, addressing the limitations of systemic antibiotic therapy in poorly vascularized regions [110]. By maintaining high local antibiotic concentrations, CLAP effectively treats biofilm-associated infections that would otherwise require minimal biofilm eradication concentrations (MBEC) exceeding 100–1000 times the minimal inhibitory concentration (MIC) [111]. Techniques such as iMAP (intra-Medullary Antibiotics Perfusion) for bone and iSAP (intra-Soft tissue Antibiotics Perfusion) for soft tissue have been developed. These technique has shown promise in managing PJI after TKA [112–114] and fracture-related infections

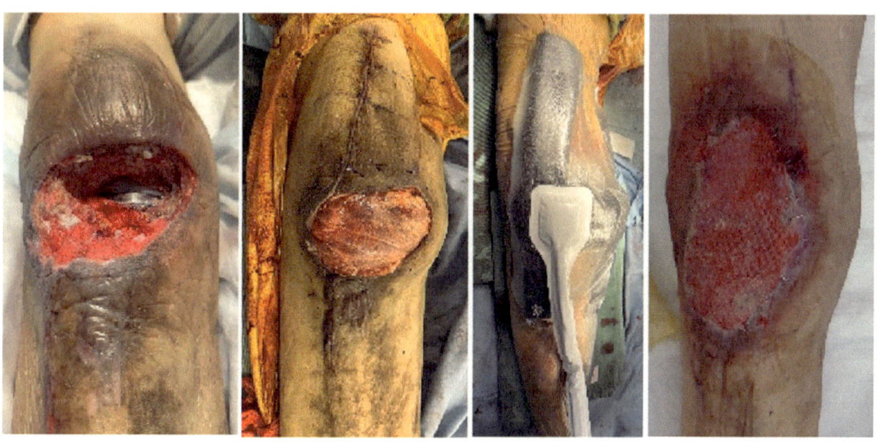

Figure 5.
After extensive debridement of PJI following TKA, the medial gastrocnemius flap for soft tissue reconstruction, postoperative management with NPWT, and split thickness skin grafting after soft tissue recovery.

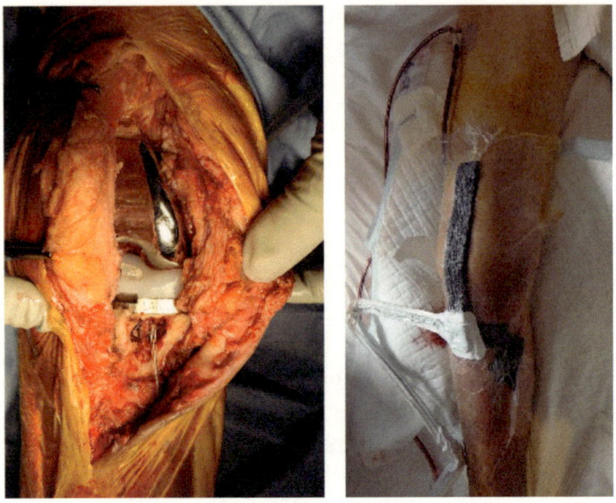

Figure 6.
PJI following TKA in an elderly patient with medical complications. Implant loosening was not observed, and infection control was achieved using CLAP with (iSAP) without removing the implant. The antibiotic delivery tube was positioned to ensure targeted flow to the debrided area.

(FRI) [110, 115–120]. Additionally, CLAP offers potential as a novel treatment for refractory infections following osteotomy (**Figure 6**).

4.6 Future perspectives

While research on HTO is extensive, studies focusing on the management of deep SSI and infectious nonunion are scarce. Various approaches for managing infections and nonunion after AKO exist, but no universal treatment strategy has been established. Treatment plans must balance stability with infection control and be tailored to the individual patient and the stage of infection. Early diagnosis and intervention, combined with appropriate antibiotic selection and surgical techniques, are critical for improving recovery rates in these complex cases. Future studies are needed to develop standardized treatment protocols.

5. Conclusion

AKO, including HTO, is an effective treatment for osteoarthritis of the knee, especially in younger active patients. Despite advances in surgical techniques and infection prevention, SSI remains a significant challenge. Although a combination of early intervention and DAIR is recommended for the management of deep SSIs, the treatment approach must be flexible and tailored to individual patient conditions. In addition to infection control, the treatment of infectious complications requires a multifaceted approach that includes bone and soft tissue reconstruction.

The identification and prevention of risk factors are important for reducing the incidence of complications. Furthermore, the accumulation of data from large multicenter studies is essential to establish more robust evidence-based treatment protocols. Further improvement in the long-term clinical outcome following AKO, particularly through enhanced infection control strategies, is expected.

Acknowledgements

The authors express their gratitude to Editage for their support in editing and language refinement.

Conflict of interest

The authors declare that they have no competing financial interests or personal relationships that may have influenced the findings reported in this study.

Author details

Munehiro Ogawa[1*] and Yasuhito Tanaka[1,2]

1 Nara Medical University, Department of Sports Medicine, Nara, Japan

2 Nara Medical University, Department of Orthopedic Surgery, Nara, Japan

*Address all correspondence to: mogawa@naramed-u.ac.jp

References

[1] Zampogna B, Vasta S, Papalia R. Patient evaluation and indications for osteotomy around the knee. Clinics in Sports Medicine. 2019;**38**:305-315. DOI: 10.1016/j.csm.2019.02.011

[2] Brinkman JM, Lobenhoffer P, Agneskirchner JD, Staubli AE, Wymenga AB, van Heerwaarden RJ. Osteotomies around the knee: Patient selection, stability of fixation and bone healing in high tibial osteotomies. Journal of Bone and Joint Surgery. British Volume (London). 2008;**90**:1548-1557. DOI: 10.1302/0301-620X.90B12.21198

[3] Duivenvoorden T, Brouwer RW, Baan A, Bos PK, Reijman M, Bierma-Zeinstra SM, et al. Comparison of closing-wedge and opening-wedge high tibial osteotomy for medial compartment osteoarthritis of the knee: A randomized controlled trial with a six-year follow-up. The Journal of Bone and Joint Surgery. American Volume. 2014;**96**:1425-1432. DOI: 10.2106/JBJS.M.00786

[4] Konopka JF, Gomoll AH, Thornhill TS, Katz JN, Losina E. The cost-effectiveness of surgical treatment of medial unicompartmental knee osteoarthritis in younger patients: A computer model-based evaluation. The Journal of Bone and Joint Surgery. American Volume. 2015;**97**:807-817. DOI: 10.2106/JBJS.N.00925

[5] Rossi R, Bonasia DE, Amendola A. The role of high tibial osteotomy in the varus knee. The Journal of the American Academy of Orthopaedic Surgeons. 2011;**19**:590-599. DOI: 10.5435/00124635-201110000-00003

[6] Coventry MB. Osteotomy of the upper portion of the tibia for degenerative arthritis of the knee. A preliminary report. The Journal of Bone and Joint Surgery. American Volume. 1965;**47**:984-990

[7] Kayaalp ME, Apseloff NA, Lott A, Kaarre J, Hughes JD, Ollivier M, et al. Around-the-knee osteotomies part 1: Definitions, rationale and planning-state of the art. Journal of ISAKOS. 2024;**9**:645-657. DOI: 10.1016/j.jisako.2024.02.017

[8] Peng H, Ou A, Huang X, Wang C, Wang L, Yu T, et al. Osteotomy around the knee: The surgical treatment of osteoarthritis. Orthopaedic Surgery. 2021;**13**:1465-1473. DOI: 10.1111/os.13021

[9] Takeuchi R, Ishikawa H, Miyasaka Y, Sasaki Y, Kuniya T, Tsukahara S. A novel closed-wedge high tibial osteotomy procedure to treat osteoarthritis of the knee: Hybrid technique and rehabilitation measures. Arthroscopy Techniques. 2014;**3**:e431-e437. DOI: 10.1016/j.eats.2014.04.004

[10] Hernigou P, Medevielle D, Debeyre J, Goutallier D. Proximal tibial osteotomy for osteoarthritis with varus deformity. A ten to thirteen-year follow-up study. The Journal of Bone and Joint Surgery. American Volume. 1987;**69**:332-354

[11] Staubli AE, De Simoni C, Babst R, Lobenhoffer P. TomoFix: A new LCP-concept for open wedge osteotomy of the medial proximal tibia--early results in 92 cases. Injury. 2003;**34**(Suppl. 2):B55-B62. DOI: 10.1016/j.injury.2003.09.025

[12] Kawata M, Sasabuchi Y, Inui H, Taketomi S, Matsui H, Fushimi K, et al. Annual trends in knee arthroplasty and tibial osteotomy: Analysis of a national database in Japan. The Knee.

2017;**24**:1198-1205. DOI: 10.1016/j.knee.2017.06.005

[13] Anagnostakos K, Mosser P, Kohn D. Infections after high tibial osteotomy. Knee Surgery, Sports Traumatology, Arthroscopy. 2013;**21**:161-169. DOI: 10.1007/s00167-012-2084-5

[14] Kawata M, Jo T, Taketomi S, Inui H, Yamagami R, Matsui H, et al. Type of bone graft and primary diagnosis were associated with nosocomial surgical site infection after high tibial osteotomy: Analysis of a national database. Knee Surgery, Sports Traumatology, Arthroscopy. 2021;**29**:429-436. DOI: 10.1007/s00167-020-05943-4

[15] Liu X, Chen Z, Gao Y, Zhang J, Jin Z. High tibial osteotomy: Review of techniques and biomechanics. Journal of Healthcare Engineering. 2019;**2019**:8363128. DOI: 10.1155/2019/8363128

[16] Smith TO, Sexton D, Mitchell P, Hing CB. Opening- or closing-wedged high tibial osteotomy: A meta-analysis of clinical and radiological outcomes. The Knee. 2011;**18**:361-368. DOI: 10.1016/j.knee.2010.10.001

[17] Wang Z, Zeng Y, She W, Luo X, Cai L. Is opening-wedge high tibial osteotomy superior to closing-wedge high tibial osteotomy in treatment of unicompartmental osteoarthritis? A meta-analysis of randomized controlled trials. International Journal of Surgery. 2018;**60**:153-163. DOI: 10.1016/j.ijsu.2018.10.045

[18] Faber S, Zellner J, Angele P, Spahn G, Loer I, Zinser W, et al. Decision making for concomitant high tibial osteotomy (HTO) in cartilage repair patients based on a nationwide cohort study of 4968 patients. Archives of Orthopaedic and Trauma Surgery. 2020;**140**:1437-1444. DOI: 10.1007/s00402-020-03476-6

[19] Schuster P, Schulz M, Mayer P, Schlumberger M, Immendoerfer M, Richter J. Open-wedge high tibial osteotomy and combined abrasion/microfracture in severe medial osteoarthritis and varus malalignment: 5-year results and arthroscopic findings after 2 years. Arthroscopy. 2015;**31**:1279-1288. DOI: 10.1016/j.arthro.2015.02.010

[20] Wang H, Man Q, Gao Y, Xu L, Zhang J, Ma Y, et al. The efficacy of medial meniscal posterior root tear repair with or without high tibial osteotomy: A systematic review. BMC Musculoskeletal Disorders. 2023;**24**:464. DOI: 10.1186/s12891-023-06520-9

[21] Amendola A, Bonasia DE. Results of high tibial osteotomy: Review of the literature. International Orthopaedics. 2010;**34**:155-160. DOI: 10.1007/s00264-009-0889-8

[22] Darees M, Putman S, Brosset T, Roumazeille T, Pasquier G, Migaud H. Opening-wedge high tibial osteotomy performed with locking plate fixation (TomoFix) and early weight-bearing but without filling the defect. A concise follow-up note of 48 cases at 10 years' follow-up. Orthopaedics & Traumatology, Surgery & Research. 2018;**104**:477-480. DOI: 10.1016/j.otsr.2017.12.021

[23] Sawaguchi T, Takeuchi R, Nakamura R, Yonekura A, Akiyama T, Kerstan M, et al. Outcome after treatment of osteoarthritis with open-wedge high-tibial osteotomy with a plate: 2-year results of a Japanese cohort study. Journal of Orthopaedic Surgery (Hong Kong). 2020;**28**:2309499019887997. DOI: 10.1177/2309499019887997

[24] Seki K, Sakka A, Tokushige A, Imagama T, Mutou M, Taguchi T. Treatment for Staphylococcus aureus infection following open wedge high

tibial osteotomy using antibiotic-impregnated calcium phosphate cement. Knee Surgery, Sports Traumatology, Arthroscopy. 2014;**22**:2614-2617. DOI: 10.1007/s00167-013-2460-9

[25] Guo H, Song B, Zhou R, Yu J, Chen P, Yang B, et al. Risk factors and dynamic nomogram development for surgical site infection following open wedge high tibial osteotomy for varus knee osteoarthritis: A retrospective cohort study. Clinical Interventions in Aging. 2023;**18**:2141-2153. DOI: 10.2147/CIA.S436816

[26] Liu TW, Chiu CH, Chen AC, Chang SS, Chan YS. Risk factor analysis for infection after medial open wedge high tibial osteotomy. Journal of Clinical Medicine. 2021;**10**:1727. DOI: 10.3390/jcm10081727

[27] Kucirek NK, Anigwe C, Zhang AL, Ma CB, Feeley BT, Lansdown DA. Complications after high tibial osteotomy and distal femoral osteotomy are associated with increasing medical comorbidities and tobacco use. Knee Surgery, Sports Traumatology, Arthroscopy. 2022;**30**:4029-4045. DOI: 10.1007/s00167-022-06865-z

[28] Woodacre T, Ricketts M, Evans JT, Pavlou G, Schranz P, Hockings M, et al. Complications associated with opening wedge high tibial osteotomy--a review of the literature and of 15 years of experience. The Knee. 2016;**23**:276-282. DOI: 10.1016/j.knee.2015.09.018

[29] Jia G, Sun C, Xie J, Li J, Liu S, Dong W, et al. Incidence and risk factors for surgical site infection after medial opening-wedge high tibial osteotomy using a locking T-shape plate. International Wound Journal. 2023;**20**:2563-2570. DOI: 10.1111/iwj.14124

[30] Allegranzi B, Bischoff P, de Jonge S, Kubilay NZ, Zayed B, Gomes SM, et al. New WHO recommendations on preoperative measures for surgical site infection prevention: An evidence-based global perspective. The Lancet Infectious Diseases. 2016;**16**:e276-e287. DOI: 10.1016/S1473-3099(16)30398-X

[31] Guo S, Dipietro LA. Factors affecting wound healing. Journal of Dental Research. 2010;**89**:219-229. DOI: 10.1177/0022034509359125

[32] Reischl N, Wahl P, Jacobi M, Clerc S, Gautier E, Jakob RP. Infections after high tibial open wedge osteotomy: A case control study. Archives of Orthopaedic and Trauma Surgery. 2009;**129**:1483-1487. DOI: 10.1007/s00402-008-0773-9

[33] Spahn G. Complications in high tibial (medial opening wedge) osteotomy. Archives of Orthopaedic and Trauma Surgery. 2004;**124**:649-653. DOI: 10.1007/s00402-003-0588-7

[34] Sidhu R, Moatshe G, Firth A, Litchfield R, Getgood A. Low rates of serious complications but high rates of hardware removal after high tibial osteotomy with tomofix locking plate. Knee Surgery, Sports Traumatology, Arthroscopy. 2021;**29**:3361-3367. DOI: 10.1007/s00167-020-06199-8

[35] Cotter EJ, Gowd AK, Bohl DD, Getgood A, Cole BJ, Frank RM. Medical comorbidities and functional dependent living are independent risk factors for short-term complications following osteotomy procedures about the knee. Cartilage. 2020;**11**:423-430. DOI: 10.1177/1947603518798889

[36] Delva ML, Samuel LT, Roth A, Yalcin S, Kamath AF. Contemporary knee osteotomy in the United States: High Tibial osteotomy and distal femoral osteotomy have comparable

complication rates despite differing demographic profiles. The Journal of Knee Surgery. 2021;**34**:816-821. DOI: 10.1055/s-0039-3400742

[37] Hancock G, Martin R, Bell L, Broderick J, Dawson M. Infection in osteotomy around the knee: Incidence, management and outcomes in a high-volume case series. Knee Surgery, Sports Traumatology, Arthroscopy. 2024;**32**:1000-1007. DOI: 10.1002/ksa.12119

[38] Jain RK, Shukla R, Singh P, Kumar R. Epidemiology and risk factors for surgical site infections in patients requiring orthopedic surgery. European Journal of Orthopaedic Surgery and Traumatology. 2015;**25**:251-254. DOI: 10.1007/s00590-014-1475-3

[39] Karlsson J. Quit smoking and reduce surgical complications. Knee Surgery, Sports Traumatology, Arthroscopy. 2011;**19**:331-332. DOI: 10.1007/s00167-010-1385-9

[40] Li J, Zhu Y, Liu B, Dong T, Chen W, Zhang Y. Incidence and risk factors for surgical site infection following open reduction and internal fixation of adult tibial plateau fractures. International Orthopaedics. 2018;**42**:1397-1403. DOI: 10.1007/s00264-017-3729-2

[41] Meidinger G, Imhoff AB, Paul J, Kirchhoff C, Sauerschnig M, Hinterwimmer S. May smokers and overweight patients be treated with a medial open-wedge HTO? Risk factors for non-union. Knee Surgery, Sports Traumatology, Arthroscopy. 2011;**19**:333-339. DOI: 10.1007/s00167-010-1335-6

[42] Namba RS, Inacio MC, Paxton EW. Risk factors associated with deep surgical site infections after primary total knee arthroplasty: An analysis of 56,216 knees. The Journal of Bone and Joint Surgery. American Volume. 2013;**95**:775-782. DOI: 10.2106/JBJS.L.00211

[43] Nasell H, Ottosson C, Tornqvist H, Linde J, Ponzer S. The impact of smoking on complications after operatively treated ankle fractures--a follow-up study of 906 patients. Journal of Orthopaedic Trauma. 2011;**25**:748-755. DOI: 10.1097/BOT.0b013e318213f217

[44] Novikov DA, Swensen SJ, Buza JA, Gidumal RH, Strauss EJ. The effect of smoking on ACL reconstruction: A systematic review. The Physician and Sportsmedicine. 2016;**44**:335-341. DOI: 10.1080/00913847.2016.1216239

[45] Patel RA, Wilson RF, Patel PA, Palmer RM. The effect of smoking on bone healing: A systematic review. Bone and Joint Research. 2013;**2**:102-111. DOI: 10.1302/2046-3758.26.2000142

[46] Schroter S, Freude T, Kopp MM, Konstantinidis L, Dobele S, Stockle U, et al. Smoking and unstable hinge fractures cause delayed gap filling irrespective of early weight bearing after open wedge osteotomy. Arthroscopy. 2015;**31**:254-265. DOI: 10.1016/j.arthro.2014.08.028

[47] Scolaro JA, Schenker ML, Yannascoli S, Baldwin K, Mehta S, Ahn J. Cigarette smoking increases complications following fracture: A systematic review. The Journal of Bone and Joint Surgery. American Volume. 2014;**96**:674-681. DOI: 10.2106/JBJS.M.00081

[48] Seo SS, Kim OG, Seo JH, Kim DH, Kim YG, Lee IS. Complications and short-term outcomes of medial opening wedge high tibial osteotomy using a locking plate for medial osteoarthritis of the knee. Knee Surgery and Related Research. 2016;**28**:289-296. DOI: 10.5792/ksrr.16.028

[49] van Houten AH, Heesterbeek PJ, van Heerwaarden RJ, van Tienen TG, Wymenga AB. Medial open wedge high tibial osteotomy: Can delayed or nonunion be predicted? Clinical Orthopaedics and Related Research. 2014;**472**:1217-1223. DOI: 10.1007/s11999-013-3383-y

[50] Chen Y, Guo Q, Pan X, Qin L, Zhang P. Smoking and impaired bone healing: Will activation of cholinergic anti-inflammatory pathway be the bridge? International Orthopaedics. 2011;**35**:1267-1270. DOI: 10.1007/s00264-011-1243-5

[51] Rahman MM, Laher I. Structural and functional alteration of blood vessels caused by cigarette smoking: An overview of molecular mechanisms. Current Vascular Pharmacology. 2007;**5**:276-292. DOI: 10.2174/157016107782023406

[52] Park HJ, Kang SB, Chang MJ, Chang CB, Jung WH, Jin H. Association of gap healing with angle of correction after opening-wedge high tibial osteotomy without bone grafting. Orthopaedic Journal of Sports Medicine. 2021;**9**:23259671211002289. DOI: 10.1177/23259671211002289

[53] Jensen JA, Goodson WH, Hopf HW, Hunt TK. Cigarette smoking decreases tissue oxygen. Archives of Surgery. 1991;**126**:1131-1134. DOI: 10.1001/archsurg.1991.01410330093013

[54] Porter SE, Hanley EN Jr. The musculoskeletal effects of smoking. The Journal of the American Academy of Orthopaedic Surgeons. 2001;**9**:9-17. DOI: 10.5435/00124635-200101000-00002

[55] Sorensen LT, Jorgensen S, Petersen LJ, Hemmingsen U, Bulow J, Loft S, et al. Acute effects of nicotine and smoking on blood flow, tissue oxygen, and aerobe metabolism of the skin and subcutis. The Journal of Surgical Research. 2009;**152**:224-230. DOI: 10.1016/j.jss.2008.02.066

[56] Agos F, Shoda C, Bransford D. Part II: Managing perioperative hyperglycemia in total hip and knee replacement surgeries. The Nursing Clinics of North America. 2014;**49**:299-308. DOI: 10.1016/j.cnur.2014.05.004

[57] Ahmad MA, Ab Rahman S, Islam MA. Prevalence and risk of infection in patients with diabetes following primary total knee arthroplasty: A global systematic review and meta-analysis of 120,754 knees. Journal of Clinical Medicine. 2022;**11**:3752. DOI: 10.3390/jcm11133752

[58] Bozic KJ, Lau E, Kurtz S, Ong K, Berry DJ. Patient-related risk factors for postoperative mortality and periprosthetic joint infection in medicare patients undergoing TKA. Clinical Orthopaedics and Related Research. 2012;**470**:130-137. DOI: 10.1007/s11999-011-2043-3

[59] Chan VWK, Chan PK, Woo YC, Fu H, Cheung A, Cheung MH, et al. Universal haemoglobin A1c screening reveals high prevalence of dysglycaemia in patients undergoing total knee arthroplasty. Hong Kong Medical Journal. 2020;**26**:304-310. DOI: 10.12809/hkmj208459

[60] Everhart JS, Altneu E, Calhoun JH. Medical comorbidities are independent preoperative risk factors for surgical infection after total joint arthroplasty. Clinical Orthopaedics and Related Research. 2013;**471**:3112-3119. DOI: 10.1007/s11999-013-2923-9

[61] Teo BJX, Yeo W, Chong HC, Tan AHC. Surgical site infection

after primary total knee arthroplasty is associated with a longer duration of surgery. Journal of Orthopaedic Surgery (Hong Kong). 2018;**26**:2309499018785647. DOI: 10.1177/2309499018785647

[62] Kurtz SM, Lau E, Schmier J, Ong KL, Zhao K, Parvizi J. Infection burden for hip and knee arthroplasty in the United States. The Journal of Arthroplasty. 2008;**23**:984-991. DOI: 10.1016/j.arth.2007.10.017

[63] Reaven PD, Emanuele NV, Wiitala WL, Bahn GD, Reda DJ, McCarren M, et al. Intensive glucose control in patients with type 2 diabetes - 15-year follow-up. The New England Journal of Medicine. 2019;**380**:2215-2224. DOI: 10.1056/NEJMoa1806802

[64] Goodson WH, Hung TK. Studies of wound healing in experimental diabetes mellitus. The Journal of Surgical Research. 1977;**22**:221-227. DOI: 10.1016/0022-4804(77)90137-8

[65] Tomic D, Shaw JE, Magliano DJ. The burden and risks of emerging complications of diabetes mellitus. Nature Reviews. Endocrinology. 2022;**18**:525-539. DOI: 10.1038/s41574-022-00690-7

[66] Pennington Z, Lubelski D, Westbroek EM, Ahmed AK, Passias PG, Sciubba DM. Persistent postoperative hyperglycemia as a risk factor for operative treatment of deep wound infection after spine surgery. Neurosurgery. 2020;**87**:211-219. DOI: 10.1093/neuros/nyz405

[67] de Boer AS, Mintjes-de Groot AJ, Severijnen AJ, van den Berg JM, van Pelt W. Risk assessment for surgical-site infections in orthopedic patients. Infection Control and Hospital Epidemiology. 1999;**20**:402-407. DOI: 10.1086/501640

[68] Fisichella L, Fenga D, Rosa MA. Surgical site infection in orthopaedic surgery: Correlation between age, diabetes, smoke and surgical risk. Folia Medica. 2014;**56**:259-263. DOI: 10.1515/folmed-2015-0005

[69] Wang T, Wang H, Yang DL, Jiang LQ, Zhang LJ, Ding WY. Factors predicting surgical site infection after posterior lumbar surgery: A multicenter retrospective study. Medicine (Baltimore). 2017;**96**:e6042. DOI: 10.1097/MD.0000000000006042

[70] Duchman KR, Pugely AJ, Martin CT, Gao Y, Bedard NA, Callaghan JJ. Operative time affects short-term complications in total joint arthroplasty. The Journal of Arthroplasty. 2017;**32**:1285-1291. DOI: 10.1016/j.arth.2016.12.003

[71] Kong L, Cao J, Zhang Y, Ding W, Shen Y. Risk factors for periprosthetic joint infection following primary total hip or knee arthroplasty: A meta-analysis. International Wound Journal. 2017;**14**:529-536. DOI: 10.1111/iwj.12640

[72] Li H, Li Y, Wang D, Huang Q, Liu D. Evaluation of risk factors for surgical site infections in osteoarthritis patients undergoing total knee arthroplasty. International Wound Journal. 2024;**21**:e14521. DOI: 10.1111/iwj.14521

[73] Tayton ER, Frampton C, Hooper GJ, Young SW. The impact of patient and surgical factors on the rate of infection after primary total knee arthroplasty: An analysis of 64,566 joints from the New Zealand joint registry. The Bone and Joint Journal. 2016;**98-B**:334-340. DOI: 10.1302/0301-620X.98B3.36775

[74] Chen H, Chen S, Shi Y, Lu Y, Yu B. Children with open tibial fractures show significantly lower infection rates than adults: Clinical comparative study.

International Orthopaedics. 2019;**43**:713-718. DOI: 10.1007/s00264-018-3996-6

[75] Ives CL, Harrison DK, Stansby GS. Tissue oxygen saturation, measured by near-infrared spectroscopy, and its relationship to surgical-site infections. The British Journal of Surgery. 2007;**94**:87-91. DOI: 10.1002/bjs.5533

[76] Stall A, Paryavi E, Gupta R, Zadnik M, Hui E, O'Toole RV. Perioperative supplemental oxygen to reduce surgical site infection after open fixation of high-risk fractures: A randomized controlled pilot trial. Journal of Trauma and Acute Care Surgery. 2013;**75**:657-663. DOI: 10.1097/TA.0b013e3182a1fe83

[77] Sun Y, Wang H, Tang Y, Zhao H, Qin S, Xu L, et al. Incidence and risk factors for surgical site infection after open reduction and internal fixation of ankle fracture: A retrospective multicenter study. Medicine (Baltimore). 2018;**97**:e9901. DOI: 10.1097/MD.0000000000009901

[78] Kaye KS, Schmit K, Pieper C, Sloane R, Caughlan KF, Sexton DJ, et al. The effect of increasing age on the risk of surgical site infection. The Journal of Infectious Diseases. 2005;**191**:1056-1062. DOI: 10.1086/428626

[79] Schenke M, Dickschas J, Simon M, Strecker W. Corrective osteotomies of the lower limb show a low intra- and perioperative complication rate-an analysis of 1003 patients. Knee Surgery, Sports Traumatology, Arthroscopy. 2018;**26**:1867-1872. DOI: 10.1007/s00167-017-4566-y

[80] Aghdassi SJS, Schroder C, Gastmeier P. Gender-related risk factors for surgical site infections. Results from 10 years of surveillance in Germany. Antimicrobial Resistance Infection Control. 2019;**8**:95. DOI: 10.1186/s13756-019-0547-x

[81] Chen J, Cui Y, Li X, Miao X, Wen Z, Xue Y, et al. Risk factors for deep infection after total knee arthroplasty: A meta-analysis. Archives of Orthopaedic and Trauma Surgery. 2013;**133**:675-687. DOI: 10.1007/s00402-013-1723-8

[82] Kawata M, Sasabuchi Y, Taketomi S, Inui H, Matsui H, Fushimi K, et al. Atopic dermatitis is a novel demographic risk factor for surgical site infection after anterior cruciate ligament reconstruction. Knee Surgery, Sports Traumatology, Arthroscopy. 2018;**26**:3699-3705. DOI: 10.1007/s00167-018-4958-7

[83] Murphy MV, Du DT, Hua W, Cortez KJ, Butler MG, Davis RL, et al. Risk factors for surgical site infections following anterior cruciate ligament reconstruction. Infection Control and Hospital Epidemiology. 2016;**37**:827-833. DOI: 10.1017/ice.2016.65

[84] Bei T, Yang L, Huang Q, Wu J, Liu J. Effectiveness of bone substitute materials in opening wedge high tibial osteotomy: A systematic review and meta-analysis. Annals of Medicine. 2022;**54**:565-577. DOI: 10.1080/07853890.2022.2036805

[85] Fucentese SF, Tscholl PM, Sutter R, Brucker PU, Meyer DC, Koch PP. Bone autografting in medial open wedge high tibial osteotomy results in improved osseous gap healing on computed tomography, but no functional advantage: A prospective, randomised, controlled trial. Knee Surgery, Sports Traumatology, Arthroscopy. 2019;**27**:2951-2957. DOI: 10.1007/s00167-018-5285-8

[86] Chen X, Wang J, Yu L, Zhou J, Zheng D, Zhang B. Effect of concentrated growth factor (CGF)

on the promotion of osteogenesis in bone marrow stromal cells (BMSC) in vivo. Scientific Reports. 2018;**8**:5876. DOI: 10.1038/s41598-018-24364-5

[87] Han JH, Kim HJ, Song JG, Yang JH, Bhandare NN, Fernandez AR, et al. Is bone grafting necessary in opening wedge high tibial osteotomy? A meta-analysis of radiological outcomes. Knee Surgery and Related Research. 2015;**27**:207-220. DOI: 10.5792/ksrr.2015.27.4.207

[88] Koshino T, Murase T, Saito T. Medial opening-wedge high tibial osteotomy with use of porous hydroxyapatite to treat medial compartment osteoarthritis of the knee. The Journal of Bone and Joint Surgery. American Volume. 2003;**85**:78-85. DOI: 10.2106/00004623-200301000-00013

[89] Saito T, Kumagai K, Akamatsu Y, Kobayashi H, Kusayama Y. Five- to ten-year outcome following medial opening-wedge high tibial osteotomy with rigid plate fixation in combination with an artificial bone substitute. The Bone and Joint Journal. 2014;**96-B**:339-344. DOI: 10.1302/0301-620X.96B3.32525

[90] Takeuchi R, Ishikawa H, Aratake M, Bito H, Saito I, Kumagai K, et al. Medial opening wedge high tibial osteotomy with early full weight bearing. Arthroscopy. 2009;**25**:46-53. DOI: 10.1016/j.arthro.2008.08.015

[91] Chae DJ, Shetty GM, Wang KH, Montalban AS Jr, Kim JI, Nha KW. Early complications of medial opening wedge high tibial osteotomy using autologous tricortical iliac bone graft and T-plate fixation. The Knee. 2011;**18**:278-284. DOI: 10.1016/j.knee.2010.05.009

[92] Ollivier M, Claes S, Mabrouk A, Elson D, Espejo-Reina A, Predescu V, et al. Surgical strategy and complication management of osteotomy around the painful degenerative varus knee: ESSKA formal consensus part II. Knee Surgery, Sports Traumatology, Arthroscopy. 2024;**32**:2194-2205. DOI: 10.1002/ksa.12273

[93] Karatosun V, Demir T, Unver B, Gunal I. A brief report on managing infected nonunion of a high tibial osteotomy in two stages: A case series involving seven knees. Journal of Bone and Joint Surgery. British Volume (London). 2011;**93**:904-906. DOI: 10.1302/0301-620X.93B7.25833

[94] Mariaux S, Borens O. Management of an infected nonunion of an opening-wedge high tibial osteotomy with 2-stage implantation of rotating hinge knee prosthesis. Case Reports in Orthopedics. 2018;**2018**:2493095. DOI: 10.1155/2018/2493095

[95] McHale KA, Ross AE. Treatment of infected tibial nonunions with debridement, antibiotic beads, and the Ilizarov method. Military Medicine. 2004;**169**:728-734. DOI: 10.7205/milmed.169.9.728

[96] Patzakis MJ, Zalavras CG. Chronic posttraumatic osteomyelitis and infected nonunion of the tibia: Current management concepts. The Journal of the American Academy of Orthopaedic Surgeons. 2005;**13**:417-427. DOI: 10.5435/00124635-200510000-00006

[97] Nishitani K, Sutipornpalangkul W, de Mesy Bentley KL, Varrone JJ, Bello-Irizarry SN, Ito H, et al. Quantifying the natural history of biofilm formation in vivo during the establishment of chronic implant-associated Staphylococcus aureus osteomyelitis in mice to identify critical pathogen and host factors. Journal of Orthopaedic Research. 2015;**33**:1311-1319. DOI: 10.1002/jor.22907

[98] Ring D, Jupiter JB, Gan BS, Israeli R, Yaremchuk MJ. Infected nonunion of the tibia. Clinical Orthopaedics and Related Research. 1999;**369**:302-311. DOI: 10.1097/00003086-199912000-00032

[99] Urabe K, Naruse K, Hattori H, Hirano M, Uchida K, Onuma K, et al. In vitro comparison of elution characteristics of vancomycin from calcium phosphate cement and polymethylmethacrylate. Journal of Orthopaedic Science. 2009;**14**:784-793. DOI: 10.1007/s00776-009-1397-9

[100] Sasaki T, Ishibashi Y, Katano H, Nagumo A, Toh S. In vitro elution of vancomycin from calcium phosphate cement. The Journal of Arthroplasty. 2005;**20**:1055-1059. DOI: 10.1016/j.arth.2005.03.035

[101] McNally MA, Ferguson JY, Lau AC, Diefenbeck M, Scarborough M, Ramsden AJ, et al. Single-stage treatment of chronic osteomyelitis with a new absorbable, gentamicin-loaded, calcium sulphate/hydroxyapatite biocomposite: A prospective series of 100 cases. The Bone and Joint Journal. 2016;**98-B**:1289-1296. DOI: 10.1302/0301-620X.98B9.38057

[102] Bezstarosti H, Metsemakers WJ, van Lieshout EMM, Voskamp LW, Kortram K, McNally MA, et al. Management of critical-sized bone defects in the treatment of fracture-related infection: A systematic review and pooled analysis. Archives of Orthopaedic and Trauma Surgery. 2021;**141**:1215-1230. DOI: 10.1007/s00402-020-03525-0

[103] Buck B, Murtha YM. The management of bone defects in periarticular knee injuries: A review article. The Journal of Knee Surgery. 2017;**30**:194-199. DOI: 10.1055/s-0037-1598076

[104] Masquelet AC, Fitoussi F, Begue T, Muller GP. Reconstruction of the long bones by the induced membrane and spongy autograft. Annales de Chirurgie Plastique et Esthétique. 2000;**45**:346-353

[105] Morelli I, Drago L, George DA, Gallazzi E, Scarponi S, Romano CL. Masquelet technique: Myth or reality? A Systematic Review and Meta-Analysis. Injury. 2016;**47**(Suppl. 6):S68-S76. DOI: 10.1016/S0020-1383(16)30842-7

[106] Gandhi R, Alomran A, Mahomed N. Bilateral non-union of high tibial osteotomies treated by total knee arthroplasty: A case report. The Knee. 2008;**15**:242-245. DOI: 10.1016/j.knee.2008.01.011

[107] Yoshino N, Takai S, Watanabe Y, Nakamura S, Kubo T. Total knee arthroplasty with long stem for treatment of nonunion after high tibial osteotomy. The Journal of Arthroplasty. 2004;**19**:528-531. DOI: 10.1016/j.arth.2003.12.068

[108] Blum ML, Esser M, Richardson M, Paul E, Rosenfeldt FL. Negative pressure wound therapy reduces deep infection rate in open tibial fractures. Journal of Orthopaedic Trauma. 2012;**26**:499-505. DOI: 10.1097/BOT.0b013e31824133e3

[109] Zhang X, Chen Y, Xiao X, Wang Z, Yang X, Zhao Z. Application of VSD technique in adults with chronic osteomyelitis of the extremities combined with soft tissue defects. International Wound Journal. 2023;**20**:768-773. DOI: 10.1111/iwj.13921

[110] Maruo A, Oda T, Mineo R, Miya H, Muratsu H, Fukui T, et al. Continuous local antibiotic perfusion: A treatment strategy that allows implant retention in fracture-related infections. Journal of Orthopaedic Surgery (Hong

Kong). 2022;**30**:10225536221111902. DOI: 10.1177/10225536221111902

[111] Ceri H, Olson ME, Stremick C, Read RR, Morck D, Buret A. The calgary biofilm device: New technology for rapid determination of antibiotic susceptibilities of bacterial biofilms. Journal of Clinical Microbiology. 1999;**37**:1771-1776. DOI: 10.1128/JCM.37.6.1771-1776.1999

[112] Miyake Y, Takagi T. Treatment experience with continuous local antibiotic perfusion for periprosthetic joint infection. Journal of Orthopaedic Science. 2024;**29**:1469-1476. DOI: 10.1016/j.jos.2023.12.001

[113] Rodriguez-Merchan EC. Biofilm related total knee arthroplasty infection: Prevention, diagnosis and treatment. The Archives of Bone and Joint Surgery. 2024;**12**:531-534. DOI: 10.22038/ABJS.2024.77560.3583

[114] Zenke Y, Motojima Y, Ando K, Kosugi K, Hamada D, Okada Y, et al. DAIR in treating chronic PJI after total knee arthroplasty using continuous local antibiotic perfusion therapy: A case series study. BMC Musculoskeletal Disorders. 2024;**25**:36. DOI: 10.1186/s12891-024-07165-y

[115] Kosugi K, Zenke Y, Sato N, Hamada D, Ando K, Okada Y, et al. Potential of continuous local antibiotic perfusion therapy for fracture-related infections. Infectious Disease and Therapy. 2022;**11**:1741-1755. DOI: 10.1007/s40121-022-00653-5

[116] Minehara H, Zenke Y, Maruo A, Matsushita T, Miclau T 3rd. Management of open fracture and related complications: The Japanese way. OTA International. 2024;7:e325. DOI: 10.1097/OI9.0000000000000325

[117] Mineo R, Oe K, Niikura T, Muratsu H, Kuroda R, Maruo A. Continuous local antibiotic perfusion (CLAP) for post-operative infection of open tibial fractures: A case report. Journal of Orthopaedic Case Reports. 2022;**12**:18-22. DOI: 10.13107/jocr.2022.v12.i02.2648

[118] Oe K, Maruo A, Fukui T, Muratsu H, Kuroda R, Niikura T. Treatment of chronic osteomyelitis of the femur by intramedullary antibiotic perfusion (iMAP): A case report. Journal of Orthopaedic Case Reports. 2021;**11**:35-38. DOI: 10.13107/jocr.2021.v11.i12.2556

[119] Sawauchi K, Fukui T, Oe K, Kuroda R, Niikura T, Muratsu H, et al. Management of infected tibial nonunion: Combining synthetic bone grafting with continuous local antibiotic perfusion (CLAP). American Journal of Case Reports. 2024;**25**:e945023. DOI: 10.12659/AJCR.945023

[120] Takahara S, Maruo A, Takayama H, Harada T. Continuous local antibiotics perfusion therapy for acute deep infections after open fractures. Case Reports in Orthopedics. 2022;**2022**:2563939. DOI: 10.1155/2022/2563939

Section 2

Osteotomies in the Hip and Foot

Chapter 7

Osteotomy Techniques in Total Hip Arthroplasty for Severe Dysplasia

Mehmet Faruk Çatma

Abstract

Femoral osteotomy is a common procedure used in total hip replacement for patients with severe hip dysplasia. In this chapter, fixation methods could be discussed for total hip replacement using transverse femoral shortening osteotomy for patients with Crowe type IV developmental hip dysplasia. Fixation of the removed femoral segment could be achieved with cable or plate techniques. In the chapter assigned, these two techniques could be discussed in detail, stating the pros and the cons in comparison to other available techniques. The clinical and functional outcomes of the patients who underwent femoral osteotomy with cable or plate techniques can be debated based on their radiological images and hip scores.

Keywords: hip dysplasia, fixation, total hip replacement, femoral osteotomy, arthroplasty

1. Introduction

Femoral osteotomies in patients with Developmental Dysplasia of the Hip are difficult and prone to complications due to femoral hypoplasia, narrow femoral medullary canal, increased anteversion of the femoral head, valgus femoral neck, posterior location of the trochanter major and previous femoral osteotomies. Femoral reconstruction should be planned considering the severity of the femoral deformity and the placement of the acetabular component.

The most important problem on the femoral side is the reduction of the hip when the acetabular component is lowered to the true acetabulum. In such cases, femoral shortening is necessary in order to prevent excessive stretching of the vessels and nerves, to create the joint in the hip in its true place and to correct additional deformities caused by previous surgeries. Femoral osteotomies also help to correct rotation deformity and eliminate the length difference in the lower limb.

2. Osteotomy techniques

Numerous techniques for femoral shortening have been described. While some surgeons shorten only at the level of the trochanter major, most surgeons prefer shortening at the proximal metaphysis.

2.1 Trochanter major osteotomy

The technique of trochanter major osteotomy was described by H.K. Dunn and W.E. Hess in 1976. The trochanter major osteotomy technique described in the literature is performed by resecting the proximal femur until reduction is achieved and the trochanter major is fixed to the lateral aspect of the remaining proximal femur with screws and cerclage wires (**Figure 1**).

Surgeons who prefer trochanteric osteotomy to subtrochanteric osteotomy claim that in addition to the possibility of advancing the trochanter laterally and distally during the surgical intervention, the acetabular exposure is better, the reaming of the femoral canal can be performed with less access and the components are placed more easily and accurately. In addition to these advantages of the trochanter major osteotomy, there are some disadvantages. These disadvantages include bone loss in the proximal femur especially in the medial region, having to choose a small and flat stem because the medulla under the trochanter minor is narrow and flat, failure of the implant placed on the osteotomy line, loss of strength in the abductor force arm, rotational and axial stability may not be provided well, nonunion of the trochanter major and trochanteric bursitis [1–4]. It should not be forgotten that nonunion of the trochanter major may cause dislocation at high rates [5]. In addition, abductor muscles play an important role in balancing the pelvis while standing and walking. If the pelvis is in balance while the patient is standing on one leg, the abductor muscle strength is considered normal on the side on which the patient is standing. On the contrary, if the pelvis falls to the opposite side while the patient is standing, muscle weakness is detected on this side. Trendelenburg gait may occur in these patients. Trendelenburg gait may be seen more frequently in patients who have undergone trochanteric osteotomy.

Subtrochanteric osteotomy has been preferred to trochanteric osteotomy in recent years because it allows the structure of the femur to be closer to normal and provides better fixation in the metaphyseal region. Nowadays, subtrochanteric osteotomy, which replaced trochanteric osteotomy, has gained popularity for the reasons mentioned. There are important points to be considered when performing arthroplasty with both osteotomy methods. In order to reconstruct the center of rotation in the arthroplasty, the elevated femoral head should be lowered inferiorly. The femoral

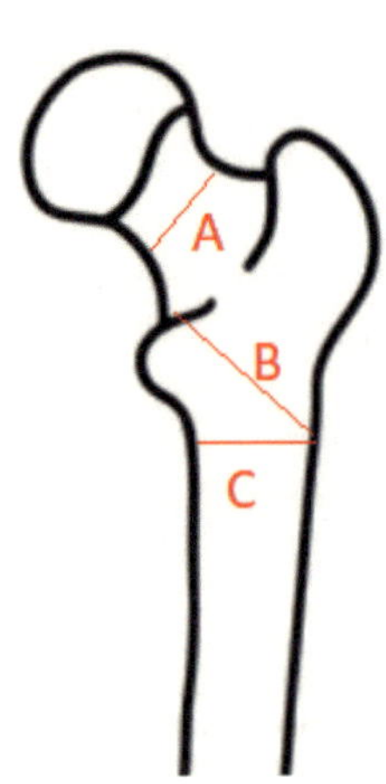

Figure 1.
Lines A and B are osteotomy lines for the trochanter incision, line C is the metaphyseal osteotomy line.

shortening osteotomy technique is used to bring the femur to the true acetabulum and to prevent neurologic damage due to overstretching. It should be kept in mind when performing arthroplasty in cases with developmental dysplasia of the hip that surgeries performed far from the anatomical center of rotation have a short implant life and are biomechanically disadvantageous.

2.2 Subtrochanteric osteotomy

The subtrochanteric osteotomy technique used in patients with developmental dysplasia of the hip with high hip dislocation was first described by P.D. Sponseller and A.A. McBeath in 1988 and was created with the idea of intramedullary fixation of the osteotomy line with an uncemented stem [6]. This technique is considered one of the most challenging surgeries in the field of orthopedics due to the center of rotation reconstruction, risk of neurovascular injury, femoral shortening osteotomy technique, severe muscle and bone deformity and the need to eliminate the limb length difference (**Figure 2**) [7, 8].

Different bone incision techniques have been described in subtrochanteric osteotomy. These incisions are basically divided into four groups. These are transverse, oblique, chevron and step-cut incisions. There is no significant difference in stability between the techniques and they have some advantages and disadvantages compared

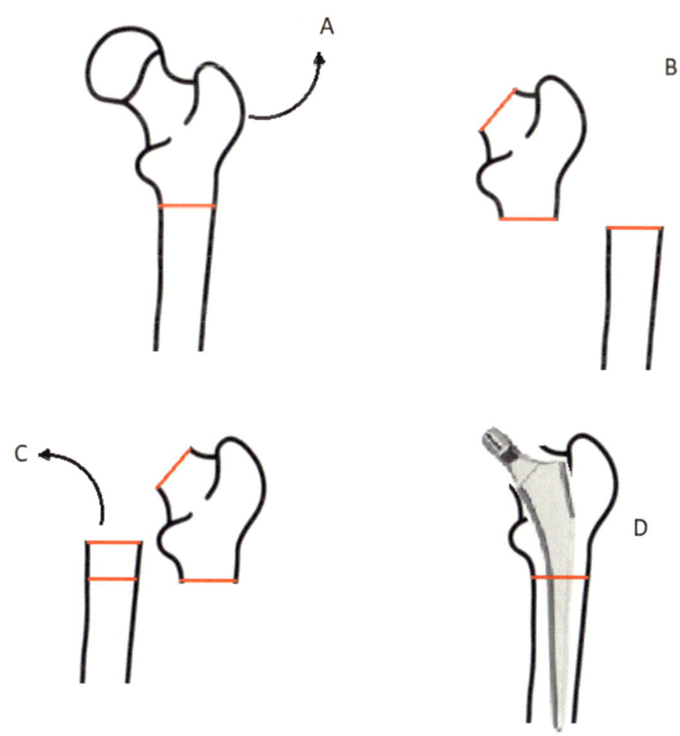

Figure 2.
Subtrochanteric osteotomy. (A) Location of the initial osteotomy, (B) The proximal femur is excised to find the level of the true acetabulum and the component is placed on the true acetabulum, (C) The proximal femoral fragment is lowered opposite the true acetabulum, while minimal traction is applied to the distal femur. The overlapping part of the femur is resected, and (D) The femoral fragment is reduced and the increased femoral anteversion is corrected. Provides intramedullary fixation of the femoral component osteotomy.

to each other. Transverse incisions, which are the least rotationally stable but the easiest methods in terms of ease of application, are more widely used [9]. More rotational stability is achieved in more complex osteotomy types [10]. Additional fixation techniques such as cable or plate/screw fixation can be used to provide rotational stability (**Figure 3**).

2.2.1 Femoral shortening with transverse osteotomy

Transverse osteotomy, which is one of the subtrochanteric osteotomy methods for Developmental Hip Dysplasia, is an osteotomy method that is easier to perform and can be performed in a shorter time. The operation time is shorter and the risk of intraoperative complications is lower. The version problem in the proximal femur can be solved most easily with this osteotomy. However, the nonunion rate is higher than other types of osteotomy due to insufficient contact surface and biomechanical stability at the osteotomy line [11].

2.2.2 Femoral shortening with oblique osteotomy

Oblique osteotomies applied from the subtrochanteric region can also be used as a femoral shortening method in patients with Developmental Hip Dysplasia. This type of osteotomy has higher stability and more contact surface than the transverse osteotomy. Oblique osteotomies are more commonly used than transverse osteotomies because they are considered to be more stable and the rotation can be adjusted better [11].

2.2.3 Femoral shortening with step-cut osteotomy

The stability of femoral shortening using this osteotomy technique is even higher. With the step-cut osteotomy method, it is seen that the existing deformity in the patient can be corrected more easily. With this technique, the deformity in the proximal femur can be corrected more easily with appropriate angular rotations [12]. In this technique, the circumferential contact between the endosteal cortex and the femoral stem is less, so unstable femoral stem press-fit and femoral stem inversion deformity can be seen [13]. In the step-cut osteotomy technique, a transverse incision is made lateral to the proximal fragment. Then, a transverse incision is made medial to the distal fragment and these fragments are brought together in the appropriate rotation.

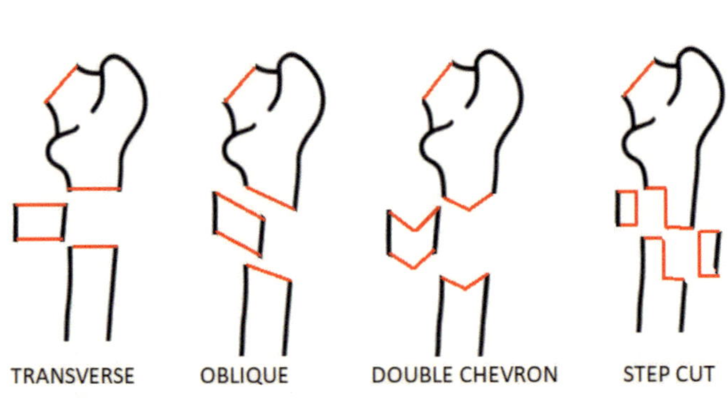

Figure 3.
Types of femoral osteotomy.

Subtrochanteric osteotomy method	Advantages	Disadvantages
Transverse osteotomy	Easier technique	Higher risk of nonunion
Oblique Double Chevron Step-cut osteotomy	Greater rotational stability More bone surface contact	More difficult technique Longer learning curve

Table 1.
Comparison of osteotomy types.

As indicated in **Table 1**, each osteotomy technique has differing pros and cons.

In our clinic, the transverse osteotomy technique was used as a femoral shortening method for total hip arthroplasty in many patients with developmental dysplasia of the hip who had complaints and clinical findings that were indications for total hip arthroplasty. After this technique was applied, two different methods were used for osteotomy fixation. The first method is fixation with dynamic compression plate (DCP) and screws after placement of the femoral stem. The other method is the fixation of two segments obtained from the osteotomy line, which are not separated from the soft tissue, with a cable after placement on the osteotomy line.

3. Examples from our cases

See **Figures 4–7**.

4. Discussion

Developmental dysplasia of the hip is one of the most difficult types of surgery and the complication rate is very high. Therefore, preoperative planning should be done carefully and possible risks should be evaluated. In order to achieve the desired level of union after femoral osteotomy, measures should be taken to facilitate union. Care should be taken to ensure rotational stability. In a cadaveric study, transverse, oblique, double

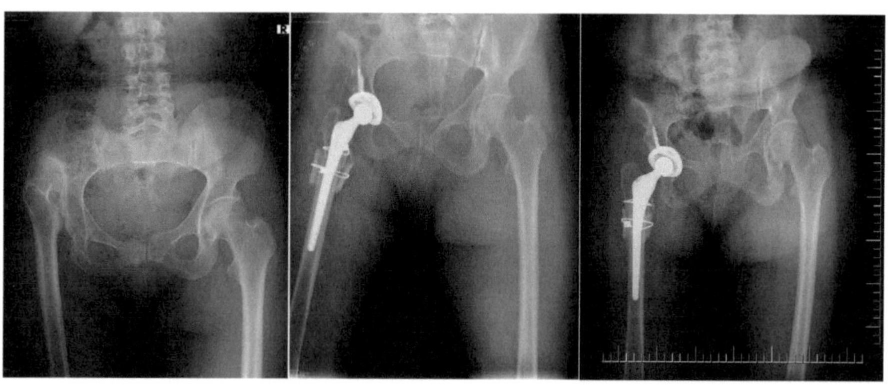

Figure 4.
A 49-year-old female patient with right Crowe Type 4 hip dysplasia underwent subtrochanteric osteotomy and was fixed with a cable.

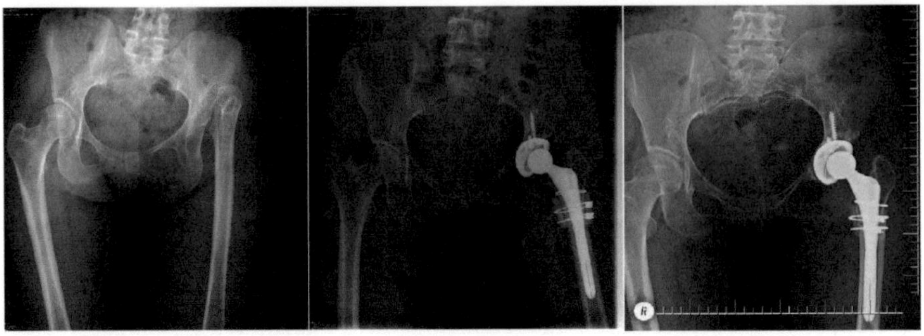

Figure 5.
A 36-year-old female patient with Crowe Type 3 hip dysplasia underwent subtrochanteric osteotomy and was fixed with a cable.

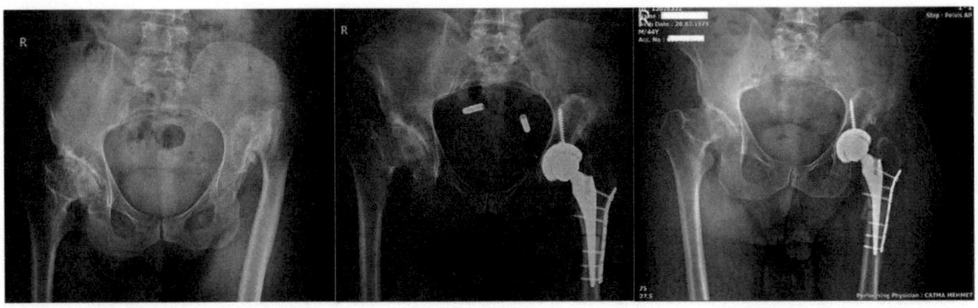

Figure 6.
A 44-year-old male patient with Crowe Type 4 hip dysplasia underwent subtrochanteric osteotomy and was fixed with plate-screw.

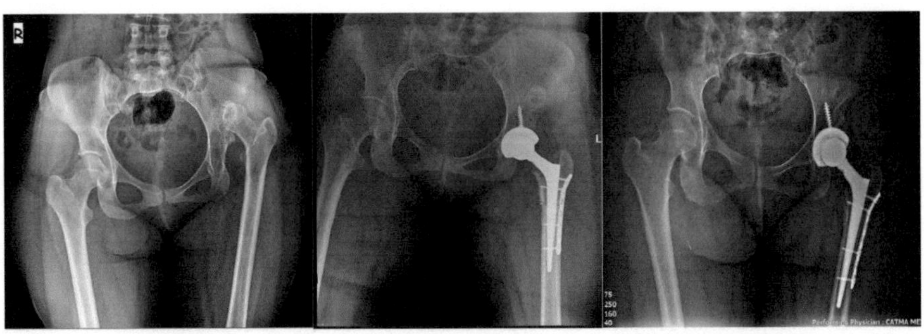

Figure 7.
A 30-year-old female patient with Crowe Type 3 hip dysplasia underwent subtrochanteric osteotomy and was fixed with plate-screw.

chevron and step-cut osteotomy types were compared biomechanically and it was found that step-cut surgical technique was more successful in antetorsion, rotation and angulation in patients with good bone stock and body mass index below 28 [14].

Transverse osteotomy is one of the most commonly used osteotomy methods due to its ease of application and short operation time [15]. In their study, Mu et al.

performed transverse osteotomy on 71 patients with developmental dysplasia of the hip and found nonunion in two hips (3.3%) [16]. In their study, Sofu et al. performed the combination of transverse osteotomy and osteotomy fixation with cable and plate on 73 patients with developmental dysplasia of the hip and found nonunion in four hips (5.5%) at the end of five-year follow-up period [17]. In their study, Şener et al. performed osteotomy fixation with step-cut osteotomy and graft-cable on 28 patients with developmental dysplasia of the hip and found nonunion in two hips at four-year follow-up [18].

Although the transverse osteotomy method is frequently used, there is no significant difference between osteotomy methods when radiographic imaging and clinical results are considered [19]. Since there is no significant difference between these osteotomy methods in the literature, the type of osteotomy to be chosen is usually the choice of the operating surgeon [20]. There are many publications comparing cemented and uncemented femoral stems that can be used after osteotomy. The nonunion rate can be seen more frequently in follow-ups after surgery with cemented femoral stems [21]. Akiyama et al. reported high rates of nonunion in a study of 15 cemented total hip arthroplasties with subtrochanteric femoral shortening [22]. Rotational correction is more easily achieved with the use of a cemented component after subtrochanteric osteotomy, but there is a risk of cement entering the osteotomy line and negatively affecting the union. Since these patients are young, it is suggested that uncemented components may last longer, the results of uncemented components are better, rotational stability is better because the metaphyseal region is preserved, anteversion and the use of an uncemented femoral stem for osteotomy fixation under appropriate conditions.

After osteotomy, graft-cable and plate-screw fixation are frequently used for fixation of the osteotomy line. There are many publications comparing these two methods. In their study, Çaylak et al. reported nonunion in only two patients in a 10-year follow-up of 50 patients and 67 hips [23]. In other studies in which plate-screw fixation was performed for fixation of the osteotomy line, the rate of nonunion was reported to be 5.5% by Charity et al. [24]; 3.3% by Çağlar et al. [25] and 5.4% by Sofu et al. [17]. When these publications and the literature are analyzed, it is seen that there is no clear opinion in terms of fixation after osteotomy and it is shaped according to the surgeon's preference.

Even if trochanteric osteotomy or subtrochanteric osteotomy is preferred in cases with developmental Hip dysplasia, it is necessary to lower the superior femoral head inferiorly in order to reconstruct the center of rotation in the arthroplasty. The femoral shortening osteotomy technique is used in such cases to lower the femoral head to the true acetabulum and to prevent the development of neurologic deficit due to overstretching. One of the important complications that can be seen after femoral shortening osteotomy in cases with developmental dysplasia of the hip is peroperative fracture. In the literature, it is observed that it can be seen between 5 and 22%. The most important reason for this is the anatomical structure of the femur. In the proximal part of the femur, the trochanter major is small, posteriorly located and osteoporotic. The intertrochanteric region is narrow and osteoporotic. In addition, since the medulla of the femur is narrow, a trochanter major fracture line, metaphyseal fissure in the intertrochanteric region and femoral shaft fractures may occur during the reaming of the medulla of the femur and proximal metaphysis [15]. According to the literature, the incidence of fracture during surgery is 0.1–3.2% when cemented prosthesis is used, while the incidence of fracture during surgery is between 3 and 28% when cementless prosthesis is used. This increases the complication rate when using a cementless prosthesis, as a tighter fit between the prosthesis and bone is desired [26].

As mentioned before, nerve lesion is the most important complication of total hip arthroplasty and its incidence has been reported between 0.8% and 3.7% in the literature [27, 28]. In addition, female gender, surgical technique, fixation of the trochanter with cerclage wire, dislocation of the hip during surgery, direct compression of the retractors used, damage to the cement and polymerization heat and hematoma have been held responsible. One of the most important points of these techniques is the adjustment of the amount of shortening. Lengthening more than 3–4 cm is considered to be the most important factor in the sciatic nerve injury. However, there are different opinions in the literature. Eggli did not find a statistically significant relationship between the frequency of nerve lesions after arthroplasty and the amount of lengthening and stated that the cause of nerve lesions was due to direct and indirect mechanical trauma during surgery [29]. Schmalzride, on the other hand, found nerve lesions in six patients with more than 3 cm of lengthening but emphasized that these nerve lesions were due to indirect compression of the prosthesis or bone fragments rather than the amount of lengthening [30]. Edwards emphasized that there was a direct relationship between the amount of lengthening and nerve lesions [31].

In addition, the risk of neurovascular damage increases if insufficient shortening is performed. If excessive shortening is performed, shortening of the leg and weakness in the muscles around the hip occur. Osteotomy should be performed by evaluating the sciatic nerve tension with the appropriate measurement method. We should not forget that neurological damage will be minimized by making incisions carefully during surgery to avoid nerve damage, placing the retractors in the appropriate position and determining the tension of the sciatic nerve after the surgical procedure. For all these reasons, soft tissue should be respected as much as possible [8, 32].

Author details

Mehmet Faruk Çatma
Ankara Etlik City Hospital, Turkey

*Address all correspondence to: farukcatma@hotmail.com

References

[1] Dunn HK, Hess WE. Total hipreconstruction in chronicallydislocatedhips. Journal of Bone and Joint Surgery. 1976;**58-A**:838-845

[2] Mendes DG. Total hiparthroplasty in congenitaldislocatedhips. Clinical Orthopaedics. 1981;**161**:163-179

[3] Chougle A, Hemmady MV, Hodgkinson JP. Long-termsurvival of the acetabular component after total hiparthroplasty with cement in patients with developmental dysplasia of the hip. Journal of Bone and Joint Surgery. 2006;**88-A**:71-79

[4] Paavilainen T, Hoikka V, Solonen KA. Cementless total replacement for severely dysplastic or dislocated hips. Journal of Bone and Joint Surgery. 1990;**72-B**:205-211

[5] Nercessian OA, Newton PM, Joshi RP, Sheikh B, Eftekhar NS. Trochanteric osteotomy and wire fixation: A comparison of 2 techniques. Clinical Orthopaedics. 1996;**333**:208-216

[6] Sponseller PD, McBeath AA. Subtrochanteric osteotomy with intramedullary fixation for arthroplasty of the dysplastic hip. A case report. The Journal of Arthroplasty. 1988;**3**(4):351-354

[7] Ollivier M, Abdel MP, Krych AJ, Trousdale RT, Berry DJ. Long-termresults of Total hip arthroplasty with shortening subtrochanteric osteotomy in Crowe IV developmental dysplasia. The Journal of Arthroplasty. 2016;**31**(8):1756-1760

[8] Erdemli B, Yilmaz C, Atalar H, Güzel B, Cetin I. Total hiparthroplasty in developmental high dislocation of the hip. The Journal of Arthroplasty. 2005;**20**(8):1021-1028

[9] Muratli KS, Karatosun V, Uzun B, Celik S. Subtrochanteric shortening in total hiparthroplasty: Biomechanical comparison of four techniques. The Journal of Arthroplasty. 2014;**29**(4):836-842

[10] Sanchez-Sotelo J, Berry DJ, Trousdale RT, Cabanela ME. Surgical treatment of developmental dysplasia of the hip in adults: II. Arthroplasty options. Journal of the American Academy of Orthopaedic Surgeons. 2002;**10**(5):334-344

[11] Necas L, Hrubina M, Melisik M, Cibula Z, Chmurny M, et al. Cementless hiparthroplasty and transverse shortening femoral osteotomy with the S-ROM stem for Crowe type IV developmental dysplasia. European Journal of Orthopaedic Surgery and Traumatology. 2019;**29**(5):1025-1033

[12] Russotti GM, Harris WH. Proximal placement of the acetabular component in total hiparthroplasty. A long-termfollow-up study. The Journal of Bone and Joint Surgery. American Volume. 1991;**73**:587-592

[13] Yalcin N, Kilicarslan K, Karatas F, Mutlu T, Yildirim H. Cementless total hip arthroplasty with subtrochanteric transverse shortening osteotomy for severely dysplastic or dislocated hips. Hip International. 2010;**20**:87-93

[14] Cashman J, Goyal N, Parvizi J. The Hip: Preservation. Replacement and Revision. United States of America: Data Trace Publishing Company; 2015

[15] Krych AJ, Howard JL, Trousdale RT, Cabanela ME, Berry DJ. Total

hip arthroplasty with shortening subtrochanteric osteotomy in Crowe type-IV developmental dysplasia. Journal of Bone and Joint Surgery. 2009;**91**:2213-2221

[16] Mu W, Yang D, Xu B, Mamtimin A, Guo W, Cao L. Mid term outcome of Cementless Total hip arthroplasty in Crowe IV-Hartofilakidis type III developmental dysplasia of the hip. The Journal of Arthroplasty. 2016;**31**(3):668-675

[17] Sofu H, Kockara N, Gursu S, Issin A, Oner A, Sahin V. Transverse subtrochanteric shortening osteotomy during Cementless Total hip arthroplasty in Crowe type-III or IV developmental dysplasia. The Journal of Arthroplasty. 2015;**30**(6):1019-1023

[18] Sener N, Tozun IR, Asik M. Femoral shortening and cementless arthroplasty in high congenital dislocation of the hip. The Journal of Arthroplasty. 2002;**17**(1):41-48

[19] Li C, Zhang C, Zhang M, Ding Y. Comparison of transverse and modified subtrochanteric femoral shortening osteotomy in total hip arthroplasty for developmental dysplasia of hip: A meta-analysis. BMC Musculoskeletal Disorders. 2014;**15**:331

[20] Kiliçoğlu OI, Türker M, Akgül T, Yazicioğlu O. Cementless total hip arthroplasty with modified oblique femoral shortening osteotomy in Crowetype IV congenital hip dislocation. The Journal of Arthroplasty. 2013;**28**:117-125

[21] Gong S, Xu W, Wang R, Liu S, Han L, Chen G, et al. The causes and management of nonunion of femoral subtrochanteric shortening osteotomy in a THA patient: A casereport. BMC Musculoskeletal Disorders. 2019;**20**:203

[22] Akiyama H, Kawanabe K, Yamamoto K, Kuroda Y, So K, Goto K, et al. Cemented total hip arthroplasty with subtrochanteric femoral shortening transverse osteotomy for severely dislocated hips: Outcome with a 3- to 10-year follow-up period. Journal of Orthopaedic Science. 2011;**16**:270-277

[23] Caylak R, Ors C, Togrul E. Minimum 10-year results of Cementles sCeramic- on-ceramic Total hip arthroplasty performed with transverse subtrochanteric osteotomy in Crowe type IV hips. The Journal of Arthroplasty. 2021;**36**(10):3519-3526

[24] Charity JA, Tsiridis E, Sheeraz A, Howell JR, Hubble MJ, Timperley AJ, et al. Treatment of Crowe IV high hip dysplasia with total hip replacement using the Exeter stemand shortening derotational subtrochanteric osteotomy. Journal of Bone and Joint Surgery (British). 2011;**93**:34-38

[25] Çağlar Ö, Özdemir E, Tokg Özoğlu AM, Atilla B. Use of proximal humerus plates for the fixation of the subtrochanteric femoral shortening osteotomy during total hip arthroplasty for Crowe type IV developmental dysplasia of the hip patients. Joint Diseases and Related Surgery. 2020;**31**:306-311

[26] Khanuja HS, Mekkawy KL, MacMahon A, McDaniel CM, Allen DA, Moskal JT. Revisiting cemented femoral fixation in hip arthroplasty. Journal of Bone and Joint Surgery. Jun 2022

[27] Eskelinen A, Remes V, Ylinen P, Helenius I, Tallroth K, Paavilainen T. Cementless total hip arthroplasty in patients with severely dysplastic hip sand aprevious Schanz osteotomy of the femur. Acta Orthopaedica. 2009;**80**(3):263-269

[28] Holtgrewe JL, Hungerford DS. Primaryandrevision total hip replacement without cement and with associated femoral osteotomy. Journal of Bone and Joint Surgery. 1989;**71-A**:1487-1495

[29] Eggli SH, Müller S, M. Nervepalsy after leg lengthening in total replacement arthroplasty fo rdevelopmental dysplasia of the hip. Journal of Bone and Joint Surgery: British Volume. 1999;**81**(5):843-845

[30] Schmalzried TP, Amstutz HC, Dorey FJ. Nervepalsy associatedwith total hipreplecament: Risk factors and prognosis. Journal of Bone and Joint Surgery. 1991;**73-A**:1074-1080

[31] Edwards BN, Tallos RS, Noble PC. Contributory factors and etiology of sciatic nevre palsy with total hip arthroplasty. Clinical Orthopaedics. 1987;**218**:136-141

[32] Paavialinen T. Total hip replacement for developmental dysplasia of the hip. Acta Orthopaedica Scandinavica. 1997;**68**:77-84

Chapter 8

Surgical Correction of the Cavovarus Foot Deformity with Utilization of Osteotomy and Arthrodesis Technique

Harry John Visser and Kyle Williams

Abstract

Cavovarus is a complex deformity characterized by a high arch and overall cavus foot deformity resulting from plantar flexion and adduction of the forefoot, increased calcaneal pitch, and most importantly hindfoot varus. There is a common misconception that all cavovarus foot types are derived from neuromuscular causes manifested in childhood. Due to this misconception the diagnosis of cavovarus foot is often overlooked in adults, particularly if it is a subtle deformity. This chapter will discuss the multiple non-neurologic and neurologic causes behind a cavovarus foot deformity in the adult patient. We will also demonstrate how to recognize and treat those difficult deformities using surgical techniques. Discussion should be centered around tendon and capsular balancing, muscle transfer, osteotomy, and arthrodesis.

Keywords: adductocavovarus foot deformity, chronic varus deformity, foot deformity, osteotomy, Charcot, reconstruction

1. Introduction

The impending discussion will encompass the utilization of osteotomy and arthrodesis and will center on conditions producing an adductocavovarus foot deformity. Recently a new encompassing classification has been established for flatfoot conditions called progressive collapsing foot deformity. This allows numerous conditions to fall into the category, which was an extension of the commonly used adult acquired flat foot deformity (AAFD) including posterior tibial tendon dysfunction. In this discussion, we will center on the more opposite deformity termed progressive elevating foot deformity. This will center on a group of bipedal conditions that will be primarily discussed such as:

1. Idiopathic non-neurologic adductocavovarus foot deformity.

2. Rheumatoid arthritis, a mononeuritis affecting the subtalar joint creating an elevating progressive foot deformity

3. Mueller Weiss disease

4. Charcot Marie Tooth disease

5. Talar neck malunion

6. Charcot osteoarthropathy

7. Traumatic or neuromuscular loss of function of the peroneal tendons, and neuro-musculature

Included in these discussions will be the utilization of osteotomy, arthrodesis, and soft tissue techniques to manage the resultant progressive deformities.

2. Idiopathic non-neurologic adductocavovarus deformity

This form of cavus foot represents a non-neurologic condition, recognized only in recent years by a loss of equilibrium and balance. This mild form most possibly represents the cavus end of the normal distribution of arch height. No neuromuscular weakness is found as noted, but arch structure leads to an unstable platform. This leads to many common conditions encountered in foot and ankle such as frequent ankle sprains, achilles tendinopathy and ankle impingement. Also, 28% have underlying stress fractures of metatarsals four and five. Peroneal tendinopathy is seen in 33% of patients.

Radiographically, Meary's angle will be slightly greater than negative, 0–5 degrees. Metatarsals will appear stacked, calcaneal inclination, which runs 25 degrees normally, will be increased to 30 degrees. The fibula will be posterior to the tibia as a

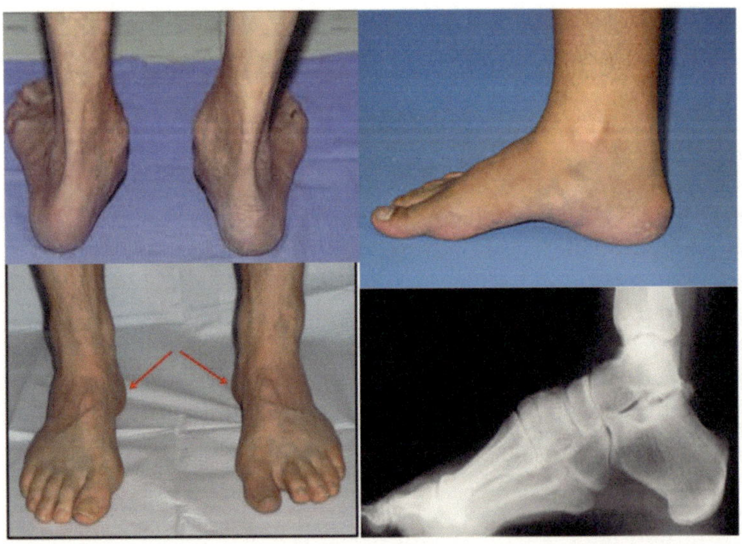

Figure 1.
Top left, too many toes sign. Bottom left, peek-a-boo heel sign of cavovarus foot. Top right, subtle cavovarus foot deformity with radiographic images below showing, increased calcaneal pitch, increased Meary's angle, and stacked metatarsals.

DOI: http://dx.doi.org/10.5772/intechopen.1008511

result of external rotation generated by the supinated subtalar joint. Also, the sinus tarsi will exhibit a bullet hole sign due the dorsiflexed and abducted position of the talus. The subtle radiographic changes represent the term subtle cavovarus foot deformity (**Figure 1**) [1].

On clinical exam, the neuromuscular exam notes no signs of weakness or abnormality. The presence of a peekaboo heel sign is present when viewing the foot and ankle from the front. The opposite is noted in the AAFD, where from behind the foot and ankle will show the too many toes sign. When performing the Coleman block test the rearfoot remains in a fixed varus position when the first metatarsal is dropped out. This indicates a rearfoot driven cavus. In most cases, the facets of the subtalar joint are congenitally aberrant. As stated previously, the condition of the peroneals, 4th and 5th metatarsal stress fractures, and ankle instability complaints focus on the need for surgical intervention. The subtle structure of the foot must be carefully assessed. This begins from posterior to anterior similar to flatfoot reconstruction. Firstly, the Silverskold test is used to evaluate for the presence of equinus deformity. With the fixed varus heel position this can lead to contracture. In most cases, a gastrocnemius equinus may be present. As a result of the Coleman block test, a fixed heel varus is noted. Attention is turned to the heel varus deformity which is corrected with a Dwyer calcaneal osteotomy [2]. The Dwyer osteotomy can be utilized in a biplane fashion by a superior shift of the tuber fragment. Occasionally, depending on deformity, a STJ arthrodesis correcting the varus deformity may be needed. Once this is performed, attention should be directed to the midfoot and forefoot. Three particular scenarios can occur. One, The first ray and midfoot can be restored completely to its normal functional position, this notes no further surgical intervention is needed. In the second scenario, the first ray remains plantar flexed but can be pushed in a dorsiflexed correct position. In this case, a transfer of the peroneus longus to the brevis can be done in the area of the peroneal groove. The first ray will then become neutral and the peroneus longus now acts with peroneus brevis to add a pronatory force to the subtalar and midtarsal joints. In the third scenario, the first ray remains

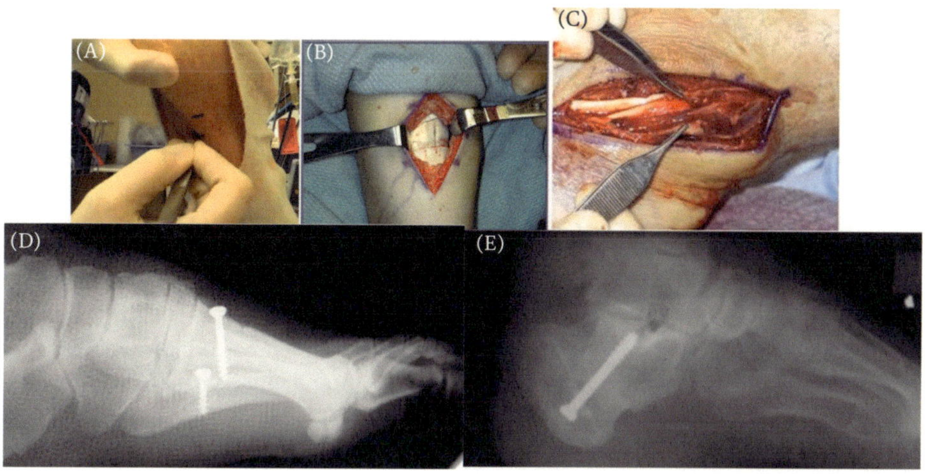

Figure 2.
Stepwise approach to treating Idiopathic cavovarus foot: (A) step 1: intra-op Silverskold test, gastroc recession, percutaneous TAL; (B) step 2: rearfoot varus, if there is a positive Coleman block test then perform a Dwyer osteotomy; (C) addressing the forefoot varus. If 1st ray remains plantarflexed then you can perform a (D) DFWO of the 1st metatarsal or a (E) peroneus longus to brevis tendon transfer.

plantarflexed and cannot be brought to the level of the lateral metatarsals. In this case, a DFWO of the first metatarsal or a first metatarsal medial cuneiform arthrodesis is performed. Once the procedures have been performed, adjunct procedures such as repair of peroneus brevis and retinaculum, delayed nonunion of a Jones fracture, or a Brostrum repair for ankle instability can be done. On average the post operative protocol is 4 weeks NWB, 4 weeks of WB and transition walking boot as needed. The patient will return to normal activity levels at 6–8 months (**Figure 2**).

3. Rheumatoid arthritis

Forefoot changes in the rheumatoid foot occur often before any associated hindfoot changes. Both the subtalar joint and the talonavicular joint are rarely affected in early rheumatoid pathogenesis [3]. When the rearfoot does become involved it affects primarily the talonavicular and subtalar joints. With talonavicular joint involvement, there is little deformity but shortening of the medial column can be produced by loss of cartilage and subchondral bone. Involvement of the pedis acetabuli can produce an adductovarus deformity. When performing surgical intervention by arthrodesis, grafting of the STJ is needed to restore proper length to the medial column. Also, the possibility exists of a cuboid osteotomy to correct further adduction. Involvement of the tarsometatarsal joints lead to destruction of the bases of the 2nd and 3rd metatarsals and a portion of their respective cuneiforms. The remaining TMT joints are unaffected. This then leads to the peroneus longus to maintain the longitudinal arch and transverse arch at the first ray. This leads to retrograde closed kinetic chain supination of the subtalar joint. Management of this condition includes arthrodesis of the tarsometatarsal joints 2 and 3 with interpositional bone graft. A peroneus longus lengthening or transfer to the brevis or even elevational osteotomy of the first metatarsal may be needed. A Dwyer calcaneal osteotomy may also be needed in these cases. Involvement of the subtalar joint leads to a collapsing foot deformity and thus is mentioned for that reason but is not part of developmental adductocavovarus foot deformity. The case study will demonstrate rheumatoid disease affecting the STJ.

3.1 Case study

56 year old white caucasian female with a long history of pedal rheumatoid arthritic changes that primarily centered in the forefoot some 10 years prior. The patient had been maintained on biologics but in the past 2 months began noticing a change in the position of her foot. A progressive adductocavovarus deformity began to occur with associated ankle instability. A revealing CT scan indicated extensive involvement of rheumatic panic disease in the medial talar and calcaneal portions of the STJ, involving the facets. The loss of bone lead to lateral transference and dorsiflexion abduction of the talus producing a closed kinetic chain supination (**Figure 3**).

The decision was made to perform a reconstruction of the medial side of the STJ utilizing a bioengineered titanium strut. This was filled with cortical cancellous autograft impregnated with bone marrow aspirate from the distal tibia. Some bone remodeling was performed to allow for a perfect fit to bring the calcaneus back to a vertical position. The talus also underwent positional change of adduction and plantarflexion. A percutaneous TAL was performed to unload the strain on the tubercle

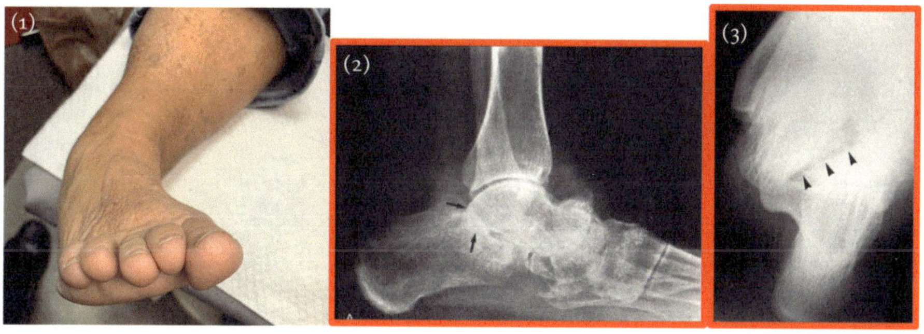

Figure 3.
Images moving from left to right: (1) clinical image of patients progressive adductocavovarus deformity and associated ankle instability; (2 and 3) initial radiographs showing collapse of calcaneus into valgus, talonavicular joint fault with subluxation, and development of advanced arthritis of the subtalar joint.

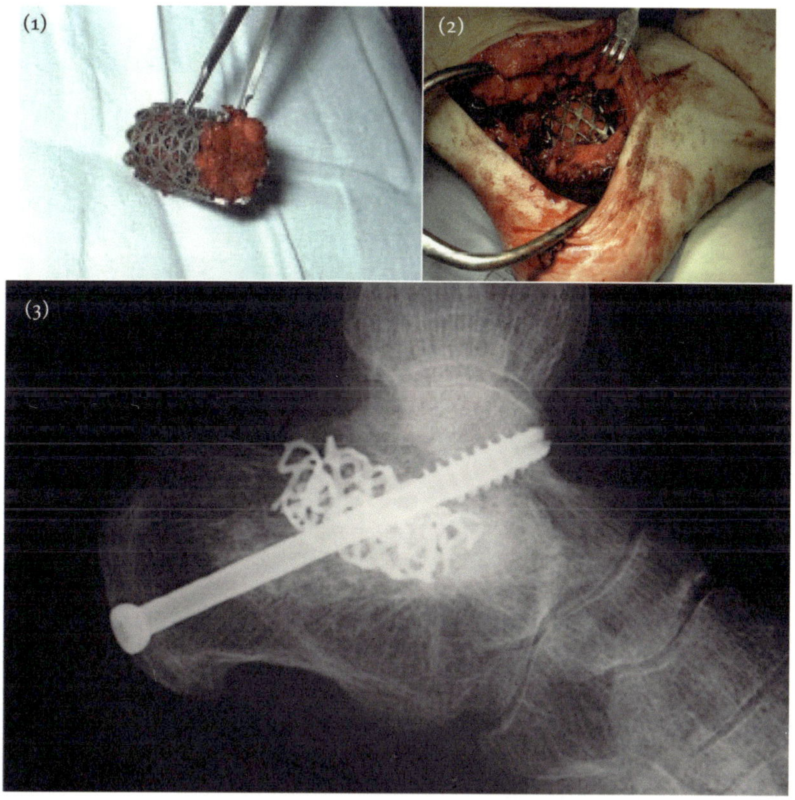

Figure 4.
From left to right. (1) Bioengineered titanium strut filled with cortical and cancellous calcaneal autograft and impregnated with bone marrow aspirate; (2) place of the strut in the medial side of the STJ for reconstruction and (3) postoperative X-rays.

of the calcaneus but with STJ stabilization, the decision was made to forego a lateral ankle stabilization. Patient was kept NWB 8 weeks, followed by 4 weeks in a walking CAM boot. Transition to shoewear by 12 weeks followed by 3 months of physical therapy. Full recovery time took approximately 1 year (**Figure 4**).

4. Mueller Weiss disease

Mueller Weiss disease is characterized by a dysplastic navicular. Konrad Weiss believed mueller weiss disease was due to osteonecrosis [4]. Several entities have been proposed but most agree on some form of traumatic event as the etiology. The condition affects the dorsal lateral aspect of the navicular with loss of volume. This leads to a lateral shift of the talus noted on a radiographic DP view as talocalcaneal convergence. The compression affects the three radial vessels passing through the central lateral body. This produces ischemia leading to secondary fragmentation and ultimate collapse of this portion of the navicular. The tuberosity is well preserved due to its rich blood supply coming from the posterior tibial artery. The result of this produces a c-shaped peri navicular condition. This leads to talonavicular and/or naviculo-cuneiform arthritis and produces midfoot collapse. Flattening of the medial arch occurs as the talus plantarflexes into the defect of the lateral central navicular. The talus also shifts lateral creating a rearfoot varus via closed kinetic chain supination [4]. This pathomechanical complex is referred to as a "paradoxical pes plano varus". Clinically, examination often relates swelling and tenderness over the dorsal medial midfoot. There is a normal or low medial longitudinal arch depending on disease severity [5]. The paradoxical nature of pes planus and hindfoot varus suggests advanced disease. Plain radiographs note a comma shape to the navicular on the DP view. On the lateral view, arthritic changes in the midfoot with fractured cancellous bone is often noted. This represents the remnants of the central-lateral pole (**Figure 5**). A radiographic classification was proposed by Maceira et al. [6].

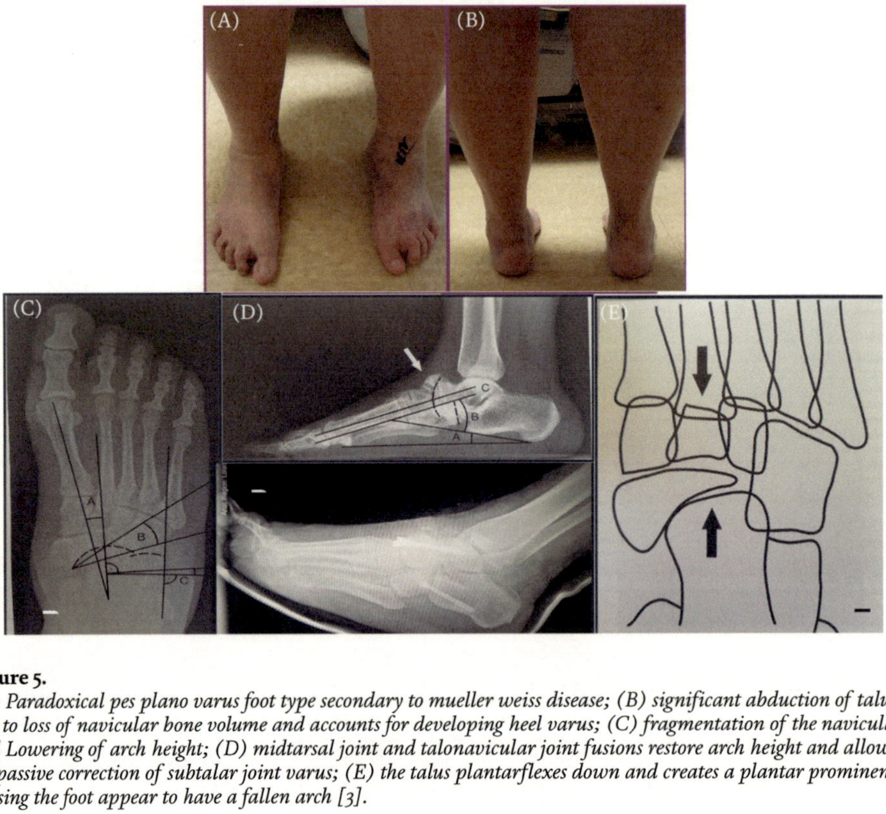

Figure 5.
(A) Paradoxical pes plano varus foot type secondary to mueller weiss disease; (B) significant abduction of talus due to loss of navicular bone volume and accounts for developing heel varus; (C) fragmentation of the navicular and Lowering of arch height; (D) midtarsal joint and talonavicular joint fusions restore arch height and allows for passive correction of subtalar joint varus; (E) the talus plantarflexes down and creates a plantar prominence causing the foot appear to have a fallen arch [3].

4.1 Surgical management of Mueller Weiss disease

See **Table 1**.

Stages (Maceira classification)	Deformity	Surgical treatment
Early Stages 0 and 1	Mild to moderate collapse of the body	Osteotomy can be considered. Evans calcaneal lengthening and Koutsogiannis posterior displaced osteotomy. Each move the talus medially to re-articulate with the remaining talonavicular joint creating closed kinetic chain pronation to the subtalar joint
Stage 2	Severe collapse of the lateral navicular body	Arthrodesis of the talonavicular joint with debridement and grafting of the lateral body. A truss bioengineered navicular
Stage 3	Advanced collapse of the navicular body with significant arthrosis of the talo cuneiform joint	Consider talonavicular joint arthrodesis which may need to include the subtalar joint and calcaneocuboid joint as a modified Charcot triple arthrodesis [5]
Stage 4	Advance collapse including the ankle joint	A modified Charcot pan arthrodesis, which is a triple arthrodesis, with a talo-cuneiform arthrodesis and ankle arthrodesis. A total ankle replacement is another viable option

Table 1.
The Maceira classification was proposed by Maceira and Rochera detailing Mueller Weiss disease based solely on Meary's angle on plain radiographs. This classification system helps explain the pathomechanics behind the disease and the pathomechanics can help guide the surgical correction of the disease.

5. Talar neck malunion

Talus fractures account for less than 1% of all fractures [7]. Malunion rates vary from 9 to 47% [8]. The most common malunion deformity is malalignment of the talar neck. This can lead to substantial shortening of the medial column. The result creates closed kinetic chain supination locking the STJ and thus rearfoot calcaneal varus. The midtarsal joint is also affected creating a forefoot varus at the TNJ and lateral column overload at the CCJ. The peroneus longus plantarflexes the first ray to keep the forefoot in contact with the ground. A malalignment of 2 mm leads to considerable load redistribution at the three STJ facets. Also one must be aware that the talus can become mal-aligned within the ankle joint created by abnormal axial rotation. This results in an adductocavovarus foot deformity.

The key falls in the initial talar neck fracture reduction which requires both a medial and lateral talar incision. The medial neck most often suffers comminution. This is why it is critical to address the lateral neck which is an isolated linear fracture. Once the lateral neck is reduced the medial side will then be brought into its normal anatomic length. The comminuted fragments then can fill the fracture defect and a solitary 4.0 or 3.5 screw or anatomic locking plate can be used for fixation.

Surgical options:

1. Corrective osteotomy with auto/allograft of talar neck.

2. Release of adhesions of the ankle, subtalar, and midtarsal joints with revision of the sinus tarsi.

3. Posterior calcaneal osteotomy.

4. Triple arthrodesis.

5. Supramalleolar osteotomies which include an opening wedge of the medial malleolus and decompression osteotomy of the fibula.

5.1 Case study

A 52 year old female presented to the clinic as a referral from the ER after a twisting type injury where X-rays did not reveal a fracture. She was treated conservatively for

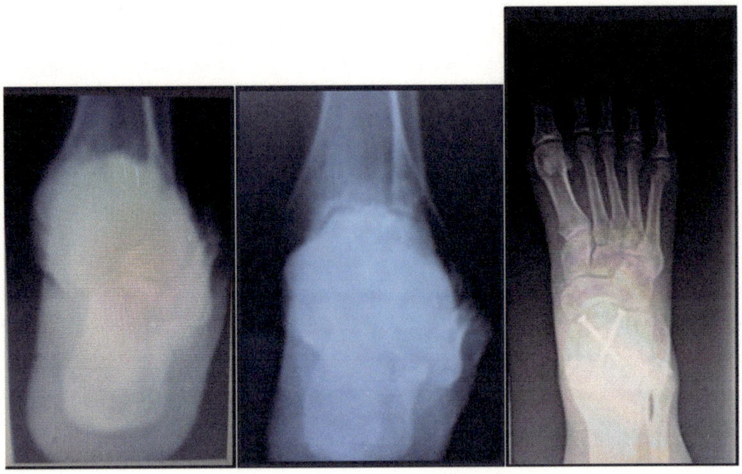

Figure 6.
Radiographs showing two screw fixation of the talar neck and the progressive heel varus from the following nonunion. The Nonunion causes shortening and gradual varus deformity of the rearfoot.

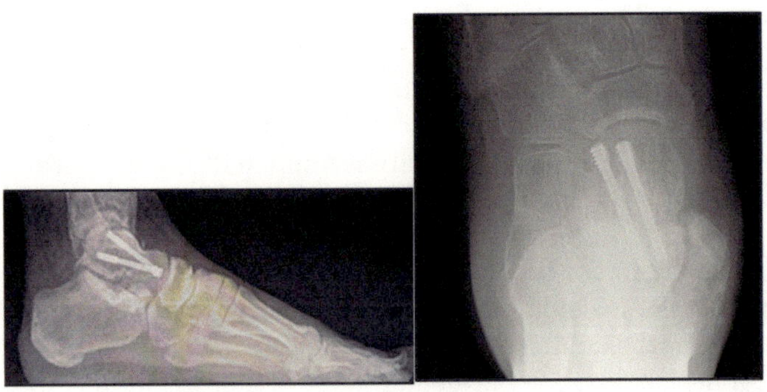

Figure 7.
Radiographic images of correction 1 year post operatively. There was Insertion of intra-articular subcapital compression screws with oblique lateral orientation of screws so as not to directly compress the bone graft. Note reduction of subtalar joint position created by lengthening of the medial neck and thus medial column. If this fails to completely reduce will need to consider dwyer calcaneal osteotomy or subtalar arthrodesis. Similarly lack of reduction of forefoot adduction may require triple arthrodesis.

the next couple of months consisting of rest, ice, elevation, NSAIDS, CAM boot and physical therapy with little improvement of pain. MRI was performed and showed talar neck fracture with medial comminution. Patient proceeded with surgical intervention at this time with two screw fixation medial and lateral. Over the next 2 years, the patient had continued pain and noted her foot beginning to turn inwards (**Figure 6**).

2 years post op the talus was healed. However, developmental subtalar joint varus secondary to talar neck malunion was occurring. Compression on the medial talar neck where comminution was present led to shortening and a developmental adductovarus. The proposed surgical management was an opening wedge osteotomy of the talar neck with interpositional bone graft. Lengthening of the talus medially leads to closed kinetic chain pronation and restoration of subtalar joint position as well as reduction of forefoot adduction. In cases where the STJ and MTJ are "locked" an aggressive soft tissue release with a Cobb elevator may be needed. In this failure, a triple arthrodesis is usually required. Occasionally, residual calcaneal varus can persist. This can be addressed by a Dwyer calcaneal osteotomy (**Figure 7**).

6. Charcot Marie Tooth

Of all conditions producing a progressive adductocavovarus foot deformity, Charcot Marie Tooth disease serves as the prototype as a neurologic condition. CMT is known as a hereditary motor sensory neuropathy associated with progressive peroneal muscular atrophy [9]. It was first described by Marie and Tooth in 1865. Patients demonstrate cavus foot forefoot adduction, midfoot pronation, and rearfoot supination. Its progression normally begins with the forefoot and also encompasses the midfoot. The STJ and ankle become involved later in progression.

A scenario that can be seen depends on the progression of weakness which can be variable [10]. In general, the forefoot is involved by intrinsic atrophy of the hallux creating a hallux malleus deformity as well as the lesser digits beginning as hammertoes that can progress to a mallet position. The tibialis anterior tendon and muscle can become involved leading to an overpowering of the peroneus longus. This brings the pronated midfoot to the floor medially. The weak peroneus brevis and strong tibialis posterior lead to the pronated midfoot and supinated STJ. The STJ then reaches end ROM in supination. This creates a fixed heel varus noted on the lateral radiograph as a bullet hole sign involving the sinus tarsi. Also, external rotation of the fibula is noted in reference to the tibia. The varus heel position leads to contracture of the achilles tendon. The results of this on lateral X-rays show increased calcaneal pitch and an increase in the Meary's angle which is demonstrated by the bisection of the talus to the first metatarsal [9]. This angle is critical in determining the apex of the deformity. Lateral tibiocalcaneal angle also shows an increase. DP radiographs show gun barrel sign at the proximal interphalangeal joints of the digits, mild to moderate forefoot adductus, decrease in the talocalcaneal angle, and talar convergence. Initial radiographs usually do not show signs of degenerative osteoarthritis (**Figure 8**).

On clinical examination, there is often lack of dorsiflexion at the ankle secondary to achilles tendon contracture. Range of motion of the subtalar joint appears to be fixed. Minimal pronatory ability is also observed at the midtarsal joint. Forefoot deformities are not fully reducible and the metatarsals are prominent plantarly. The first metatarsal position is often covered by the peroneus longus. Clinically, the result is considerable instability, a pronated MTJ, and a supinated STJ with an equinus

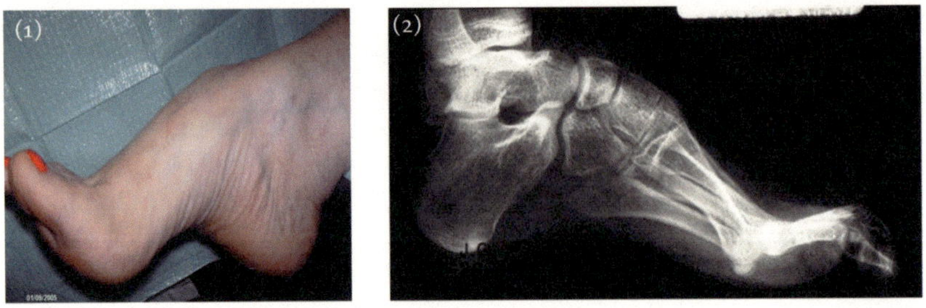

Figure 8.
Left to right. (1) Clinical images of a CMT affected foot; (2) radiographs showing increased calcaneal pitch, increased Meary's angle, and increased lateral tibiocalcaneal angle.

contracture at the ankle joint. The first metatarsal brought to the ground by the peroneus longus can also add a re-supinatory force.

The surgical approach to this condition attempts to establish a plantigrade foot. A major factor that is not often considered is the contractures brought on by the soft tissues. There are three main contractures that must be addressed. First the achilles, second, peroneus longus, and third, the tibialis posterior muscle tendon. A gastroc recession or an achilles lengthening will bring the foot underneath the ankle and allow better heel contact. The varus condition of the heel will need to be addressed by a Dwyer biplanar osteotomy. The tibialis posterior by being released from the navicular tuberosity down to the cuneiform will help release the pronatory force at the STJ. If lack of talo-calcaneal correction is noted at this juncture, a full talonavicular capsulotomy with release of the spring ligament and deltoid ligament must be considered. The TP tendon is then transferred to the dorsal foot through the interosseous membrane (Watkins procedure) to the intermediate cuneiform as a non-phasic transfer [11]. This leads to a considerable release of deformity at the midfoot correcting its pronatory position. It can also offer dorsiflexion power to the ankle. Next the peroneus longus is transferred to the brevis in the area of the cuboid tunnel which also helps in forefoot and midtarsal joint alignment correcting midfoot pronation and forefoot abduction. Once the soft tissue contractures and tendon transfers are performed, correction of the foot deformity appears to

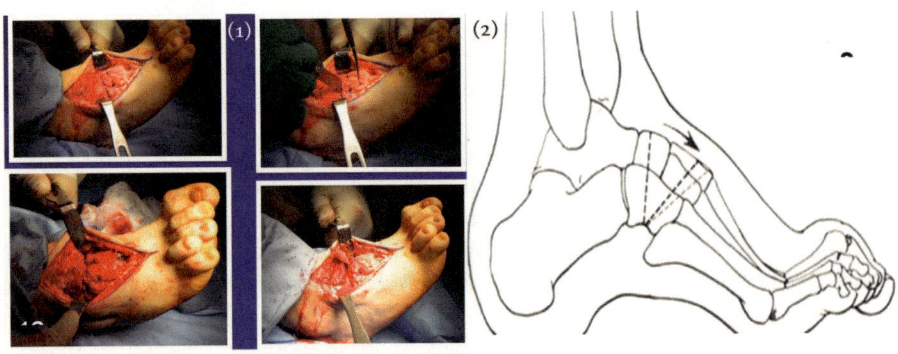

Figure 9.
*Example of the Cole midfoot osteotomy used to correct the Meary's angle in cavus deformity. A dorsal curvilinear incision is made over the midfoot in order to expose the navicular and cuboid (1). A dorsal and slightly laterally based transverse-wedge osteotomy (2) is made through the naviculo-cuneiform joints medially and the cuboid laterally. After the bony wedge is removed the osteotomy is reduced into the corrected position and fixated using Steinman pins, staples, screws, or even external fixation techniques (**Figure 10**).*

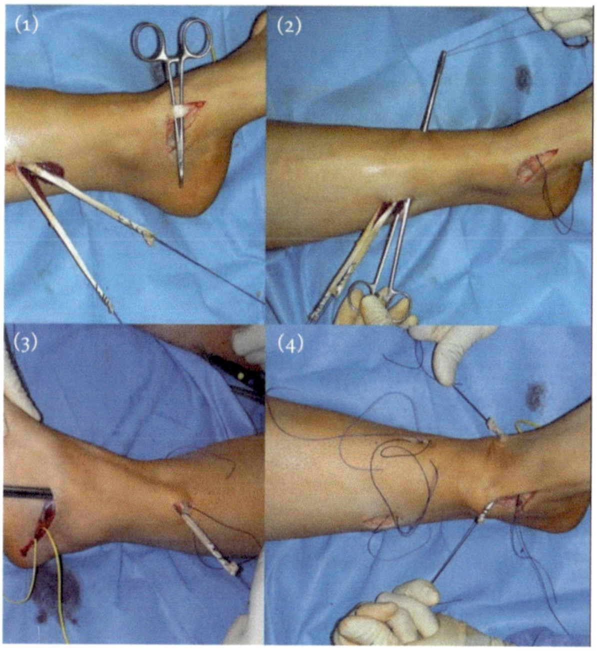

Figure 10.
Top left moving left to right describing a tibialis posterior tendon transfer. (1) Harvesting TP at the Master Knot of Henry; (2) harvest the second tendon approximately 9 cm above the ankle joint; (3) incision created by transfer of the tendon medial to lateral directly posterior on the tibia creating a generous window in the IO membrane and (4) insertion of the TP in the lateral cuneiform with biotenodesis screw.

be much improved. The midfoot, where Meary's angle intersects in the area of the TN and CC joints, can be addressed with a midfoot Cole osteotomy. If residual 1st metatarsal plantarflexion exists a 1st metatarsal osteotomy can be performed for further elevation. This then leads to a functional plantigrade foot. The forefoot is then addressed in a second stage, including a Jones sling procedure with hallux interphalangeal joint arthrodesis. The digits are then addressed by proximal interphalangeal joint arthrodesis (Taylor type). If metatarsal declination persists, consider a Hibbs EDL tendon transfer (forefoot suspension) to the intermediate cuneiform. Thus one can see that with a seemingly rigid foot correction can be attained with soft tissue release, tendon transfer, and osteotomy with avoidance of arthrodesis (**Figure 9**).

7. Loss of peroneal function

This is a condition where both peroneal tendons (cables) are severely damaged and cannot be repaired. Two scenarios can occur. In the first scenario, the peroneal musculature is still intact. On MRI, there is no significant sign of fibrosis or fatty infiltration. In this scenario an allograft can be used to replace one or both tendons (see case). In the second condition, there are signs of loss of muscle mass forming a myopathy. Fibrosis and fatty infiltration will be noted. Here one cannot depend on an allograft for reconstruction. An active motor unit will need to be utilized. The following case study demonstrates an FDL transfer to peroneus brevis insertion. This provides an active motor to the damaged end.

Adjunctive procedures performed:

1. Complete excision of both peroneal tendons, with preservation of the distal peroneal insertion for utilization of pulver-taft technique. Utilized in conjunction with the FDL transfer.

2. Dwyer Calcaneal osteotomy or possible STJ arthrodesis for the fixed heel varus condition.

3. Z-plasty lengthening of the tibialis posterior tendon with possible excision.

4. Possible split or total transfer of tibialis anterior tendon to the lateral foot for cases of residual forefoot varus creating by loss of peroneus longus function.

7.1 Case study

A 60 year old female presented with a history of pain in the anterior lateral aspect of her left foot. She sought medical care initially, but no presumptive diagnosis was made. Patient eventually received an MRI which revealed rupture of the peroneus brevis tendon at the area of the peroneal tubercle. The imaging also showed advanced peroneus longus tendinopathy with a high grade tear inferior to the cuboid. MRI also revealed fatty and fibrous infiltration of the peroneal musculature with loss of girth. As a consequence, the patient had developed a significant varus deformity (**Figure 11**) [1].

Given the fatty infiltration along the course of the peroneal musculature this is indicating that the peroneus brevis is no longer contractile. The decision was made to proceed with a transfer of the flexor digitorum longus tendon to the fifth metatarsal base (pictured below). The tendon was transferred behind the tibia and allows the foot to maintain primary eversion function for the foot. To counteract the anterior forces, a functional lengthing of the posterior tibial tendon was also performed. Finally, a Dwyer calcaneal osteotomy was done in order to correct the varus and to stabilize the

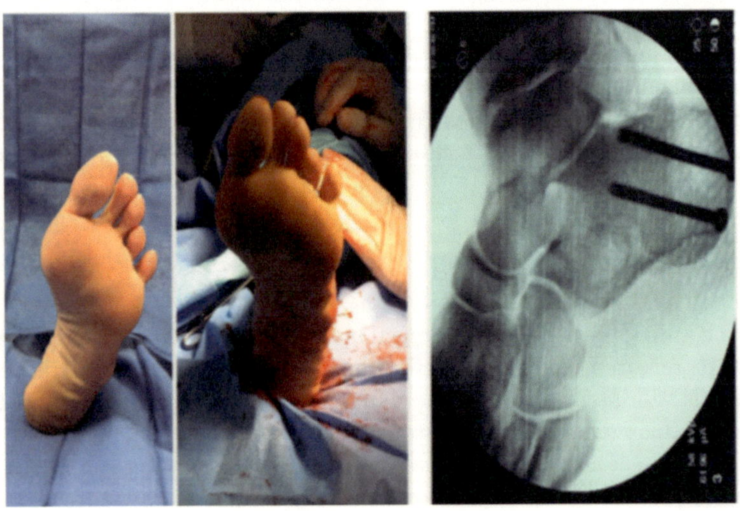

Figure 11.
Immediate post operative images following FDL transfer, PT tendon lengthening, and calcaneal Dwyer osteotomy. Immediate correction of the varus deformity is seen.

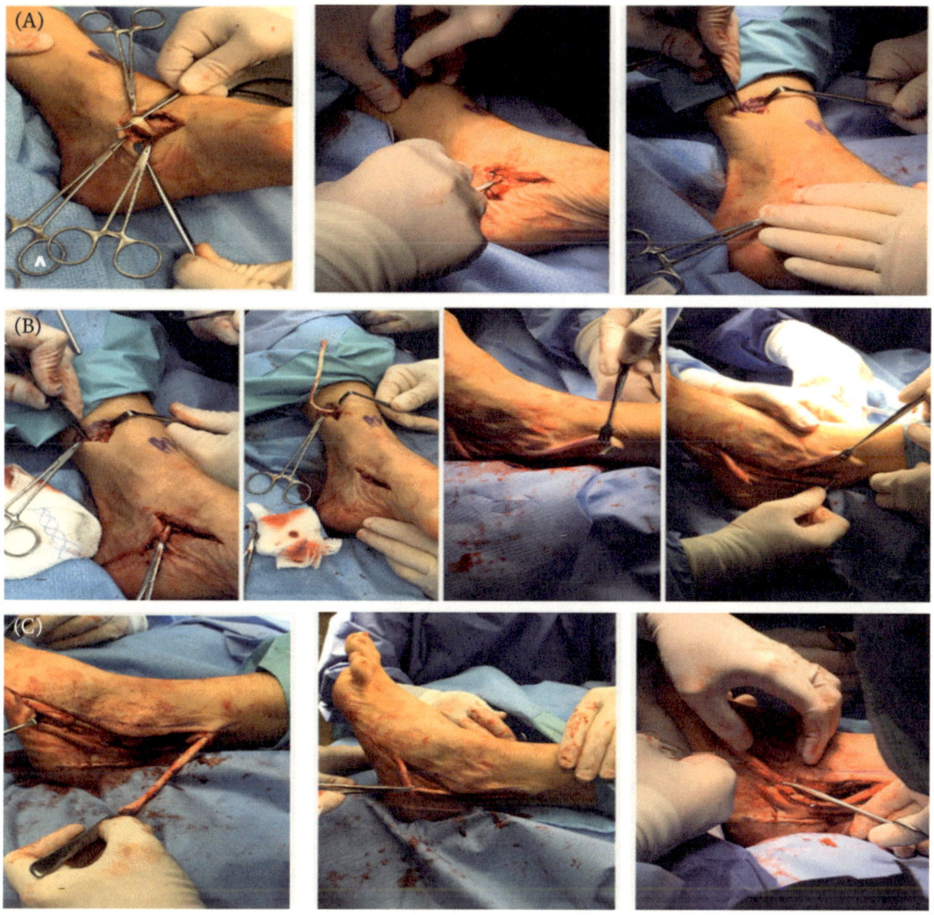

Figure 12.
Series of photos depicting FDL tendon transfer (A) harvesting the FDL from the Master Knot of Henry; (B) harvesting FDL 7–9 cm proximal to the ankle joint and bringing the tendon behind the posterior tibial tendon; (C) using the Pulver-Taft technique to transfer the FDL into the peroneus brevis insertion with the foot in maximal dorsiflexion and abduction.

subtalar joint. This correction allows an immediate improvement of the varus deformity and most importantly treats the underlying etiology preventing any recurrence. Postoperative management is 4 weeks NWB, followed by 4 weeks in a weight bearing boot and conversion to shoewear with 2–3 months of physical therapy (**Figure 12**).

8. Charcot neuroarthropathy

Charcot neuroarthropathy, although quite common in the diabetic population, has become more commonplace in the non-diabetic population. As is known, stages have been described by Eichenholtz and more recently modified by Shibata [12] which can help guide treatment. Controversy is still very prominent concerning when best to intercede surgically or pursue a conservative non-weight bearing course in the fragmentation phase. Often however, stage 2 and 3, are when the patient presents with significant deformity making surgical intervention more difficult. Midfoot involvement is quite common in this condition (**Figure 13**) [13].

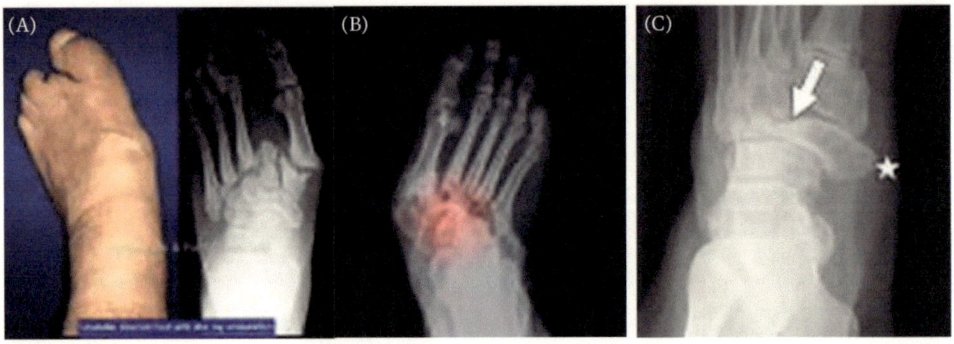

Figure 13.
Three cases of the most common form of Charcot which is the midfoot type. Radiographic changes can indicate significant instability and corresponding deformity. (A) Represents an Schon 2 classification of Charcot. With the position of the talus heading straight to the cuneiforms. Operative intervention will not be needed in Eichenholtz stage 1. This pattern leads to usually a plantigrade weight bearing foot; (B) this represents a Schon 4 classification involvement of the TN joint. This does best by being managed during Eichenholtz stage 1. This leads to an unstable pronatory condition with the talus head becoming weight bearing by stage 3; (C) this represents Koenig stage 3 which is the peri-navicular form. This also requires operative intervention during the fragmentation phase. The result is that the navicular becomes convergent and abducted leading to a varus foot overload. Thus, the cuboid, 4th, and 5th metatarsals become dislocated by Eichenholtz stage 3.

Schon classified this by 3 patterns in the stage 1 and 2 cases [12]. The first pattern involves the TMT and Cuneiform joints. This leads to developing a stage 3 condition often due to a plantigrade foot. What is noticed is that the talus remains in the central foot. The next pattern type noted the talus adducting medial to the navicular. This represented a broken down midfoot with the medial portion superiorly pronating the talus. This requires early intervention to prevent this rapidly developing rocker bottom condition. A Charcot type of triple arthrodesis utilizing beaming screws is utilized. In stage 1 conditions (fragmentation stage) a static external fixator is used. The third pattern is the peri-navicular type. In this case the talus will shift lateral and thus produce a varus deformity and unstable subtalar joint. This unstable subtalar joint leads to the very difficult plantar cuboid ulceration. Early intervention is also required here and will need to be addressed with a charcot triple arthrodesis again with an external fixator, another option includes a subtalar joint arthrodesis with an open Z-plasty of the achilles tendon.

9. Conclusion

In conclusion, this discussion encompasses a myriad of deformities. It is important that one carefully evaluate and diagnose each condition. Biomechanical abnormalities are the hallmark of each, but because of the areas of involvement, each deformity can present in a different fashion. Our approach addresses the pathobiomechanics of each of these conditions involving the adductocavovarus foot. Once recognized the surgical approach will vary but the use of osteotomy, arthrodesis, and even soft tissue release will be paramount.

Conflicts of interest

None to report.

Author details

Harry John Visser* and Kyle Williams
SSM Health DePaul Hospital Foot and Ankle Surgery Residency, St. Louis, MO, United States

*Address all correspondence to: tsarhjv@aol.com

References

[1] Deben SE, Pomeroy GC. Subtle cavus foot: Diagnosis and management. Journal of the American Academy of Orthopaedic Surgeons. 2014;**22**(8):512-520. DOI: 10.5435/JAAOS-22-08-512

[2] Dwyer FC. Osteotomy of the calcaneum for pes cavus. Journal of Bone and Joint Surgery. British Volume (London). 1959;**41**:80-86

[3] Wakabayashi H, Nakata K, Nishimura A, Hasegawa M, Sudo A. The onset of subtalar joint monoarthritis in a patient with rheumatoid arthritis. Diagnostics (Basel). 2022;**12**(10):2311. DOI: 10.3390/diagnostics12102311

[4] Angthong C, Younger ASE, Chuckpaiwong B, Harnroongroj T, Veljkovic A. A novel update on the management of Müller-Weiss disease: Presentation of a treatment algorithm. Cartilage. 2024;**15**(1):65-71. DOI: 10.1177/19476035231205684. Epub 2023 Oct 18

[5] Zhang H, Li J, Qiao Y, et al. Open triple fusion versus TNC arthrodesis in the treatment of Mueller-Weiss disease. Journal of Orthopaedic Surgery and Research. 2017;**12**:13. DOI: 10.1186/s13018-017-0513-3

[6] Maceira E et al. Müller-Weiss disease: Clinical and biomechanical features. Foot and Ankle Clinics. 2004;**9**(1):105-125

[7] Chen G, Hu M, Xu Y, Zhen YH, Hong Y, Xu XY. Joint-preserving surgery for Talar Malunions or nonunions. Orthopaedic Surgery. 2017;**9**(1):34-41. DOI: 10.1111/os.12301

[8] Galanopoulos IP, Sellina D, Drakopoulos P, Psarakis SA. Posttraumatic cavovarus deformity due to a varus malunited talar neck fracture, treated with corrective talar osteotomy: A case report. Cureus. 2024;**16**(1):e52206. DOI: 10.7759/cureus.52206

[9] Bertorini T, Narayanaswami P, Rashed H. Charcot Marie-Tooth disease (hereditary motor sensory neuropathies) and hereditary sensory and autonomic neuropathies. The Neurologist. 2004;**10**(6):327-337

[10] Joo SY, Choi BO, Kim DY, Jung SJ, Cho SY, Hwang SJ. Foot deformity in Charcot Marie Tooth disease according to disease severity. Annals of Rehabilitation Medicine. 2011;**35**(4):499-506. DOI: 10.5535/arm.2011.35.4.499. Epub 2011 Aug 31

[11] Rodríguez-Argueta ME, Suarez-Ahedo C, Jiménez-Aroche CA, Rodríguez-SantamariaI, Pérez-JiménezFJ, Ibarra C, et al. Anterior tibial tendon side-to-side tenorrhaphy after posterior tibial tendon transfer: A technique to improve reliability in drop foot after common peroneal nerve injury. Arthroscopy Techniques. 2021;**10**(5):e1361-e1368. DOI: 10.1016/j.eats.2021.01.039

[12] Rosenbaum AJ, DiPreta JA. Classifications in brief: Eichenholtz classification of Charcot arthropathy. Clinical Orthopaedics and Related Research. 2015;**473**(3):1168-1171. DOI: 10.1007/s11999-014-4059-y. Epub 2014 Nov 21

[13] Schon LC, Easley ME, Cohen I, Lam PW, Badekas A, Anderson CD. The acquired midtarsus deformity classification system--interobserver reliability and intraobserver reproducibility. Foot & Ankle International. 2002;**23**(1):30-36. DOI: 10.1177/107110070202300106

Chapter 9

Proximal and Distal Osteotomies in Treatment of Hallux Valugs

Nadan Mikić, Ivan Marjanović, Aleksandar Stanković, Dragiša Stamenković, Vesna Ranković and Vladimir Gordić

Abstract

Hallux valgus is one of the most common deformities in the musculoskeletal system. It is a chronic progressive condition of the foot that is prevented by lateral deviation of the big toe and deformity of the first metatarsophalangeal joint. The complexity of the condition is reflected in the progressive development of deformities at the front of the foot, which is manifested by pain, the appearance of calluses, difficulty walking. Non-operative treatment is aimed at reducing symptoms, improving tolerance of deformities, but often does not deal with the altered mechanics of the foot. For this reason, surgical correction is often used. The existence of numerous surgical procedures indicates that there is no universally successful method for dealing with this deformity. In this chapter, we will provide a brief overview of the history, anatomy of the metatarsus, and surgical techniques of the proximal and distal osteotomies of the first metatarsal, with a particular focus on Golden and Mitches osteotomies, including the presentation of the results.

Keywords: 1st metatarsal, hallux valgus, Mitchell osteotomy, golden osteotomy, comparative analysis

1. Introduction

1.1 Hallux valgus: General part

The significance of hallux valgus deformity is that it is very common, especially in women. It is a problem for the patient due to the formation of calluses, pain, difficulty wearing shoes and difficulty walking.

Treatment of hallux valgus deformity is carried out conservatively and surgically.

Non-operative treatment has the role of reducing problems, enabling the deformity to be better tolerated, but often does not solve the essence, that is, disturbed statics in the function of the foot.

This is the reason why treatment is often carried out with surgical corrections. The existence of a large number of surgical procedures shows that there is no completely successful way to solve this deformity.

1.2 Definition and brief history

One of the most common diseases of modern man, which dominates among foot deformities, is the bunion foot.

Hallux valgus is a chronic progressive disease of the foot, represented primarily by lateral deviation of the big toe and deformity of the first metatarsophalangeal (MTF) joint. The complexity of the disease is reflected in the fact that with the progression of the disease there is a gradual formation of deformities at the front of the foot.

Valgus hallux was first described by La Forrest, Louis XVI's physician, and the term was introduced into professional use by Carl Heuter in 1871.

1.3 Frequency and etiology

Hallux valgus deformity (bunion) is highly prevalent among the population. Depending on age, the incidence rate ranges from 7.8% in young people under 18 years of age to 35.7% in people over 65 years of age. In people between the ages of 18 and 65, the deformity occurs in 27% of cases [1].

The formation of the hallux valgus is influenced by internal factors such as: heredity, pes planus-flat foot, metatarsus primus varus—varus first MT bone, length of the big toe, and external factors: uncomfortable shoes, trauma, amputation of the second toe [2].

There are three types of feet compared to the length of a big toe with another toe. The first is the Egyptian foot where the big toe is longer than the second toe, the second type is the square foot where the big toe and the second toe are the same length, and the third type of foot is the Greek foot, where the second toe is longer than the big toe (**Figure 1**).

The greatest predisposition to the formation of hallux valgus exists in the Egyptian type of foot [3].

1.4 Pathoanatomical changes

By changing the balance of bone and soft tissue of the forefoot, the development of hallux valgus deformity gradually occurs. Congenital or increased mobility

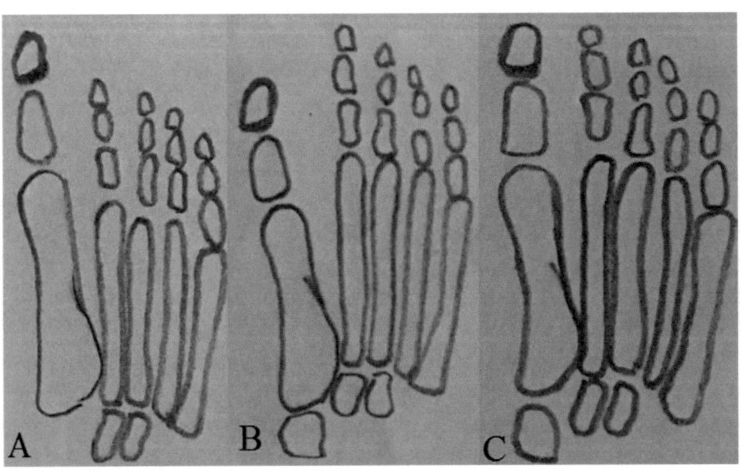

Figure 1.
Schematic representation of foot types: Egyptian foot (A), Greek foot (B), square foot (C).

of the first MT bone during life is one of the main causes of the development of hallux valgus. Wearing high-heeled shoes increases the load on the front of the foot. Under load, the first MT bone moves away from the other bones, leaving its place of the lowest bone. The base of the proximal phalanx of the thumb first shifts laterally and gradually subluxates relative to the head of the first MT bone. At the same time, the proximal phalanx rotates in a field around its axis, the muscles weaken, the fingers come closer to each other due to the narrow space and deform, and there is a lateral deviation of the thumb. Placing the thumb in the valgus position and extension leads to the fact that when supporting, the thumb separates from the ground and so that the force of the body's weight is not transferred to it. The weight of the body is transferred to the lateral part of the foot, especially to the head of the second MT bone, under which a callus forms. The pain affects the metatarsus and metatarsalgia occurs. Due to the tightening of the medial ligament of the first MT joint, inflammation is caused on the medial side of the head, which results in the formation of fibrocartilaginous prominence, which later ossifies in the form of a painful exostosis on the inside of the foot. Gradually, there is a rotation of the phalanges of the thumb around its longitudinal shaft, so that the nail looks upwards and inwards. The main cause of rotation of the thumb is the loss of balance between the abductor hallucis and m. adductor hallucis, which attach at the base of the proximal phalanx and on the sesamoid bones. Both sesamoid bones migrate toward laterally proportional to the lateral deviation of the thumb. The head of the first MT bone moves laterally. The articular capsule on the medial side is thickened, while on the lateral side it is shortened (McBride's test) and does not allow the proximal phalanx to move medially, until the tendon of the adductor hallucis, which attach both at the base of the proximal phalanx and on the outer part of the capsule, is cut. Due to weakness of the deep transverse ligament on the medial side of the medial sesamoid bone and on the lateral side of the head of the heel of the MT bone, an extension of the forefoot (splay foot) occurs. There is a change in the function of the adductor hallucis, which, with the shortening of the m. extensor hallucis longus, leads to an increase in the deformity of the thumb. It is also shortened by m. flexor hallucis brevis and m. flexor hallucis longus. The only muscle that opposes the further progression of the deformity of the thumb is the abductor hallucis, by fixing the proximal phalanx in the valgus position, the rotation of the first MT bone [4].

1.5 Diagnosis

A medical history, clinical examination, and radiographic imaging of the foot are required to make a diagnosis.

1.5.1 Anamnesis

From the anamnesis, a lot can be learned about the onset of the onset of problems, the type and severity of pain, about external factors that can affect the occurrence of deformities, heredity [2].

1.5.2 Clinical examination

The inspection determines the existence of a lateral deviation of the big toe with a wide front part of the foot in the form of a fan and deformation of the head, and the first MT bone on the medial side is observed as the most dominant signs of hallux valgus deformity. The Mc Bride test examines the correctability of deformities. The test is positive if the thumb cannot be corrected [4].

1.5.3 Radiographic diagnostics

Radiographic examination follows a detailed clinical examination (**Figure 2**). The foot is radiographed in standard positions under load from a height of 1.5 m. Radiography under load is a balance between the action of the force of the weight of the body and the reaction of the force of the surface on the foot, reflecting a realistic relationship between the position of the bones and joints when the foot is in function.

In addition to standard radiographs in the dorsoplantar and profile directions, sesamoid bones in the tangential direction are radiographed separately, and other joints and foot bones if the clinical finding requires it.

Dorsoplantar radiographs determine the hallux valgus angle (HVA), distal metatarsal articular angle (DMAA), intermetatarsal angle (IMTA), interphalangeal angle of thumb (IFA), congruence of the MTF joint, angle of inclination of the first MT bone, angle of pronation of the first MT bone, arthritic changes.

The angle that the longitudinal shafts of the first MT bone and the proximal phalanx overlap is HVA. HVA values in a healthy foot are 0–15° (**Figure 2**).

DMAA is the angle formed by a line extending along the axis of the first MT bone with a line running through the articular surface of the head of the first MT bone. In a healthy foot, DMAU is 0–15° (**Figure 2**).

IMTU is the angle that the longitudinal axes of the first and second MT bones interact. Its physiological values are 6–9°C (**Figure 3**).

The angle that the longitudinal shafts of the proximal and distal phalanx of the thumb overlap is the IFU angle. In a healthy foot, the values of the interphalangeal angle are from 0 to 5° (**Figure 4**).

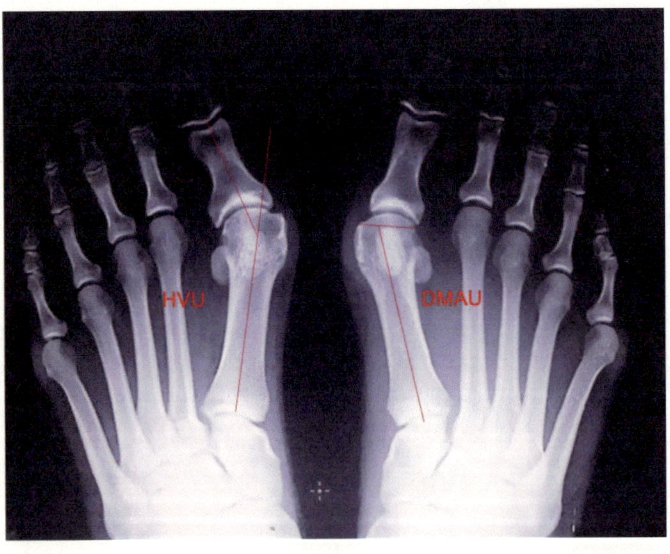

Figure 2.
Radiographic representation of HVA and DMAA.

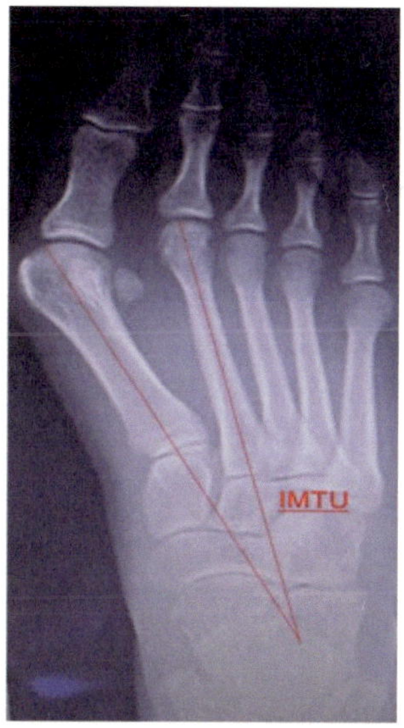

Figure 3.
Radiographic representation of IMTA.

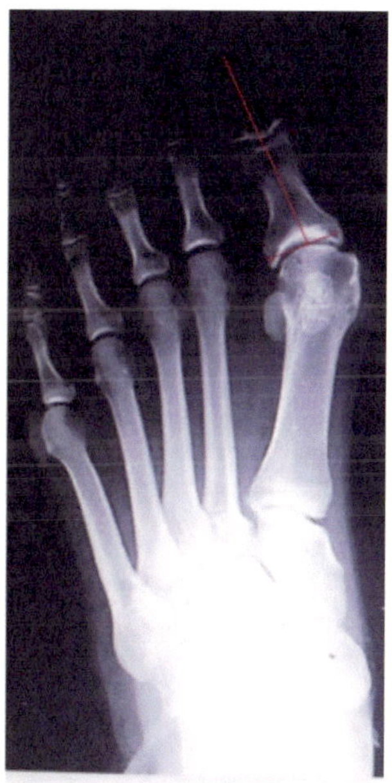

Figure 4.
Radiographic representation of IFA.

The first MTF joint is congruent in a healthy foot; that is, the concavity of the articular surface of the base of the proximal phalanx of the big toe corresponds to the convexity of the articular surface of the head of the first MT bone (**Figure 5**).

Subluxation and luxation of MTF joints is best observed on profile radiography.

The angle of inclination of the first MT bone is formed by a line extending along the axis of the MT bone with a horizontal line (**Figure 6**).

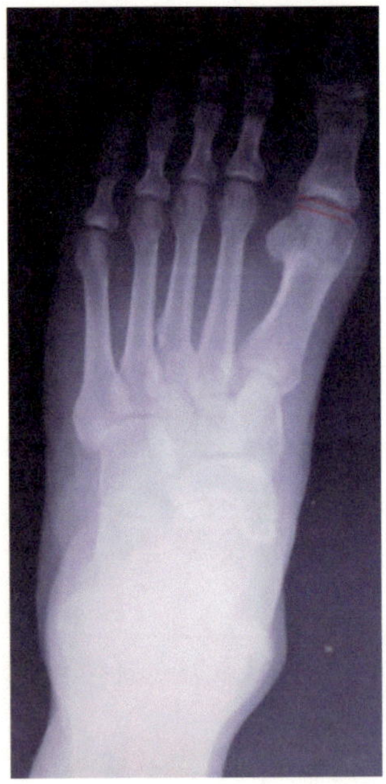

Figure 5.
Radiographic view congruence of the MTF joint of the big toe of the left foot.

Tangential or sesamoid radiography shows the position of the sesamoid bones relative to the head of the first MT bone and their degree of migration laterally. Sesamoid bones in a healthy foot are projected symmetrically onto the head of the first MT bone and do not normally emerge from the head shadow (**Figure 7**) [5, 6].

The angle of pronation of the first MT bone is the angle that closes the line extending through the dorsal surface of the medial and lateral sesamoid with a horizontal line (**Figure 8**).

1.6 Treatment

Before making any decision on operative treatment, in patients with initial and moderate hallux valgus deformity, it is necessary to try non-operative treatment.

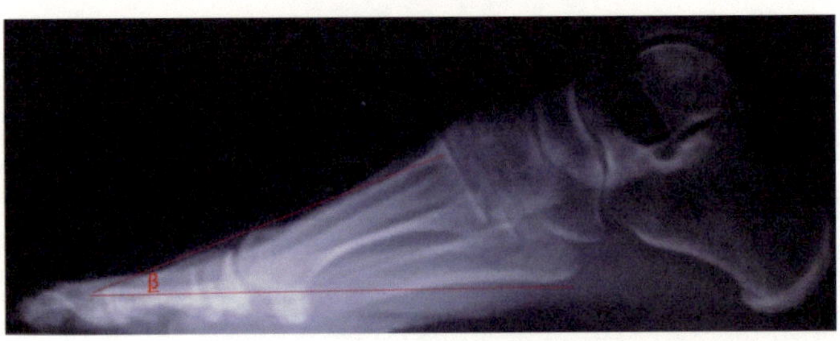

Figure 6.
Radiographic representation in the lateral projection of the angle of inclination of the first MT bone.

Figure 7.
Radiographic representation of the position of sesamoid in tangetial projection.

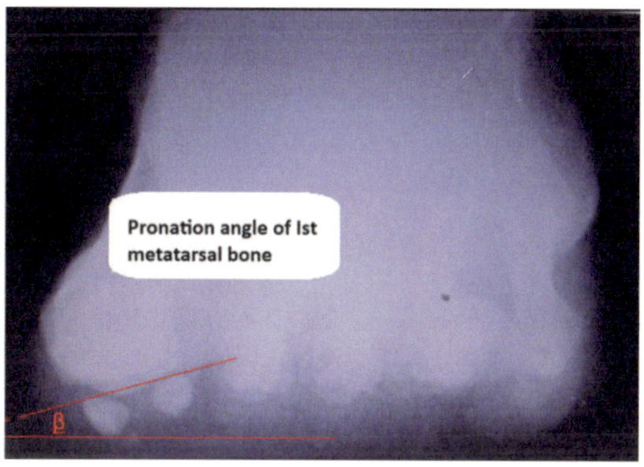

Figure 8.
Radiographic representation in tangential projection of the pronation angle of the first MT bone.

1.6.1 Non-operative treatment

Non-operative treatment of hallux valgus gives the best results at the very beginning of the formation. Treatment of bunion foot should begin with the elimination of the most common external cause that leads to the development of deformity due to uncomfortable footwear. Footwear should be suitable for the feet, made of leather with a wider rounded front and preferably laced with a heel height of 2.5 cm. The aforementioned footwear with the wearing of orthoses can somewhat slow down the development of deformities.

When the valgus hallux becomes so painful that, despite all the conservative treatments taken, it threatens the function of the foot as a whole, a plan for surgical treatment is made.

1.6.2 Operative treatment

Due to the limited effectiveness of non-surgical procedures, the treatment of deformities in most cases ends with surgery [7].

The existence of a large number of surgical methods in the treatment of bunion foot clearly shows that there is no single method that can solve all clinical variants of this disease [8]. Each patient should be observed individually, as well as the feet of the same patient. The choice of method to be used in the surgical treatment of deformities depends on several factors: the size of HVA and IMTA, the presence of arthrosis of the MTF joint, the position of sesamoids, the movement of the thumb, persistent comorbidities, the age of the patient. A very important segment when deciding on the type of surgical technique that will be applied to a given deformity is the experience of the orthopedist, that is, his mastery of certain surgical methods.

To date, a number of surgical techniques have been described, which can be divided into two basic groups of surgical interventions: surgical techniques, where only soft tissues are used to correct deformities, and surgical procedures that, in addition to soft tissues, also affect the bone and joint systems.

In 1856, Volkman described the first operative technique for the treatment of hallux valgus deformity [9]. In 1881, Reverdin used distal MT osteotomy and medial resection of the exostosis from the head of the first MT bone to solve hallux valgus deformity. As early as 1933, Verbrugge claimed that there were 152 surgical techniques for correcting deformities in hallux valgus [10].

Deformity of the valgus hallux can be divided into five main groups for the purpose of an appropriate surgical treatment strategy [2]:

1. Deformity with the congruent joint,
2. Deformity with the incongruent joint,
3. Deformity with arthritic changes in the first MTF joint,
4. Deformity with unstable (loose) first metatarsocouneiform joint, and
5. Juvenile hallux valgus.

The extent of the deformity can be further divided into three groups:

1. Initial (mild) deformity, in which HVA is 15–30°, and IMTA 9–13°
2. Moderate (medium) deformity, in which the HVA is from 31 to 40°, and the IMTA from 14 to 20°
3. A severe deformity, in which HVA > 40°, and IMTA > 20° [8]

In addition to the above classification of the hallux valgus, it should be borne in mind the possibility of the existence of only an isolated prominence of the medial part of the head of the first MT bone as well as the existence of the hallux valgus interphalangeus.

It is very important for orthopedists to follow the above indications for the surgical treatment of hallux valgus deformity, which is not always the case in practice. Often, surgeons operate on patients with the method they know best, and not with the method that, according to the algorithm recommended in the treatment of hallux valgus deformities, they should. This approach can have its ups and downs.

The bad thing is that if you do not follow the previously mentioned principles of surgical treatment, it can happen that the deformity is not corrected to the desired extent with the appearance of accompanying complications. As a possible advantage of such an approach, the surgeon has less possibility of making mistakes by doing a similar method.

When working with patients, an individual approach is very important. For each patient individually, in accordance with the set indications, an appropriate method for surgical care of the bunion foot is applied.

1.6.2.1 Soft tissue operations

If an attempt at non-surgical treatment of hallux valgus is unsuccessful, and the existing deformity is flexible, that is, it can be manually corrected, soft tissue surgical procedures are performed to achieve a satisfactory functional and esthetic result, if the following conditions are met:

- If the valgus hallux is an angle between 20° and 35°.
- An angle of less than 15°
- Valgus INTF angle less than 15°
- If the MTF of the thumb joint is without degenerative changes [11].

1.6.2.2 Operations on bone tissue

Bone surgical procedures are performed when, on the basis of a detailed clinical and radiographic examination, it is estimated that soft tissue surgical procedures cannot achieve the desired result. There are a number of surgical procedures in which osteotomy is used in the correction of deformities and which can be divided into:

- procedures performed on the proximal phalanx of the thumb,
- distal osteotomy of the first MT bone,
- osteotomy of the body of the first MT bone,
- and osteotomy of the base of the first MT bone.

1.6.2.2.1 Procedures on the proximal phalanx of the thumb

In 1904, Keller described a technique for correcting hallux valgus.

The essence of the operation itself is the resection of the medial bone prominence on the head of the first MT bone and the resection of the base of the proximal phalanx of the thumb with stabilization of the resected phalanx with Kirschner's needle (**Figure 9**) [12].

In 1925, in patients with minor deformities where the angle of the hallux valgus is 15°–30°, and the intermetatarsal angle is 9°–12°, after removal of the medial bone prominence and tenotomy of the adductor hallucis, Akin performed a wedge-shaped basal osteotomy of the proximal phalanx of the thumb with the base of the wedge toward the medial with the fixation of the fragments with Kirshner's needle [13] (**Figure 10**).

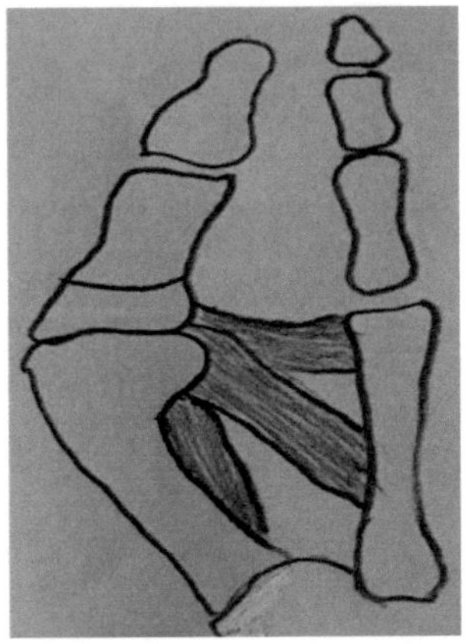

Figure 9.
Sketch of proximal phalanx resection arthroplasty (Keller).

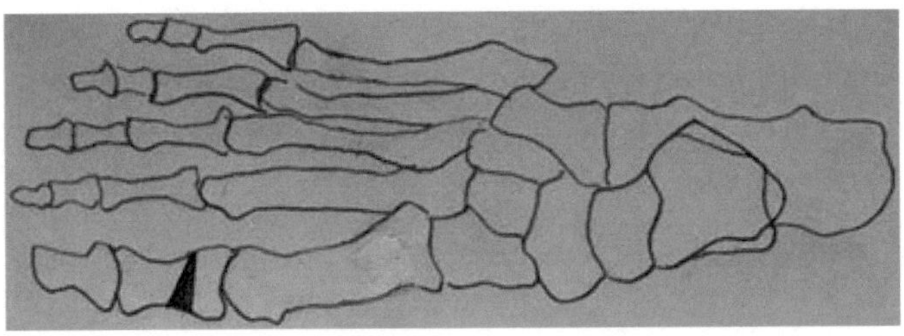

Figure 10.
Osteotomy of the proximal phalanx of the thumb according to Akin (sketch).

1.6.2.2.2 Distal osteotomy of the first metatarsal bone

There are a large number of distal metatarsal osteotomies. Indications for which they are used are initial and moderate hallux valgus deformity.

In 1881, Reverdin was the first to describe a distal, closed wedge-shaped osteotomy of the first MT bone (**Figure 11**).

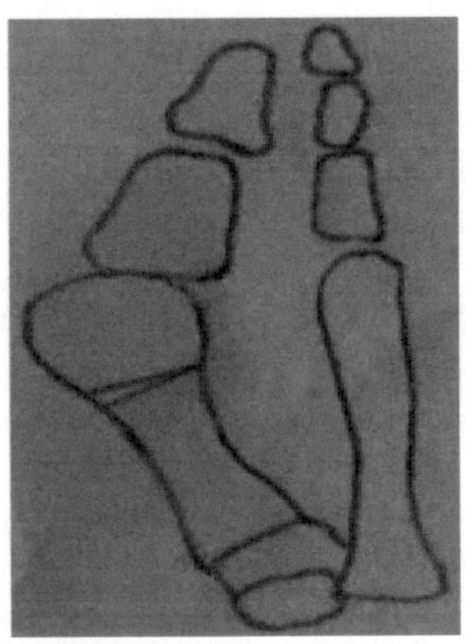

Figure 11.
Reverdin's distal osteotomy of the first MT bone (sketch).

As part of the surgical method according to Reverdin, a resection of the deformed part of the head of the first MT bone was performed, which will otherwise become a common practice in all future surgical methods in the treatment of hallux valgus [14].

In 1920, Roux described a closed distal osteotomy that has a trapezoidal shape at its base. Proximal osteotomy extends across the entire width of the MT bone, while distal osteotomy is incomplete. The formed tooth formed after these osteotomies gives stability to the osteotomized fragments (**Figure 12**) [15].

In 1931, Peabody corrected the hallux valgus by moving the closure osteotomy slightly more proximal than Reverdin did (**Figure 13**) [1].

Another modification of Reverdin's osteotomy is distal L osteotomy or Eeverdin-Green osteotomy (**Figure 14**) [16].

In 1923, Hohmann introduced a procedure that underpins trapezoidal osteotomy, but unlike the Roux procedure, the proximal and distal arms of Hohmann's osteotomy extend through the entire circumference of the MT bone (**Figure 15**) [17].

In 1974, Johnson and Smith introduced derotation, angulation, transposition osteotomy, or DRATO osteotomy (**Figure 16**) [18].

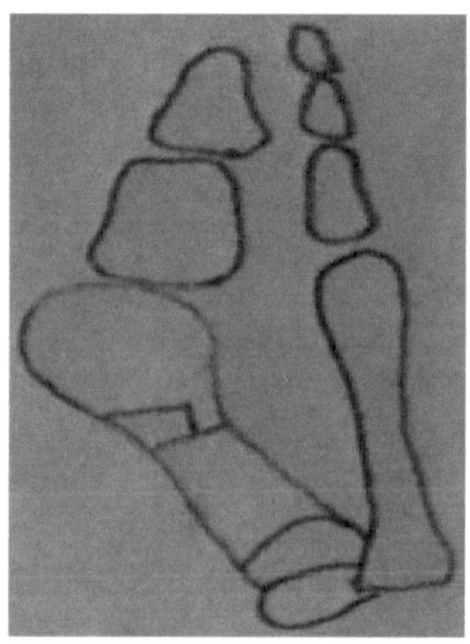

Figure 12.
Distal osteotomy of the first MT bone—Roux (sketch).

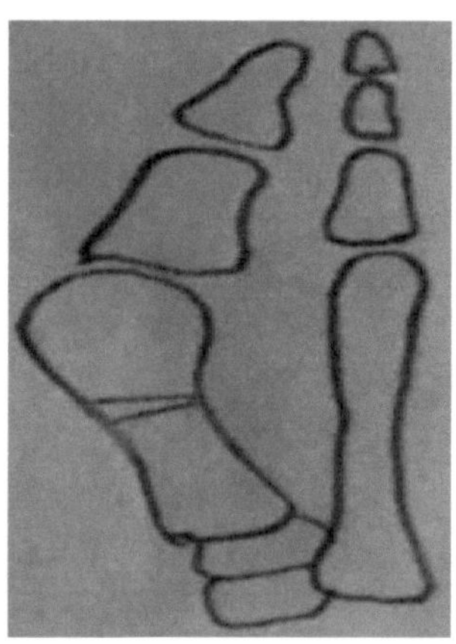

Figure 13.
Distal osteotomy of the first MT bone—Peabody (sketch).

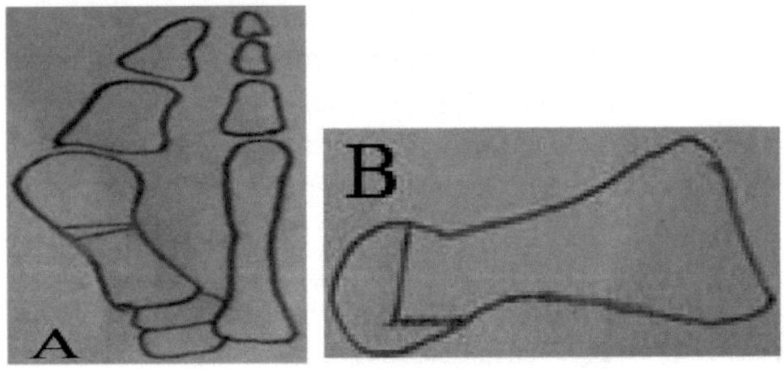

Figure 14.
(A and B) Sketch of the distal osteotomy of the first MT bone—Eeverdin-Green (A—sketch in the anteroposterior plane, B—sketch in the lateral plane).

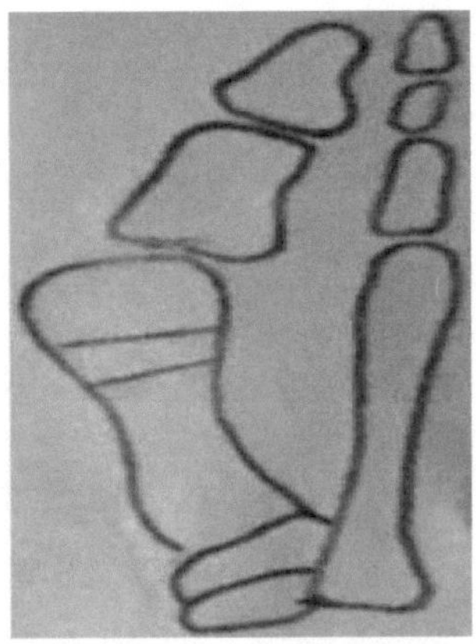

Figure 15.
Hohmann distal MT osteotomy (sketch).

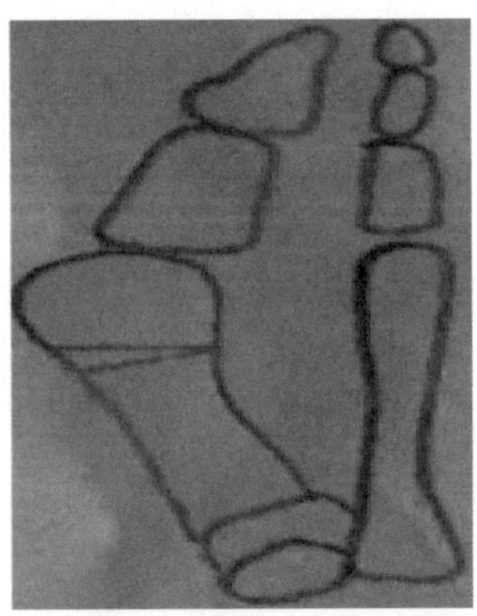

Figure 16.
DRATO osteotomy (sketch).

In 1958, Mitchell introduced his osteotomy [19], and in 1974, Miller made a modification of it. Miller performed the osteotomy in relation to the axis of the foot in contrast to Mitchell, who performed the osteotomy in relation to the axis of the first MT bone (**Figure 17**) [20].

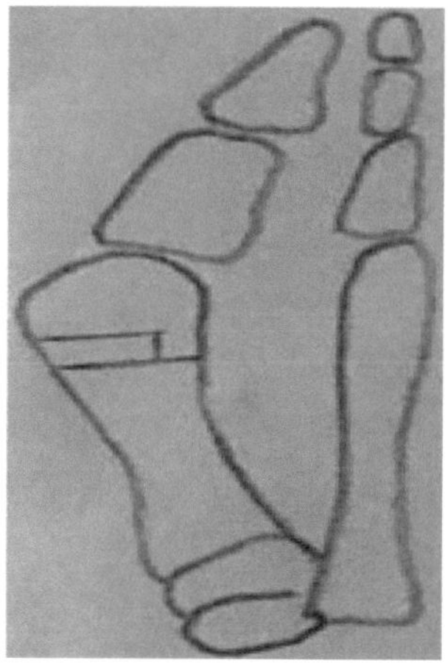

Figure 17.
Miller's distal MT osteotomy (sketch).

Lndbren and Turan described transverse osteotomy. The cutting line of the MT bone extended at an angle of 30° to the transverse line located at right angles to the line passing through the middle of the first MT bone (**Figure 18**) [21].

Austin introduced his ostetomy in 1981. The osteotomy has two horizontal sections at a cutting angle of 60° (**Figure 19**) [22].

Chervon ostcotomy is a V-shaped distal MT osteotomy with a cutting angle of 60°, whereby the arc of the angle is 10 mm from the articular surface of the head of the first MT bone. After a lateral displacement of the head of 5–7 mm and additional resection of the diaphysis of the first MT bone, the stability of the obtained position is ensured by a Kirschner needle or a resorptive screw (**Figure 20**) [23].

Johnson modified the Chervon osteotomy by lengthening its lower arm, which made it easier to place the stabilizing screw (**Figure 21**).

In valgus deformities with the congruent joint, Johnson also introduced an additional subcapital closure osteotomy with a wedge base medially of 2 mm in order to correct the distal metatarsal articular angle (DMAU) [8].

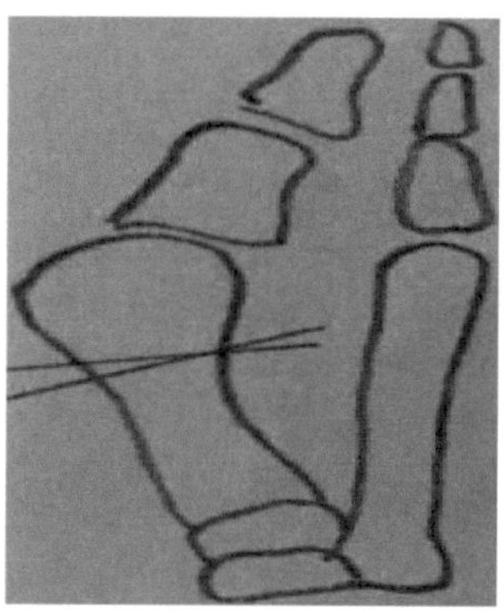

Figure 18.
Transverse distal MT osteotomy according to Lindbren and Turan (sketch).

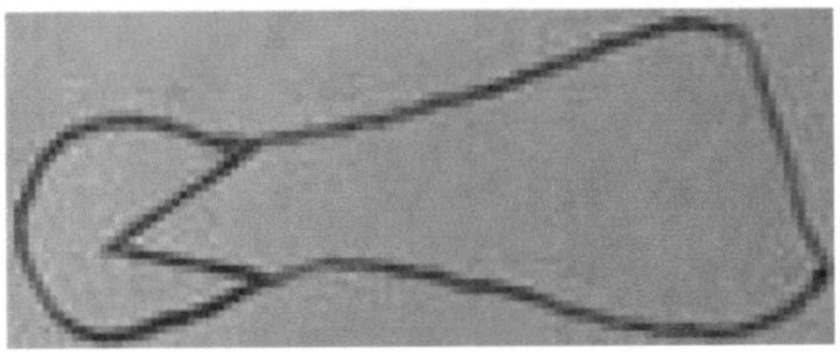

Figure 19.
Austin's distal MT osteotomy (sketch).

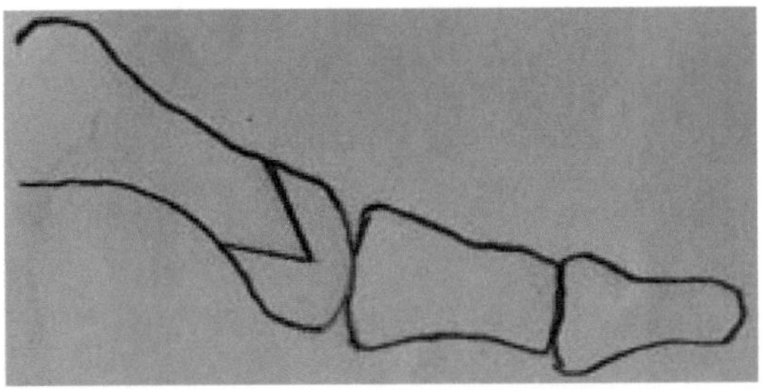

Figure 20.
Chervon distal MT osteotomy (sketch).

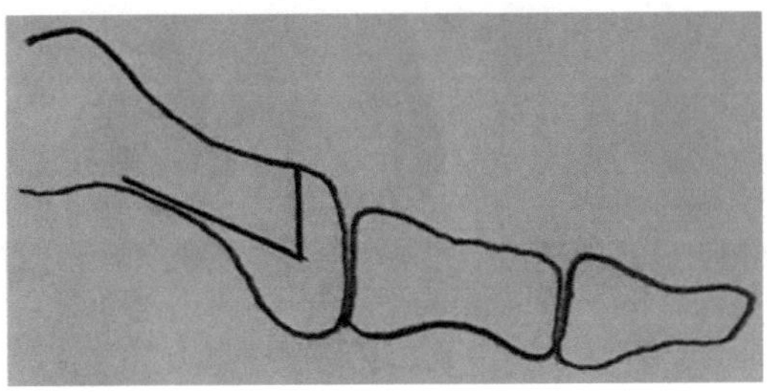

Figure 21.
Johnson modification of Chevron osteotomy (sketch).

1.6.2.2.3 Osteotomy of the body of the first metatarsal bone

Ludolph's osteotomy was described in 1918. It is an oblique osteotomy of the body of the first MT bone, where the stability of the osteotomized fragments is achieved with one screw and two Kirschner needles [24].

In 1963, Wilson introduced an oblique osteotomy in the distal part of the body of the first MT bone with a direction of extension from the distal-medial to the proximal-lateral side at an angle of 45 degrees, which, after dislocation of the fragments, corrects the varus position of the first MT bone (**Figure 22**) [25–32].

A scarf osteotomy is a Z-shaped osteotomy of the diaphysis of the first MT bone with a cutting line that runs downwards and laterally. It allows for further shortening or lengthening of the first MT bone by proximal-distal displacement of fragments. After osteotomy, the new position is secured by fixation with two screws (**Figure 23**) [11, 33].

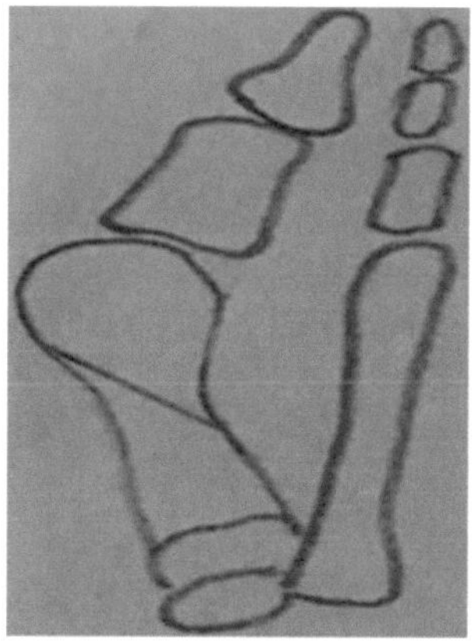

Figure 22.
Wilson's osteotomy of the body of the first MT bone (sketch).

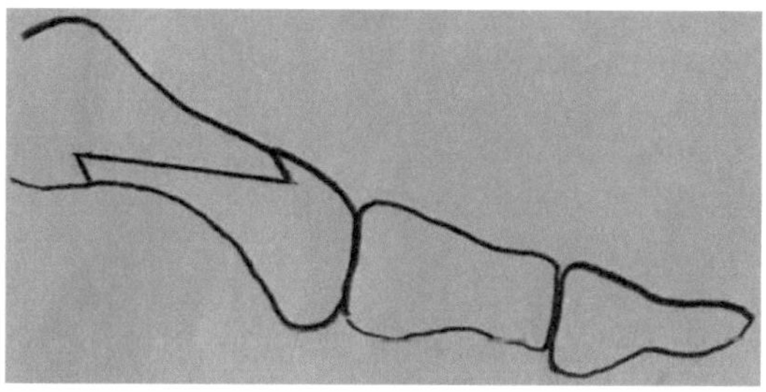

Figure 23.
Scarf osteotomy of the diaphysis of the first MT bone (sketch).

1.6.2.2.4 Proximal (basal) osteotomy of the first metatarsal bone

Basal osteotomy is used for moderate and major deformities, but only if the MTF joint is not arthrotic altered. They are operated at 10–15 mm distal to the MTF joint. A very small displacement of the first MT bone at its base after osteotomy achieves a significantly greater displacement in the distal part toward the lateral. There are several described techniques of proximal osteotomy. In all proximal osteotomies, medial resection of bone prominence should be performed with thumb adductor tenotomy and medial capsulorrhaphy. All proximal osteotomies require stabilization of the corrected position by applying Kirschner needles, screws, or specially designed plates [34–36].

In 1923, Trethowan described an open wedge-shaped osteotomy at 1 cm from the base of the first MT bone [37, 38]. In recent years, proximal chevron osteotomy [39–43] has been used in the correction of deformities.

Of the proximal osteotomies of the base of the first MT bones, in addition to open and closed wedge-shaped osteotomies, among which is Golden's osteotomy, which will be described in more detail under the subheading Material and Methods [44–52]. Osteotomies with opening lengthen and wedge-shaped osteotomies with closure lead to shortening of the first MT bone.

A semicircular proximal osteotomy of the base of the first MT bone with a convexity proximally allows for greater movement of the distal fragment than other osteotomies. After osteotomy and correction of deformities, the osteotomized fragments are fixed. Semicircular or semi-arcuate osteotomy does not result in a change in the length of the first MT bone (**Figure 24**) [53].

Arthrodesis of the MTC joint (Lapidus) is a surgical procedure that achieves correction of even the most severe deformities. After cutting the wedge with the base laterally and plantarly, stabilization, of the previously denuded surfaces of the MT and the cuneiform bone, is achieved with two screws (**Figure 25**) [54].

1.7 Distal metatarsal osteotomy according to Mitchell

The initial incision in the Mitchell method begins on the dorsomedial side of the foot, in the middle of the proximal phalanx, and is directed distally, passing through the exostosis and ending 3 cm proximal to the MTF joint on the medial side of the MT bone. Caution should be exercised to avoid the extremities of the medial part of the medial part of the peroneus superficialis. With a sharp dissection, an exostosis covered with a capsule and bursa is identified. It then begins with a Y-shaped capsule incision on the dorsomedial edge of the MT joint that points toward the medial line where the exostosis and the body of the MT bone meet. This incision arm is usually 10–15 mm long depending on the size of the exostosis and the length of the first MT bone. The plantar arm of the incision is of the same length and is directed from the plantar-medial part of the MT joint to the median line of the MT bone. The straight part of the incision is directed proximally and extends along the medial line from the junction of the head and diaphysis along the body of the MT bone in the length of 15–20 mm. Then, the resected wings of the capsule are lifted to get an insight into the MT joint.

Care should be taken not to damage or remove parts of the capsule, given the subsequent role of the capsule in stabilizing and correcting the valgus hallux.

1.7.1 Elimination of exostosis

A parasagittal depression and the junction of the exostosis with the body of the MT bone are identified, which are marked by the osteotome as an orientation point. Using the same osteotome, exostosis is removed starting from the dorsal wing of the parasagittal groove. Osteotomy is directed proximally, plantarly, and slightly medially toward a previously marked portion of bone.

Exposure of the body and neck of the MT bone and placement of orientation openings.

The periosteum is lifted dorsally and plantar to visualize the dorsal portion of the neck and the distal 2–3 cm of the body of the MT bone. The lateral part of the

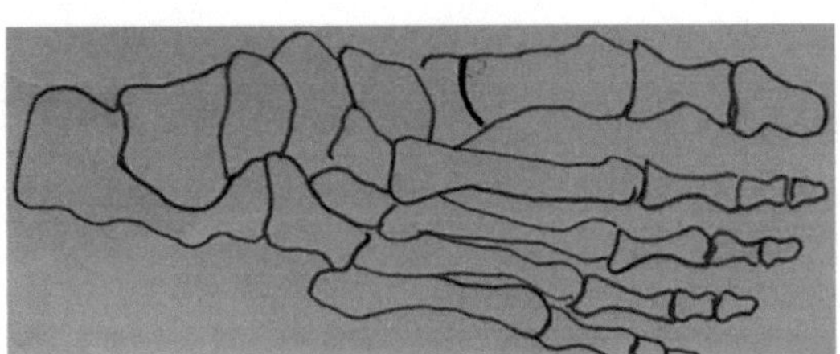

Figure 24.
Semi-arched proximal (basal) osteotomy—Mann (sketch).

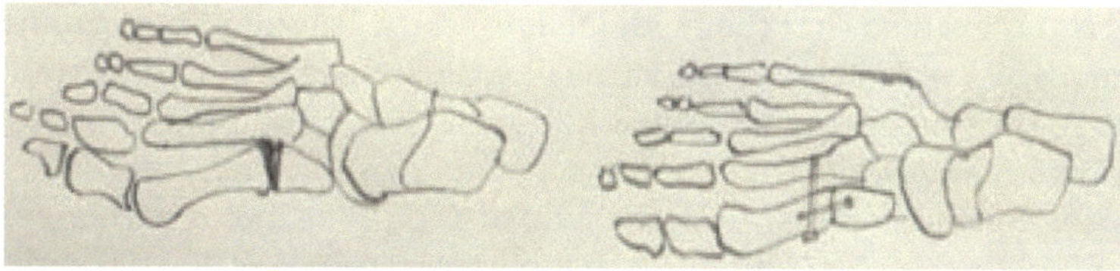

Figure 25.
Lapidus arthrodesis of the MTC joint (sketch).

capsule of the head and neck of the MT bone is not resected because it contributes to the blood supply to the head of the MT bone. With a small drill or Kirschner needle, two parallel canals are drawn through the body of the metatarsal bone, directed from dorsal to plantar, wide enough for the thread to pass 1–0. The first canal is formed on a longitudinal line representing the middle of the dorsal side of the first MT bone, approximately 1.5 cm proximal to the distal edge of the articular surface of the head of the MT bone and directed toward the medial cortex. The second canal is made 1 cm proximal to the first canal, but is directed toward the lateral cortex of the body of the MT bone. An absorbing, monofilament thread of 1–0 size is threaded through the canals so that it can be tied on the dorsal side. The first osteotomy is performed distally, parallel to the medial border of the neck of the MT bone, 3–4 mm proximal to the distal canal located 1.5 cm from the MTF joint. This osteotomy is not complete and should leave 3–6 mm of the lateral part of the body intact. The width of the lateral spike depends on the extent of correction required to relax the soft tissue structures of the MTF joint. In other words, it depends on the size of the deformity. If the IMA is 10°–12°, 3–4 mm of the width of the spike is sufficient, and if the IMTA is 13°–15°, 5–6 mm of the width of the spike is required. The second osteotomy is performed in the same direction, parallel to the first osteotomy starting medially, 3–4 mm proximal to the first incision. This osteotomy is complete and passes through the lateral cortex of the MT bone. The direction of delivery of the third osteotomy is which is done at an angle of 90° with respect to the previous two osteotomies is from the lateral end of the incomplete distal osteotomy to the proximal osteotomy. The resulting fragment 3–4 mm wide of bone is removed from the distal fragment (**Figure 26**).

Upon completion of the osteotomy and the formation of the lateral spike, the entire capital fragment is manually moved laterally until the bone spike rests against the lateral cortex of the proximal fragment. With this maneuver, the MT bone is shortened by 5–6 mm, the varus deformation of the MT bone is reduced, the articular structures are aligned, and the adductor hallucis muscle is relaxed. The capital fragment is plantarically flexed and the sutures are fixed. Before closing the capsule, the medial prominent part of the bone on the proximal side of the

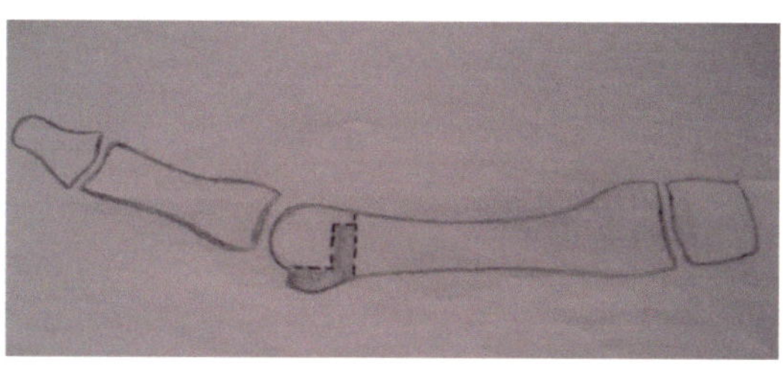

Figure 26.
Mitchell operative technique (sketch in the horizontal plan).

osteotomy is removed so that the medial edges of the fragments are in line. Medial capsulorrhaphy is performed in the varus position of the thumb of 5° and in plantar flexion. In the postoperative course, the patient is immobilized. Immobilization is placed to avoid angulation of fragments or their displacement in the dorsal direction. Standing up and walking with the help of armpit crutches without support on the operated foot is allowed on the first postoperative day. Partial support is allowed for 3 days and full support for 2 weeks after surgery. Immobilization is carried until the osteotomy heals, which is controlled by radiographic and clinical examination. Immobilization is removed 5 to 6 weeks after surgery and begins with physical rehabilitation [55]. Radiographic control of the operated foot after surgery is shown in **Figure 27**.

1.8 Proximal metatarsal osteotomy according to Golden

Proximal osteotomy according to Golden was performed according to the original technique with minimal modifications. The first longitudinal soft tissue surgical incision is made at the level of the MTF joint between the heads of the first and second MT bones and the tenotomy of the thumb is made. The second longitudinal soft tissue incision is made on the medial side at the level of the first MTF joint and continues proximal to the MTC joint, slightly moving to the dorsal side. The exostosis is removed from the head of the first MT bone, leaving the entire articular surface. Then, 10 mm distal to the MTC joint, a wedge osteotomy is made with the base outward and inferiorly. The first osteotomy is transverse and runs its entire length at 10 mm from the first MTC joint, and the second oblique shorter than the first osteotomy by 2–3 mm and with distal osteotomy forms an angle of 10° open laterally and proximally. The third osteotomy extends at right angles to the second and ends at the extreme lateral point of the first osteotomy, forming a wedge-shaped dentition on the lateral side of the base of the first MT bone, for the angle of correction of the hallux valgus (**Figure 28**).

The osteotomy site is then fixed with a Kirschner needle in the corrected position. It is placed below the medial incision through the skin into the bone, at the level of the distal part with the direction of extension from the medial side to proximal and lateral through osteotomized fragments to the cuneiform bone (**Figure 29**).

After the surgical treatment is completed, the feet are radiographically monitored (**Figure 30**).

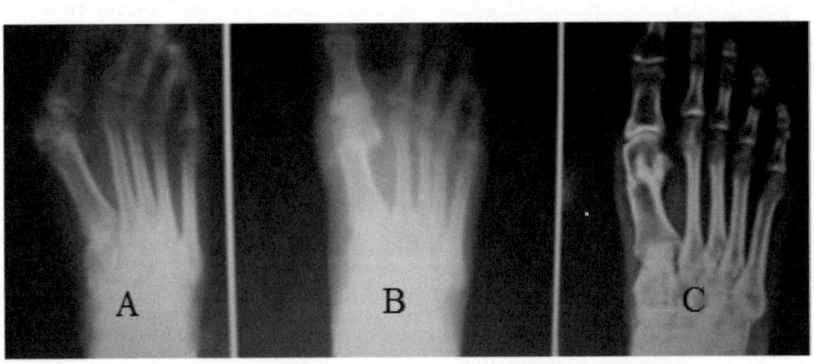

Figure 27.
Radiograph of hallux valgus before surgery (A), postoperative image of Mitchell's osteotomy (B), and image 2 years after surgery (C).

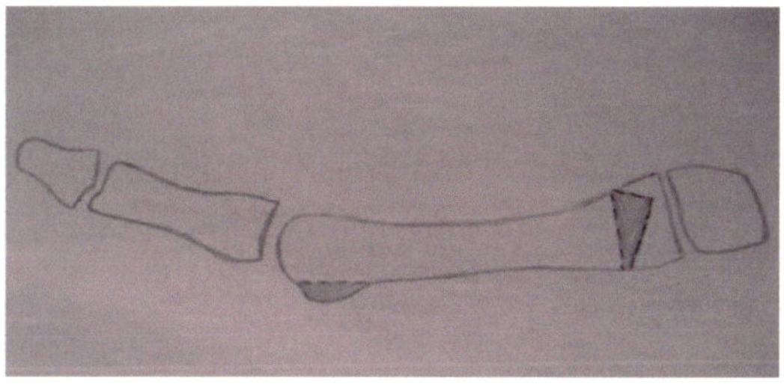

Figure 28.
Operative technique according to Golden (sketch in the horizontal plane).

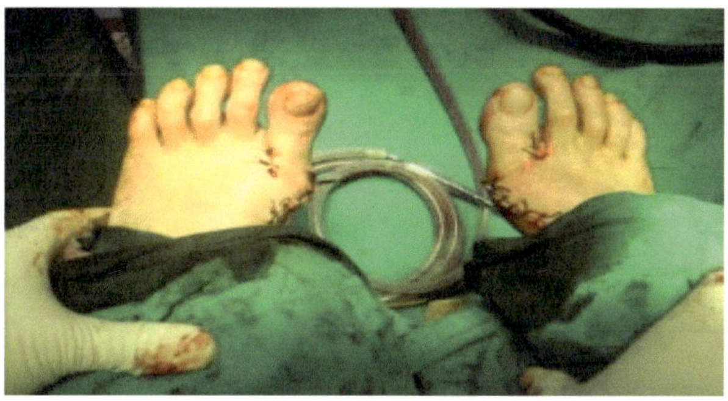

Figure 29.
Presentation of Golden's osteotomy after surgery performed on both feet in one act.

The results were also assessed according to the Hallux Metatarsophalangeal Interphalangeal Score (HMIS) [56] (Scale 1) and according to the criteria of the Bonney and Mc Nab classification modified according to Hellal [57]. Also, the analysis of the results was done on the basis of pre- and postoperative determination of HVA, IMTA, sesamoid position and length of the first MT bone, using radiographic dorsoplantar and profile images of the foot at support, and then based on the movement of the thumb in the MTF joint, the length of postoperative immobilization, the duration of treatment, and the existence of complications (infection, recurrence, and metatarsalgia).

On the radiographic image in the horizontal plane (radiographic image from the face), the position of the sesamoid is determined on the basis of the position of the medial sesamoid in relation to the longitudinal axis passing through the middle of the first MT bone and is represented by values from 0 to 3 (0—physiological position, the position of the medial sesamoid on the medial side of the longitudinal axis passing through the middle of the first MT bone, 1—less than 50% of the sesamoid bone is projected lateral to the longitudinal axis of the first MT bone, 2—more than 50% of the sesamoid bone is projected lateral to the longitudinal axis of the first MT bone, and 3—lateral luxation of the medial sesamoid is entirely lateral to the longitudinal axis of the first MT bone) (**Figure 31**) [58].

Higher values of the position of the medial sesamoid indicate a greater degree of deformity [59].

Dorsoplantar movement in the first MT joint before and after surgical treatment was determined by a goniometer.

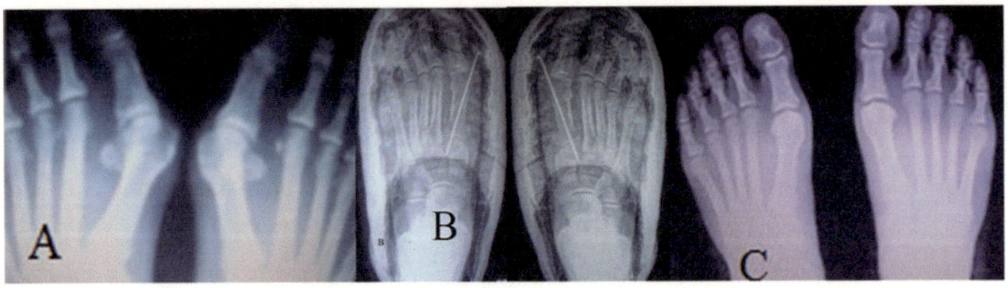

Figure 30.
Preoperative radiograph of hallux valgus (A), postoperative image of Golden osteotomy (B), image 2 years after surgery (C).

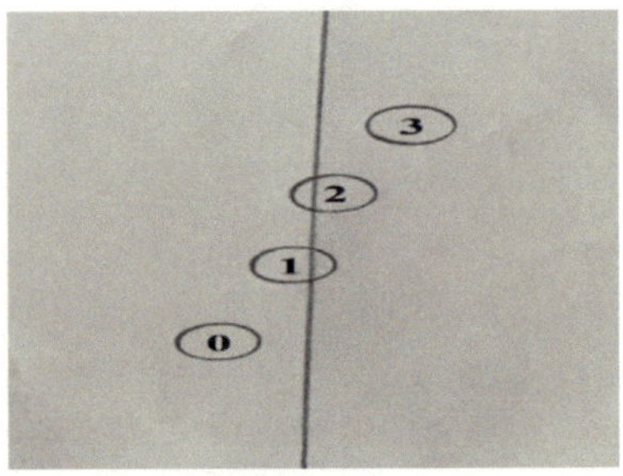

Figure 31.
Sesamoid position values.

2. Discussion

In the surgical treatment of hallux valgus with moderate deformity (HVU from 25 to 40 and IMTU from 13 to 20), distal and proximal osteotomies are used, allowing the correction of most components of the deformed foot [10]. Distal metatarsal osteotomy is very popular among orthopedic surgeons due to its simplicity, low invasiveness, and very low complication rates. Proximal metatarsal osteotomy can achieve significant correction of the deformity, but it is technically demanding to perform, and due to the presence of two surgical incisions, there is a higher risk of infection in operated patients [60]. Both distal and proximal osteotomies, which require the use of osteofixation materials such as screws, Kirschner wires, or miniplates, potentially increase the risk of infection. Reverdin was the first surgeon in 1881 to treat hallux valgus with distal MT osteotomy and medial resection of the exostosis [14]. Generally, proximal MT osteotomy is recommended for severe hallux valgus deformities (HVU greater than 40 and IMTU greater than 20). Distal metatarsal osteotomy is recommended for mild hallux valgus deformities (HVU less than 25 and IMTU less than 13) [10]. However, many researchers have reported the successful use of metatarsal osteotomies in the treatment of hallux valgus deformities outside of the recommended indications. Robinson, Sargas, and Adam reported successful and different techniques of proximal osteotomy for moderate-to-severe hallux valgus deformities [61–63]. Bai reported a series of effective distal MT osteotomies for 76 moderate-to-severe hallux valgus deformities, with a very low incidence of complications [37]. On the other hand, Saro analyzed 100 patients with moderate-to-severe hallux valgus who underwent various techniques of distal MT osteotomies and recommended the procedure only for patients with mild-to-moderate deformities [38]. Chucpaiwong states that only Deenik compared distal MT osteotomies for moderate-to-severe hallux valgus deformities in their study, but without reporting different outcomes in a randomized comparison of distal and proximal osteotomies in patients with hallux valgus [64]. According to Chucpaiwong, Deeniks conclusion regarding whether to perform distal or proximal MT osteotomy for moderate-to-severe hallux valgus deformities remains controversial due to the small sample size [60, 64]. Therefore, further research is needed to determine whether distal MT osteotomy is suitable for treating moderate-to-severe hallux valgus deformities [64].

There are a limited number of studies comparing distal with proximal MT osteotomies. Bostan and associates, in their study comparing distal and proximal osteotomies in combination with distal soft tissue procedures, concluded that, due to similar clinical results (measured by AOFAS) and similar radiological outcomes (HVA, IMTU, sesamoid position, and shortening of the first MT bone), the modified distal MT osteotomy according to Lindgren-Turan has an advantage over proximal MT osteotomy in combination with soft tissue procedures due to the use of a single incision, simpler surgical technique, and shorter operative time [65]. A prospective randomized controlled study conducted by Lee aimed to compare the outcomes of proximal and distal osteotomies with soft tissue procedures performed synchronously in one operation in patients with bilateral deformities, and found that distal Chevron osteotomy with distal soft tissue procedure is reliable for correcting moderate-to-severe hallux valgus, just as proximal Chevron osteotomy with distal soft tissue procedure is [66]. This study showed that indications for distal MT osteotomy could be extended to include moderate-to-severe deformities [67]. Although they emerged three years apart, Mitchell's method (1958) and Golden's method (1961) have not gained the same popularity in the treatment of hallux valgus, with Mitchell's method being more widely adopted [56, 67, 68]. Mitchell osteotomy is used for mild-to-moderate deformities, and the percentage of satisfactory results with this method ranges from 85% to 97% [58, 69]. Golden's osteotomy, like other osteotomies of the first MT base, combined with soft tissue procedures at the first MTP joint, achieves good to excellent results [34, 47]. There is no literature comparing these two methods directly. One limitation of this study could be that multiple surgeons performed the procedures and that two different procedures at different locations on the first MT bone were compared.

Nonoperative treatment for moderate-to-severe hallux valgus is generally insufficient, and treatment outcomes are better if the patient undergoes surgery early in the disease course, before arthritic changes occur in the first metatarsophalangeal joint. Prior to surgery, the overall status of patients in the Mitchell group, classified according to Bonney and McNab modified by Hellal, was rated as poor for all feet. Postoperatively, in the Mitchell group, the overall status improved in 78 (96%) feet ($p<0.001$). According to HMIS, improvement was observed in 79 (97.5%) feet ($p<0.001$). The improvement achieved represents a combination of excellent and good results, which correlates with the results reported by other authors [70, 71]. In the Golden group, the overall status before surgery, classified according to Bonney and McNab modified by Hellal, was poor for all feet. In that group, the overall status improved in 71 (92.2%) feet ($p<0.001$), and according to HMIS, it improved in 79 (97.4%) feet ($p<0.001$). Golden reported successful results in 78% of patients [56]. In patients treated with Mitchell's method, the average correction of HVU was 21.85±2.15° and IMTU was 7.83±1.07°, which matches the results of most authors, who report HVU correction of 10–25° and IMTU correction of 5° to 10° [69, 72–74]. In patients treated with Golden's method, the average correction of HVU and IMTU was 19.66±3.31° and 6.86±1.69°, respectively, which is 2.19° and 0.9° less than Mitchell's method. The obtained values are similar to the results reported by other authors [75, 76].

Malik and Methison emphasize that in assessing hallux valgus deformity, in addition to radiographic images and IMTU, the position of the sesamoids plays a very important role [77]. The position of the sesamoids in patients treated with Mitchell's method changed from position 2 to position 0, while in the Golden group it changed from position 2 to position 1. Some authors emphasize the very important role of shortening the first MT bone in deformity correction [78]. The shortening of the first MT bone in Mitchell's procedure was 4.87±7.20 mm, while in Golden's procedure it was 2.97±7.70 mm. According to some authors, excessive shortening of the first MT bone can be one of the most important factors in the development of metatarsalgia [79]. Merkel suggests that shortening of the bone by more than 10 mm can cause metatarsalgia [74]. Baba points out metatarsalgia in patients with shortening greater than 8 mm and persistent pain in patients with shortening greater than 10 mm [71]. Some authors disagree with the concept that metatarsalgia is linked to shortening the first MT bone [53, 78]. In this study, it was found that preoperative metatarsalgia was present in 51% of feet in the Mitchell group and in 53% of feet in the Golden group. Other authors report preoperative metatarsalgia in 33% to 40% of patients [7, 80]. Postoperatively, metatarsalgia was present in 13 feet (16%) in the Mitchell group and in 18 feet (23%) in the Golden group. Some authors report postoperative metatarsalgia in 27% of cases [81]. This study did not find a correlation between shortening of the first MT bone and the development of metatarsalgia. In patients treated with Mitchell's method, recurrence occurred in one foot, and superficial infection in two feet. Recurrence in patients treated with Golden's method occurred in three feet, and superficial infection in five feet. The use of sutures to maintain position after Mitchell's distal metatarsal osteotomy eliminates the need for a second intervention (removal of foreign body) and thus reduces the risk of infection. In Golden's method, the Kirschner wire used to stabilize the osteotomy is removed after 5 weeks, which prolongs the treatment, requires an additional intervention, and increases the risk of infection. The risk of infection is lower with Mitchell's method due to the use of a single incision for deformity correction (Golden's method uses two surgical incisions). No other complications such as nonunion of the osteotomy site, pseudoarthrosis, avascular necrosis of the first MT head, or thrombophlebitis were noted [82–85].

Pain resulting from the deformity that impedes usual life activities is the primary reason patients opt for surgical treatment. In 90% of patients treated with Mitchell's method, pain disappeared. These results are comparable to those of other authors who reported complete pain relief in 80–95% of operated patients [55, 86, 87]. In patients treated with Golden's method, pain disappeared in 78% of patients, which correlates with the results reported by Golden in his study [67].

3. Conclusion

The study showed that both Mitchell's and Golden's osteotomies achieve good clinical and radiographic results in the treatment of bunions of moderate degree of deformity.

Acknowledgements

We are grateful to "Nobel" for their generous support in making this publication possible. Their commitment to advancing scientific research has helped us share our work with the community, and we truly appreciate their encouragement and backing.

Author details

Nadan Mikić*, Ivan Marjanović, Aleksandar Stanković, Dragiša Stamenković, Vesna Ranković and Vladimir Gordić
KBC Zvezdara, Belgrade, Serbia

*Address all correspondence to: nadanmikic@gmali.com

References

[1] Nix S, Smith M, Vicenzino B. Prevalence of hallux valgus in the general population: A systematic review and meta-analysis. Journal of Foot and Ankle Research. 2010;**27**(3):21

[2] Vukašinović Z, Baščarević Z, Bumbaširević M, Butković I, Lešić A, Popović Z et al. Specijalna ortopedija. 2004;**132**:390-400

[3] Denis A. Physioparthology. Approche physiopathologique des anomalies morhphologiques de Lavant-pied. Revue de Chirurgie Orthopédique et Traumatologique. 1974;**60**(Suppl. II):117-130

[4] Krajčinović J. Hirurgija stopala i skočnog zgloba. Faculty of Medicine Novi Sad; 1995

[5] Shima H, Okuda R, Yasuda T, Jotoku T, Kitano N, Konoshita M. Radiographic measurements in patients with hallux valgus before anf after proximal cresentic osteotomy. The Journal of Bone and Joint Surgery. American Volume. 2009;**91**:1369-1376

[6] D'Arcangelo PR, Landorf KB, Munteanu SE, Zammit GV, Menz HB. Radiographic correlates of hallux valgus severity in older people. Foot & Ankle. 2010;**3**:20

[7] Robinson AH, Limbers JP. Modern concepts in the treatment of hallux valgus. Journal of Bone & Joint Surgery. 2005;**87**(8):1038-1045

[8] Butković I. Povrede i oboljenja stopala i skočnog zgloba. Naučna KMD. 2009:41-49

[9] Volkman R. Ueber die sogenannte Exostose der grossen Zehe. Archiv für pathologische Anatomie und Physiologie und für klinische Medicin. 1856;**10**:297-306

[10] Richardson EG. Disorders of the hallux valgus. Campbell's Operative Orthopaedics. 2012;**4**:3805-3891

[11] Schwartz N, Groves ER. Long-term follow-up of internal threaded Kirschner-wire fixation of the scarf bunionectomy. The Journal of Foot Surgery. 1987;**26**:313-316

[12] Henry AP, Waugth J, Wood H. The use of foot prints in assessing the results of operations for hallux valgus. A comparasion of Keller's operation and arthrodesis. The Journal of Bone & Joint Surgery British Volume. 1975;**57**:478-481

[13] Boberg JS, Menn JJ, Brown WL. The distal akin osteotomy: A new approach. Journal of Foot Surgery. 1991;**30**:131-136

[14] Reverdin J. Anatomie et operation de hallux valgus. Int Med Congr. 1881;**2**:508-512

[15] Roux C. Aux pieds sensible. Revue Médicale de la Suisse Romande. 1920;**40**:62

[16] Zyzda MJ, Hineser W. Distal L osteotomy in treatment of hallux abducto valgus. The Journal of Foot Surgery. 1989;**28**:445

[17] Hohmann G. Uber hallux und spreizfuss ihre eatstehung und physidegische behandlung. Archiv fur Orthopadische und Unfall-Chirurgie. 1923;**21**:525

[18] Johnson JB, Smith SB. Preliminary report on derotational angulational transpositional osteotomy: A new

approach to hallux valgus abducto valgus surgery. Journal of the American Podiatry Association. 1974;**64**:667

[19] Mitchell CL, Fleming JL, Allen R, Glenney C, Sanford GA. Osteotomy-bunionectomy for hallux valgus. The Journal of Bone and Joint Surgery. American Volume. 1958;**40**(1):41-60

[20] Miller JW. Distal first metatarsal displacement osteotomy. Journal of Bone and Joint Surgery. 1974;**56A**:923

[21] Lindgren U, Turan I. A new operation for hallux valgus. Clinical Orthopaedics and Related Research. 1983;**175**:179

[22] Austin DW, Leventon EO. A new osteotomy for hallux valgus: A horizontally directed "V" displacement osteotomy of the metatarsal head for hallux valgus and primus varus. Clinical Orthopaedics and Related Research. 1981;**157**:25

[23] Lambers LFO, Verburg H, Reininga IH. Chevron versus Mitchell osteotomy in hallux valgus surgery: A comparative study. Journal of Foot & Ankle Surgery. 2015;**54**(3):361-364

[24] Saxena A, McCammon D. The Ludloff osteotomy: A critical analysis. The Journal of Foot and Ankle Surgery. 1997;**36**:100-105

[25] Wilson JN. Oblique displacement osteotomy for hallux valgus. Journal of Bone and Joint Surgery. 1963;**45**:552

[26] Dooley BJ, Berryman DB. Wilson's osteotomy of the first metatarsal for hallux valgus in the adolescent and the young adult. ANZ Journal of Surgery. 1973;**43**:255

[27] Helal B, Gupta SK, Gojaseni P. Surgery for adolescent hallux valgus. Acta Orthopaedica Scandinavica. 1974;**45**:271

[28] Davis M, Litman T. Simple osteotomy for hallux valgus. Minnesota Medicine. 1976;**12**:836

[29] Allen TR, Gross M, Miller J, Lowe LW, Hulton WC. The assessment of adolescent hallux valgus before and after first metatarsal osteotomy. International Orthopaedics. 1981;**5**:111

[30] Pittman SR, Burns DE. The Wilson bunion procedure modified for improved clinical results. The Journal of Foot Surgery. 1984;**23**:314

[31] Farguharson-Roberts MA, Osborne AH. The Telfer osteotomy for hallux valgus. Journal of the Royal Naval Medical Service. 1985;**71**:15

[32] Klareskov B, Dalsgaard S, Gebuhr P. Wilson shaft osteotomy for hallux valgus. Acta Orthopaedica Scandinavica. 1988;**59**:307

[33] Suresh SS. Scarf osteotomy – Is it the procedure of choice in hallux valgus surgery. A preliminary report. Oman Medical Journal. 2007;**22**(3):47-50

[34] Thordarson DB, Leventen EO. Hallux valgus correction with proximal metatarsal osteotomy: Two-year follow-up. Foot & Ankle. 1992;**13**:321-326

[35] Morris J, Ryan M. First Metatarsal Base osteotomies for hallux valgus Abducto valgus deformities. Clinics in Podiatric Medicine & Surgery. 2014;**31**:247-263

[36] Mittag F, Leichtle U, Meisner C, Ipach I, Wulker N, Wunschel M. Proximal metatarsal osteotomy for hallux valgus: An audit of radiologic outocome after single screw fixation and full posoperative weightbearing. Journal of Foot and Ankle Research. 2013;**6**:22

[37] Bai LB, Lee KB, Seo CY, Song EK, Yoon TR. Distal chevron osteotomy with distal soft tissue procedure for moderate to severe hallux valgus deformity. Foot & Ankle International. 2010;**31**(8):683-688

[38] Saro C, Andrén B, Wildemyr Z, Felländer-Tsai L. Outcome after distal metatarsal osteotomy for hallux valgus: A prospective randomized controlled trial of two methods. Foot & Ankle International. 2007;**28**(7):778-787

[39] Johnswon K, Cofield B, Morrey B. Chervon osteotomy for hallux valgus. Clinical Orthopaedics. 1979;**142**:44-47

[40] Park CH, Ahn JY, Kim YM, Lee WC. Plate fixation for proximal chevron osteotomy has greater risk for hallux valgus recurrence than Kirschner wire fixation. International Orthopaedics. 2013;**37**:1085-1092

[41] Choi WJ, Yoon HK, Yoon HS, Kim BS, Lee JW. Comparison of the proximal chevron and Ludloff osteotomies for the correction of hallux valgus. Foot & Ankle International. 2009;**30**:1154-1160

[42] Lee KB, Cho NY, Park HW, Seon JK, Lee SH. A comparasion of proximal and distal Chervon osteotomy, both with lateral soft- tissue release, for moderate to servere hallux valgus in patiens undergoing simultaneos bilateral correction: A prospective randomised controlled trial. The Bone & Joint Journal. 2015;**97**(2):202-207

[43] Easley ME, Kiebzak GM, Davis WH, Anderson RB. Prospective, randomized comparison of proximal crescentic and proximal chevron osteotomies for correction of hallux valgus deformity. Foot & Ankle International. 1996;**17**:307-316

[44] Cooper MT, Berlet GC, Shurnas PS, Lee TH. Proximal opening-wedge osteotomy of the first metatarsal for correction of hallux valgus. Surgical Technology International. 2007;**16**:215-221

[45] Shurnas PS, Watson TS, Crislip TW. Proximal first metatarsal opening wedge osteotomy with a low profile plate. Foot & Ankle International. 2009;**30**:865-872

[46] Saragas NP. Proximal opening-wedge osteotomy of the first metatarsal for hallux valgus using a low profile plate. Foot & Ankle International. 2009;**30**:976-980

[47] Randhawa S, Pepper D. Radiographic evaluation of hallux valgus treated with opening wedge osteotomy. Foot & Ankle International. 2009;**30**:427-431

[48] Watson TS, Shurnas PS. The proximal opening wedge osteotomy for the correction of hallux valgus deformity. Techniques in Foot & Ankle Surgery. 2012;**11**:168-174

[49] Badekas A, Geogiannos D, Lampiridis V, Bisbinas I. Proximal opening wedge metatarsal osteotomy for correction of moderate to severe hallux valgus deformity using a lolocking plate. International Orthopaedics. 2013;**37**(9):1765-1770

[50] Han SH, Park EH, Jo J, Koh YG, Lee JW, Choi WJ, et al. First metatarsal proximal opening wedge osteotomy for correction of hallux valgus deformity: Comparison of straight versus oblique osteotomy. Yonsei Medical Journal. 2015;**56**(3):744-752

[51] Campbell JT, Schon LC, Parks BG, Wang Y, Berger BI. Mechanical comparison of biplanar proximal closing wedge osteotomy with plantar plate fixation versus crescentic osteotomy with screw fixation for the correction of

metatarsus primus varus. Foot & Ankle International. 1998;**19**:293-299

[52] Neese DJ, Zelichowski JE, Patton GW. Mau osteotomy: An alternative procedure to the closing abductory base wedge osteotomy. The Journal of Foot Surgery. 1989;**28**:352-362

[53] Mann RA, Rudicel S, Graves SC. Repair of hallux valgus with a distal soft –tissue procedure and proximal metatarsal osteotomy. A long- term follow-up. Journal of Bone and Joint Surgery. 1992;**74**(1):124-129

[54] Coetzee JC, Resig SG, Kuskowski M, Saleh KJ. The Lapidus procedure as salvage after failed surgical treatment of hallux valgus. Surgical technique. The Journal of Bone and Joint Surgery. American Volume. 2004;**86**:30-36

[55] Dermon H, Petrou K, Tilkeridis T, et al. Long-term results with Mitchell's Osteotomy applied for hallux valgus. The Journal of Bone & Joint Surgery. 2003;**85**:85-227

[56] Golden GN. Hallux valgus: The osteotomy operation. British Medical Journal. 5 May 1961;**1**(5236):1361-1365

[57] Kitaoka HB, Alexander IJ, Adellaar RS, Nunley JA, Myerson MS, Sanders M. Clinical rating system for ankle-hidfoot, hallux, and lasser toes. Foot & Ankle. 1994;**15**:349-353

[58] Helal B. Surgery for adolescent hallux valgus. Clinical Orthopaedics and Related Research. 1981;**157**:50-63

[59] Zettl R, Trnka HJ, Easley M, Salzer M, Ritschl P. Moderate to severe hallux valgus deformity: Correction with proximal crescentic osteotomy and distal soft-tissue release. Archives of Orthopaedic and Trauma Surgery. 2000;**120**(7-8):397-402

[60] Chuckpaiwong B. Comparing proximal and distal metatarsal osteotomy for moderate to severe hallux valgus. International Orthopaedics. 2012;**36**(11):2275-2278

[61] Robinson AH, Bhatia M, Eaton C, Bishop L. Prospective comparative study of the scarf and Ludloff osteotomies in the treatment of hallux valgus. Foot & Ankle International. 2009;**31**(10):955-963

[62] Saragas NP. Proximal opening-wedge osteotomy of the first metatarsal for hallux valgus using a low profile plate. Foot & Ankle International. 2009;**30**(10):967-980

[63] Adam SP, Choung SC, Gu Y, O'Malley MJ. Outcomes after scarf osteotomy for treatment of adult hallux valgus deformity. Clinical Orthopaedics and Related Research. 2011;**469**(3):854-859

[64] Deenik A, Mameren H, Visser E, Waal Malefijt M, Draijer F, Bie R. Equivalent correction in scarf and chevron osteotomy in moderate and severe hallux valgus: A randomized. Controlled trial. Foot & Ankle International. 2008;**29**(12):1209-1215

[65] Bostan B, Gunes T, Erden N, Asci M, Sen C, Erdogan H. Comparasion of modified Lindgren-Turan operation and proximal crescentic osteotomy combined with distal soft tissue procedure in the treatment of hallux valgus. Joint Diseases and Related Surgery. 2008;**19**(2):61-65

[66] Lee GW, Kim M, Lee KB. Comparison between proximal Chevron and distal Chevron osteotomy in moderate to severe hallux valgus patiens undergoing simultaneous bilateral correction. Foot and Ankle Surgery. 2017;**23**:8

[67] Mitchell CL, Fleming JL, Allen R, Glenning C, Sanford GA.

Osteotomy-bunionectomy for hallux valgus. Journal of Bone and Joint Surgery. 1954;**40**:41

[68] Baba AN, Bhat JA, Paljor S, Mir NA, Majid S. Mitchell's osteotomy in the management of hallux valgus: An Indian perspective. Indian Journal of Orthopaedics. 2009;**43**(1):76-81

[69] Blum JL. The modified Mitchell osteotomy-bunionectomy: Indications and technical considerations. Foot & Ankle International. 1994;**15**(3):103-106

[70] Glynn MK, Dunlop JB, Fitzpatrick D. The Mitchell distal metatarsal osteotomy for hallux valgus. The Journal of Bone & Joint Surgery British Volume. 1980;**62**(2):188-191

[71] Tan MY, Seow KH, Tay BK. The Mitchell distal metatarsal osteotomy for hallux valgus—The Singapore General Hospital experience. Singapore Medical Journal. 1998;**39**(12):547-550

[72] Briggs TW, Smith P, McAuliffe TB. Mitchell's osteotomy using internal fixation and early mobilisation. The Journal of Bone & Joint Surgery British Volume. 1992;**74**(1):137-139

[73] Wu KK. Modified Mitchell's bunionectomy (Wu's bunionectomy). Orthopedics. 1997;**20**(3):253-257

[74] Merkel KD, Katoh Y, Johnson EW, Chao EY. Mitchell osteotomy for hallux valgus: Long-term follow-up and gait analysis. Foot & Ankle. 1983;**3**(4):189-196

[75] Galaviz IVE, Marquez IXA, Penagos PJA, Young ZW. Osteoplastia de Golden modificada para la corrección de hallux valgus y metatarso primo varo. Revista Mexicana de ortopedia y Traumatología. 1999;**13**(3):219-222

[76] Matsubara N. Surgical resultats of the modified Golden method for hallux valgus. The Central Japan Yournal of Orthopaedic Surgery & Traumatology. 1999;**3**(42):611-612

[77] Malik J, Mathieson I. Clinical usage and influence of radiographs in the assessment of hallux valgus. The Journal of Foot and Ankle Surgery. 2013;**52**(3):291-294

[78] Christensen PH, Hansen TB. Hallux valgus correction using a modified Hohmann technique. Foot & Ankle International. 1995;**16**(4):177-180

[79] Broughton NS, Winson IG. Keller's arthroplasty and Mitchell osteotomy: A comparison with first metatarsal osteotomy of the long-term results for hallux valgus deformity in the younger female. Foot & Ankle. 1990;**10**(4):201-205

[80] Sarrafin SK. Method of predicting the degree of functional correction of the metatarsus primus varus with a lateral displacement osteotomy in hallux valgus. Foot & Ankle. 1985;**5**(6):322-326

[81] Lucijanić I, Bičanić G, Sonicki Z, Mirković M, Pecina M. Treatmant of hallux valgus with three-dimensional modification of Mitchell's osteotomy: Technique and results. Journal of the American Podiatric Medical Association. 2009;**99**(2):167-172

[82] Sanmarco GJ, Idusuyi OB. Complications after syrgery of the hallux. Clinical Orthopaedics and Related Research. 2001;**391**:59-71

[83] Belczuk R, Stapelton JJ, Grossman JP, Zgonis T. Comlications and revisional hallux valgus surgery. Clinics in Podiatric Medicine and Surgery. 2009;**26**(3):457-484

[84] Leutloff D, Mockel G, Perka C. Pseudoarthrosis after distal metatarsal osteotomy in hallux valgus surgery. Foot & Ankle. 2002;**8**(2):137-140

[85] Radl R, Kastner N, Aigner C, Portugaller H, Schreyer H, Windhager R. Venous thrombosis after hallux valgus surgery. Journal of Bone and Joint Surgery. 2003;**85**:1204-1208

[86] Desjardins AL, Hajj C, Racine L, Fallaha M, Bornais S. Mitchell's osteotomy in the treatment of hallux valgus. Annales de Chirurgie. 1993;**47**(9):894-899

[87] Oye C, Finsen VR. Mitchell's osteotomy of hallux valgus. Tidsskrift for den Norske Lægeforening. 1998;**118**(24):3765-3767

Section 3

Osteotomies of the Facial Bones

Chapter 10

Technological Advances in Maxillofacial Surgery: Function and Esthetics

Ji Youn Maeng and Jin Young Choi

Abstract

What defines a "naturally" esthetic face? Can natural beauty be comprehensively understood through scientific analysis? What systematic efforts can be made to ultimately achieve natural beauty? In previous years, the management of facial asymmetry to satisfy both function and esthetics has posed a paramount challenge to many maxillofacial surgeons. With the collateral developments of imaging technologies, virtual surgical technologies, and CAD/CAM technologies, unprecedented accuracy and precision have been achieved in osteotomies. With advances in maxillofacial osteotomies that have already been made, it is more important to establish different standards for application and to continuously scrutinize potential errors in current technologies.

Keywords: facial asymmetry, 3D virtual surgery, CAD/CAM technology, orthognathic surgery, contouring surgery

1. Introduction

It is of human nature to pursue attractiveness; an attractive face is a mixture of facial harmony and symmetry. Symmetry and harmony have some subjective components, and minor deviations from the norm are not always subject to change. Disharmony or asymmetry to a certain degree is accepted as normal, and cultural standards on beauty vary as well [1].

Apart from postoperative complications, the determination of surgical success relies heavily on the patient's satisfaction with his or her morphological correction. Because facial asymmetry (FA) and surgical changes from the frontal view are relatively more conspicuous than those from the lateral view, patients naturally care more about maxillofacial disproportions and asymmetry from the frontal view; improvements from the frontal view are of primary importance to patients in subjectively evaluating an esthetic aspect of the operation.

Compared to the past, patients are more demanding in perfecting symmetry or removing deformities of facial contour, and therefore so have technological advances and surgical efforts to achieve esthetically pleasing face. Treatment plans must, therefore, satisfy functional as well as esthetic demands of patients. Maxillofacial osteotomies to restore skeletal esthetics and function can be divided depending on purpose: transverse correction and vertical correction. Transverse or horizontal correction focuses on establishing symmetry of the right and left sides. Protrusion of the zygoma and frontal ramal inclination (FRI) of the mandible are important factors that determine the symmetry of the facial contour. Vertical correction makes changes to the lower thirds of the face to establish harmony among the vertical thirds of the face. Vertical correction concerns not only the comparative proportion of the mandible but also the different vertical ramal heights of the right and left mandible.

Facial asymmetry (FA) is a difference between the right and left sides. Because there are multiple aspects of FA (i.e., transverse, vertical, positional asymmetry) and different factors (i.e., soft tissue, hard tissue—zygoma, maxilla, mandible) involved, knowing what is and what is not subject to surgical correction is important. In other words, disciplined diagnosis and understanding the limitations of surgical correction are critical in establishing an appropriate treatment strategy. For example, unilateral craniosynostosis can result in horizontal asymmetry of the mandible. However, horizontal asymmetry of the mandible due to mediolaterally different positions of the right and left mandibular fossa cannot be fundamentally fixed. FA due to such difference must be compensated through contour surgery instead. In most FA cases, a similar flow of treatment strategy can be followed.

Analysis of facial asymmetry of the maxillomandibular complex should precede the asymmetry of the zygoma. Analysis of the complex can be done in a top-to-bottom manner. Maxillary dental canting and midline deviation must first be looked at. Slight deviation or asymmetry of less than 2 mm can be ignored because such insignificant differences are often inconspicuous to laypersons [2, 3]. Orthognathic surgery (OGS) should be chosen for FA involving significant positional asymmetry of the maxilla. For FA cases with insignificant maxilla asymmetry, differences in frontal ramal inclination (FRI) of the mandible should be analyzed. FRI can only be corrected through an intentional change of FRI with mandible osteotomy. For FA cases that have none of the above, simple contouring surgery can be chosen as a treatment strategy (**Figure 1**).

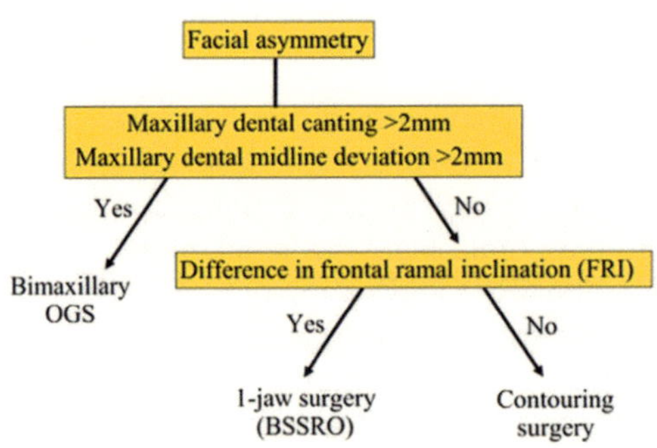

Figure 1.
Flow diagram of surgical strategy according to facial asymmetry of maxillomandibular complex.

2. Orthognathic surgery (OGS) for facial asymmetry (FA)

2.1 Adjuvant technological advances

2.1.1 Imaging and virtual surgical planning

A reproducible and objective method of measurement is necessary for accurate treatment planning. In previous years, two-dimensional radiographs were utilized for the measurement of ramal heights. Although skeletal landmarks such as gonion (Go) and highest point of condyle head (Co) were used, accurate bilateral measurements to compare ramal height differences were not easy and susceptible to inter- and intra-observer errors. Measurements on two-dimensional radiographs show limitations due to magnified and angled projection of radiographic images, leading to inaccurate diagnosis of skeletal asymmetry [4]. Technological developments in cone-beam computed tomography (CBCT) imaging provide craniofacial imaging that is not magnified or distorted. Such high-resolution imaging advancements have facilitated accurate three-dimensional evaluation of complex facial asymmetry [5]. However, because compensatory postures of patients during examination or imaging are inevitable, re-orientation of three-dimensional skull images to determine true natural head position must precede skeletal assessment or treatment planning [1].

Results of different surgical osteotomies can be explored on the virtual skull model, and the most appropriate treatment plan can be selected after comparing postoperative images of the virtual skull models. Such images can also be used as a visual aid during communication with the patient, which helps understand the patient's expectations from the surgery.

2.1.2 CAD/CAM technology (printed surgical guides and plates)

One possible problem that can be encountered in a surgery requiring osteotomy or resection is that the amount to resect can differ depending on anatomical landmarks and measuring methods set by the surgeon in the field. Printed surgical guides to mark osteotomy line can help remove human error and accurately transfer surgical plan to the field. Printed surgical guides are fabricated to reflect the exact location of osteotomy, bony amounts to be removed, and plate hole locations on adjoining bony surfaces (**Figure 2A**). In other words, all information of the surgical treatment plan is comprehensively included.

Plates for the fixation of osteotomized segments can also be customized in its design (**Figure 2B**). Hole positions of plates can be pre-determined according to surgical plan, to allow intimate fixation of osteotomized bone segments. Plate hole position can be set to avoid brittle or thin bone during the virtual surgical planning process, further allowing sturdy fixation of the osteotomized segments. Because the shape and hole locations of each individual plate reflect the contour of the specific site near osteotomized hard tissue, customized titanium plates can be utilized to confirm that surgery has been carried out as planned [6].

2.2 Frontal ramal inclination (FRI)

Differences in frontal ramal inclination (FRI) of the left and right sides are commonly observed among facial asymmetry patients. Simple bimaxillary OGS involving

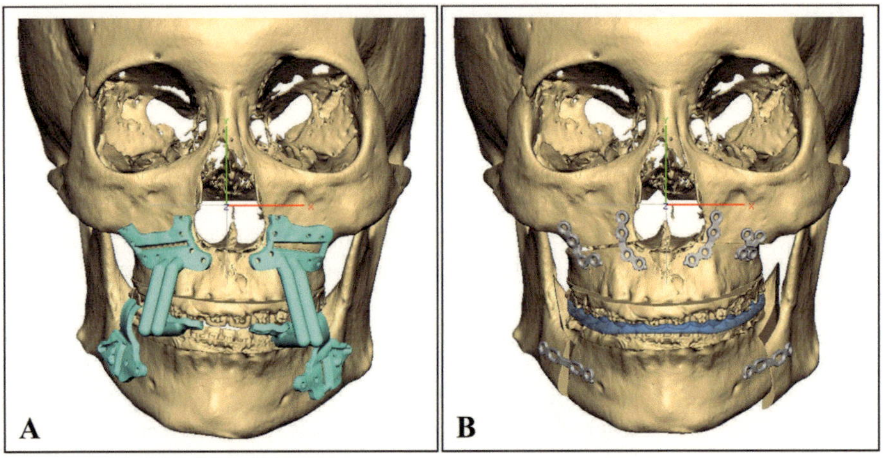

Figure 2.
Designs of surgical guides and plates on virtual skull model.

correction of maxillary canting and positional adjustment of the mandible distal segment does not solve facial asymmetry (**Figure 3A**). Intentional change of FRI can be performed for restoration of facial symmetry. FRI can be changed by medially or laterally rotating the proximal segment of the mandible, with the center of rotation fixed at the condyle head (**Figure 3B**). The amount and direction of FRI change can differ on the right and left sides depending on the type of FA.

Intentional change of FRI through conventional two-dimensional analysis or conventional OGS is extremely difficult and inaccurate. Virtual surgical planning (VSP) using a 3D virtual skull model and computer-assisted design/computer-assisted manufacturing (CAD/CAM) technology is fundamental in planning and carrying out precise restoration of facial symmetry. On a 3D virtual model, FRI can be intentionally adjusted to restore the symmetry of the right and left sides. The proximal segment of the mandible can be rotated medially or laterally, with the rotation center fixed at the most superior point of the condylar head [7].

During the actual intentional change of FRI, special attention should be paid to avoid anteroposterior or mediolateral movement of the condyle head. Large setback on the long side of the mandible, and advancement or minimal setback on the

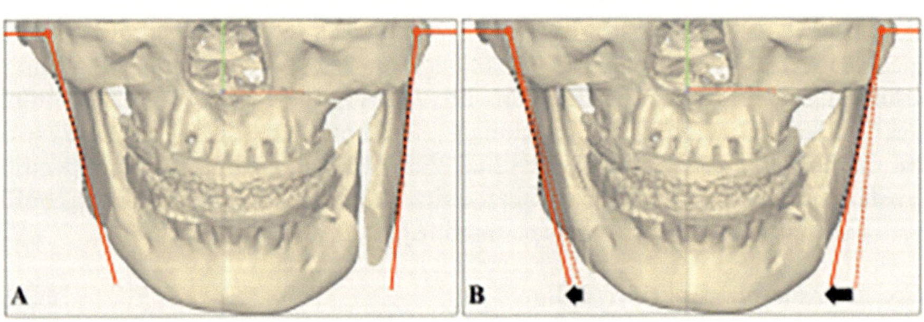

Figure 3.
Intentional change of FRI for symmetry of right and left sides. A: Different FRI of right and left sides before adjustment, B: Right proximal segment was laterally rotated for a decrease of FRI, and left proximal segment was rotated medially for an increase of FRI.

shorter side, in combination with intentional FRI change, inevitably creates bone interferences between proximal and distal segments. Most premature bone contact is observed in the posterior areas of the shorter side. Bony interferences between proximal and distal segments of the mandible prevent passive fixation of the segments, inducing lateral shift of the condylar head. Change in condylar head position can hinder accurate FRI change due to change in rotation center. Therefore, bony interferences between mandible segments must be checked before fixation, especially in FA cases where significant changes of FRI are planned.

Long-term stability of FRI change using VSP and CAD/CAM technology has been proven accurate in a number of studies [7, 8]. Both esthetic and function showed stable results; no occlusal changes due to significant bone remodeling of the condylar head were observed, and facial symmetry achieved after intentional change of FRI also showed esthetically stable morphology.

3. Contouring surgery

Contouring surgery can be performed simultaneously with OGS if necessary or in two separate operations. An expected advantage of one-time OGS and contouring surgery is a reduced amount of surgery. Postoperative skeletal changes are stably and easily predicted using VSP. If possible, both the patient and surgeon would prefer to reduce the number of surgeries. Single operations of OGS with simultaneous contouring surgery are possible for mild-to-moderate horizontal FA.

In cases where horizontal FA with different frontal ramal inclination (FRI) is due to fundamentally asymmetrical locations of the mandibular fossa or shape of the mandibular ramus, OGS alone will not completely resolve the asymmetry (**Figure 4**). For severe horizontal FA with such characteristics, separate operation of contouring surgery is preferred because (1) postoperative soft tissue response after intentional FRI may camouflage fundamental skeletal differences, removing the necessity for additional contouring surgery; (2) corticectomy cannot be done in areas where pre-fabricated plates are meant to be fixed; and (3) uneven

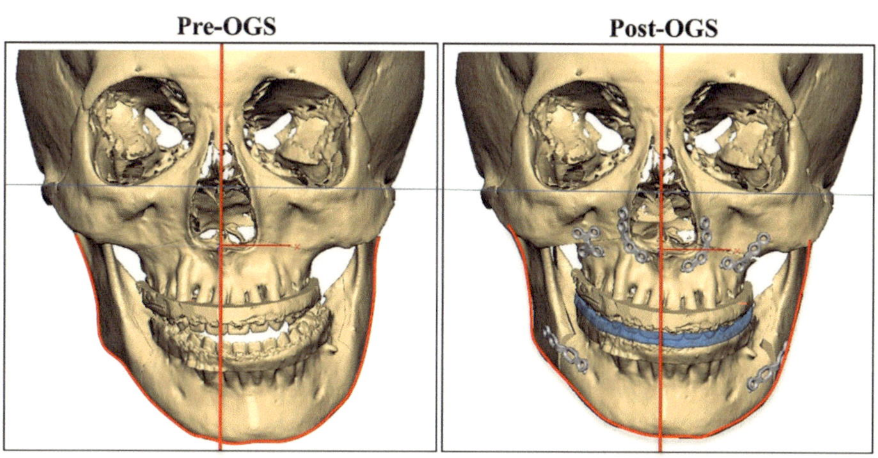

Figure 4.
Severe facial asymmetry cases will still exhibit asymmetry of skeletal contour after OGS, requiring additional contouring surgery.

postoperative soft tissue response can induce additional FA. Regarding soft tissue changes, the necessity of contouring surgery should be re-evaluated after soft tissue response becomes stable, especially in cases with non-adjustable skeletal differences [9, 10].

If the degree of facial asymmetry is severe, comparatively more postoperative soft tissue changes are expected than in minimal or no facial asymmetry cases. It takes 6–12 months for soft tissue to stabilize after surgery [9]. Likewise, it takes a similar amount of time for remodeling and stabilization of hard tissue to occur. Postoperative soft tissue changes are harder to predict than postoperative hard tissue changes [10]. Because soft tissue changes are unpredictable to a degree, precise and accurate prediction of postoperative external appearance is also very difficult. This unpredictability reduces the advantage of VSP, which helps accurate deduction of postoperative morphological changes on virtual preoperative and postoperative skeletal models. Because postoperative soft tissue changes are less predictable, additional surgery may be needed due to unexpected remnant asymmetry. Therefore, in severe FA cases, it is more stable to use two steps. Because it takes time for patients to become accustomed to their own appearance, it is recommended to evaluate the residual asymmetry and the necessity of additional treatment after 1–1.5 years postoperatively.

Contouring surgery includes the process of refining uneven contours as well as correcting residual asymmetry. It has more esthetic purpose than functional purpose. Although there may be differences in cultural standards of beauty, establishing symmetry and harmony of the face is, without a doubt, a large common factor in determining attractiveness [11]. Therefore, although contouring surgery may not have a direct correlation with function including mastication and speech, it still has a significant meaning in the psychosocial aspects of patients. Skeletal correction can be divided into horizontal skeletal correction and vertical skeletal correction. In zygoma, malarplasty is mainly performed for the purpose of horizontal skeletal correction. Because lateral protrusion is common in the Asian population, zygoma reduction is often performed.

3.1 Malarplasty

Extremely prominent or wide cheekbone is a feature that is often associated with a "strong" or "stubborn" image in many Asian faces and is often subject to reduction for esthetic purposes. Convexity of the zygomatic arch and lateral protrusion of the zygomatic body are responsible for the wide cheekbone. The prominence of the zygomatic arch can effectively be analyzed from the axial plane, and the prominence of the zygomatic body can most effectively be analyzed from a 45-degree frontal view.

The fan-shaped temporalis muscle runs medial to the zygomatic arch, originating from the temporal bone and inserting onto the coronoid process of the mandible. Bodily and rotational inward movement of the zygoma segment toward the temporalis muscle inevitably occurs during zygoma reduction. Sometimes, extreme inward movement of the zygoma arch can cause interference with the coronoid process and the temporalis muscle. This interference may result in postoperative mouth opening limitation (MOL). Analyzing comparative location of the zygomatic arch to relevant anatomy and establishing an appropriate treatment plan can effectively prevent MOL due to temporalis and/or coronoid process interference [12].

Standardized strategies for zygoma reduction depending on the amount of zygoma asymmetry are more useful nowadays because the viability of treatment plans can be tested with patients' virtual skull model, and accurate transfer of treatment plan is possible with CAD/CAM technology. The surgical strategy must consider function as well as esthetics; mouth opening limitations or unesthetically depressed zygoma bone are possible results of extreme surgical plans. If asymmetry discrepancies between the right and left sides are large, it is smarter to consider augmentation of one side and reduction of the other side instead of establishing an extreme unilateral reduction that may possibly cause complications.

Different strategies for zygoma reduction can be chosen for unilateral and bilateral zygoma protrusion, and severity of the protrusion discrepancies (**Figure 5**). For unilateral protrusion cases, only the protruded side of the zygoma is subject to change. A minor difference between the right and left sides can be simply fixed through simple grinding of the protruded portion. However, a conspicuous difference between right and left sides over 3 mm is subject to osteotomy; unilateral zygoma reduction should be performed on the protruded side.

A slightly different approach should be considered for bilateral zygoma protrusion. The bigger the amount of zygoma reduction, the higher the chances that the inwardly fixed zygoma segment will interfere with the temporalis muscle, potentially causing MOL. In addition, postoperative soft tissue changes may be more noticeable if the reduction amount of one side is too great. Therefore, in bilateral zygoma protrusion cases where discrepancies of right and left sides surpass 5 mm, unilateral zygoma reduction with a contralateral zygoma augmentation using PSI is highly recommended.

Malarplasty can be performed in conjunction with OGS. VSP can be utilized to determine the amount of zygoma asymmetry of the right and left sides by mirroring one side to another and measuring the discrepancy. The mirroring should be done with facial midline as the reference line. Once the Rt-Lt discrepancy is measured, a surgical strategy for the zygoma can be chosen. Since results of differential zygoma reduction can be seen on the virtual 3D model, the most appropriate reduction amount can be determined after comparison of multiple reduction models. In addition to the esthetic aspect, surgical stability can also be predicted on the 3D virtual model; bony contact of segments at the zygomatic arch must be confirmed. When designing the osteotomy line for zygoma reduction, it is advantageous to position the osteotomy line where the bone is thick enough for stable plate fixation but not too thick that osteotomy takes a long time and effort (**Figure 6A**).

For accurate osteotomy and reduction amounts, surgical guides can be designed and manufactured with CAD/CAM technology. Because the surgical field for zygoma body reduction is narrow and dark, the surgical guide should be designed long enough to cover two-thirds of the osteotomy line to increase the accurate transfer of the treatment plan (**Figure 6B**).

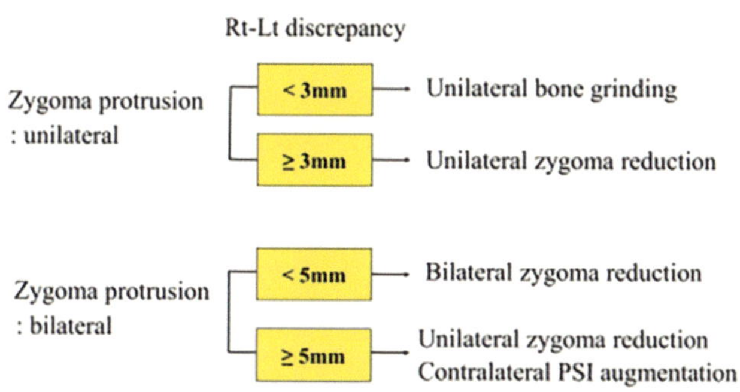

Figure 5.
Treatment strategy for restoration of zygoma symmetry according to the amount of Rt-Lt discrepancy.

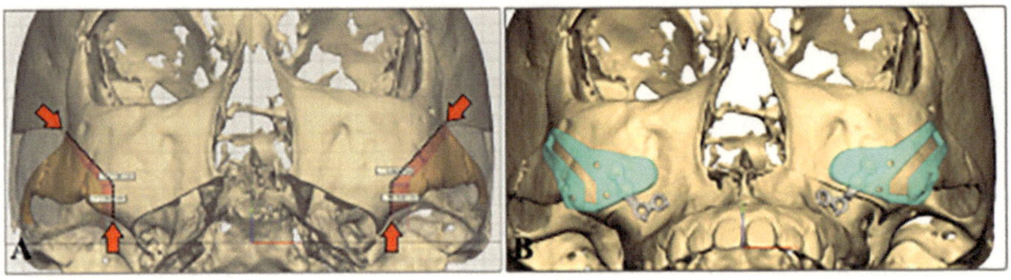

Figure 6.
VSP model for zygoma reduction for symmetry restoration. A: Bilateral zygoma reduction with differential reduction amount. Arrows indicate the most appropriate osteotomy line, B: Surgical guide design for zygoma reduction when planned in conjunction with OGS.

3.2 Corticectomy

Transverse skeletal correction of the lower one-third of the face regards horizontal width from the facial midline to gonion, measured from a frontal view. Corticectomy, which is a surgical procedure that removes cortical bone of the targeted area, is a useful method for controlling asymmetrical horizontal widths of the mandible angle.

Remnant horizontal asymmetry of the mandible may be observed even after OGS in cases of (1) significant movements of the hard tissue due to severe maxilla canting or FRI discrepancies, (2) remaining yaw asymmetry of the mandible, (3) differential soft

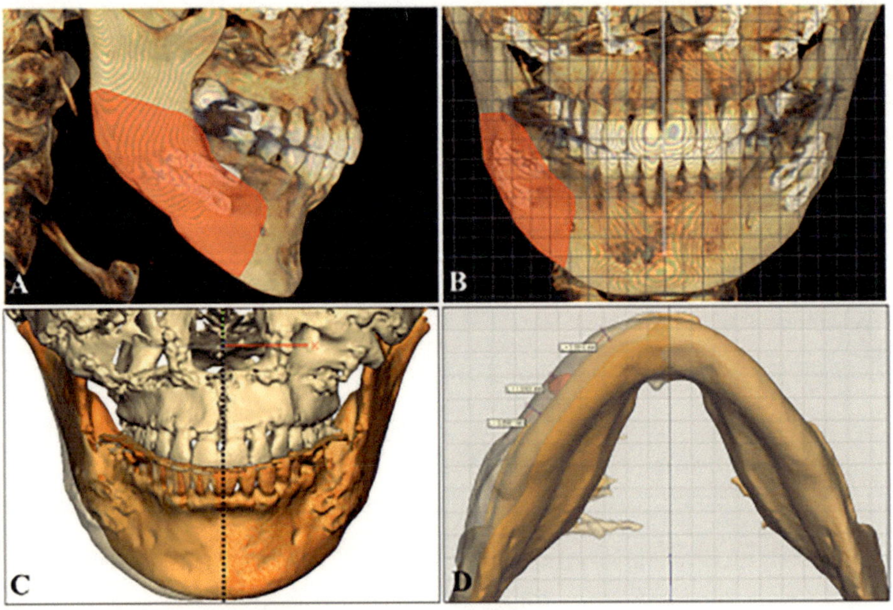

Figure 7.
VSP model for planning corticectomy. A: Area of corticectomy marked in red, B: Area of corticectomy marked in red, C: A mirror image of the left side of the mandible is overlapped with the right side of the mandible, D: Measurements and nerve marking on the virtual 3D model of the mandible.

tissue response causing facial asymmetry despite achieved skeletal symmetry. Usually, horizontally wide mandibular morphology is a combination of muscle hypertrophy and skeletal growth. If muscle hypertrophy is also an additional cause of unilaterally wide mandible, muscle hypertrophy must be treated prior to evaluation of skeletal cause.

Overlap of a mirror image of the "slimmer" side of the mandible to another helps visualize the discrepancy between the two sides (**Figure 7**). On the 3D virtual model, inferior alveolar nerves of the right and left sides are marked. The 3D virtual model helps to avoid nerve damage and adjust the surgical plan preoperatively. With VSP, therefore, viability and results of corticectomy can be predicted.

3.3 Mandibuloplasty

Mandibuloplasty can be performed simultaneously with bimaxillary OGS in cases where horizontal discrepancy involving FRI is not significant. If mandibuloplasty is planned to be performed together with mandible osteotomy, mandibuloplasty should be performed first, followed by splitting of the mandible. Separate osteotomy of proximal and distal segments is not preferred due to bone bleeding and inaccuracy. Regardless of whether mandibuloplasty is performed in conjunction with bimaxillary OGS, the virtual simulation process is identical (**Figure 8**).

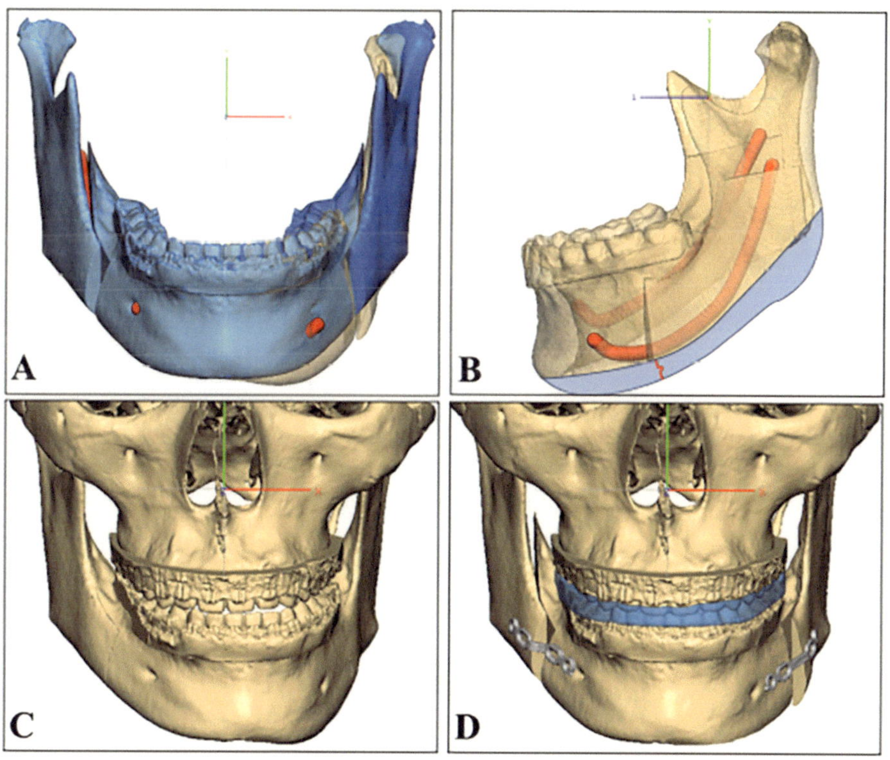

Figure 8.
VSP models for mandibuloplasty. A: mirror image (blue) of right side of mandible overlapped to left side for asymmetry analysis, B: appropriate osteotomy design to satiate symmetry and prevent nerve damage, C: preoperative asymmetry of the mandible, D: postoperative symmetry achieved after mandibuloplasty and BSSRO.

4. Conclusion

Management of facial asymmetry is like a multi-layer intricate puzzle. Considerations of skeletal, dental, and soft tissue components in horizontal and vertical planes must be considered in establishing an appropriate treatment plan. In addition, the treatment plan must satisfy both functional and esthetician objectives. Management of facial asymmetry, therefore, poses challenges to surgeons.

Various treatment modalities combining bimaxillary OGS with contouring surgery should be conjointly considered to improve treatment outcomes. Many technological advances have contributed to the precise management and prediction of surgery. However, perfect facial symmetry may not be achieved due to fundamental craniofacial asymmetries or the unknown impact of soft tissue response on treatment outcomes. Such limitations of the current management of FA leave room for improvement.

Conflict of interest

The authors declare no conflict of interest.

Author details

Ji Youn Maeng[1*] and Jin Young Choi[2]

1 Gaon Dental Hospital, Cheon-An, Republic of Korea

2 Seoul National University, Seoul, Republic of Korea

*Address all correspondence to: jymaeng@snu.ac.kr

References

[1] Jearanai T, Samruajbenjakun B, Chanmanee P. Relationship between bilateral landmarks of facial asymmetry in skeletal class II and class III in vertical dimension: 3D facial scan and cone-beam computed tomography. Diagnostics. 2024;**14**:590. DOI: 10.3390/diagnostics14060590

[2] Alrbata RH, Alfaqih AK, Almhaidat MR, Al-Tarawneh AM. Thresholds of abnormality perception in facial esthetics among laypersons and dental professionals: Frontal esthetics. International Journal of Dentistry. 2020;**2020**:8946063. DOI: 10.1155/2020/8946063

[3] Tayyebi K, Arab S, Razmara F, Geramy A, Kharazifard MJ, Kamali E. Perceptions of mandibular asymmetry among orthodontists, oral and maxillofacial surgeons, and laypersons. Dental Research Journal (Isfahan). 2023;**20**:107

[4] Kambylafkas P, Murdock E, Gilda E, Tallents RH, Kyrkanides S. Validity of panoramic radiographs for measuring mandibular asymmetry. The Angle Orthodontist. 2006;**76**:388-393. DOI: 10.1043/0003-3219(2006)076[0388:VOPRFM]2.0.CO; 2

[5] Udomlarptham N, Lin CH, Wang YC, Ko EW. Does two-dimensional vs. three-dimensional surgical simulation produce better surgical outcomes among patients with class III facial asymmetry? International Journal of Oral and Maxillofacial Surgery. 2018;**47**:1022-1031. DOI: 10.1016/j.ijom.2018.02.014

[6] Ji H, Du W, Xu C, Zhao Q, Ye B, Luo E. Computer-assisted osteotomy guides and pre-bent titanium plates improve the planning for correction of facial asymmetry. International Journal of Oral and Maxillofacial Surgery. 2019;**48**:1043-1050. DOI: 10.1016/j.ijom.2019.01.026

[7] Woo M-H, Youn S, Woo JM, Baek S-H, Choi J-Y. Accuracy of intentional change of frontal ramal inclination from virtual to actual orthognathic surgery using computer-aided design and computer-aided manufacturing-made customized metal plates. The Journal of Craniofacial Surgery. 2022;**33**:376-382. DOI: 10.1097/SCS.0000000000008174

[8] Ha S-H, Meny AH, Jeong C-G, Yeo J-H, Baek S-H, Choi J-Y. The accuracy and stability of intentional change of frontal-Ramal inclination in orthognathic surgery for facial asymmetry patients. Journal of Craniofacial Surgery. 2023;**34**:462-468. DOI: 10.1097/SCS.0000000000009306

[9] Mandrekar PN, Dhupar V, Akkara F. Prediction of soft-tissue changes following single and Bi-Jaw surgery: An evaluative study. Annals of Maxillofacial Surgery. 2021;**11**:32-36. DOI: 10.4103/ams.ams_138_20

[10] Huang L, Li Z, Yan J, Chen L, Piao ZG. Evaluation of facial soft tissue thickness in asymmetric mandibular deformities after orthognathic surgery. Maxillofacial Plastic and Reconstructive Surgery. 2021;**43**:37. DOI: 10.1186/s40902-021-00323-5

[11] Perrett DI, Burt DM, Penton-Voak IS, Lee KJ, Rowland DA, Edwards R. Symmetry and human facial attractiveness. Evolution and Human Behavior. 1999;**20**:295-307. DOI: 10.1016/S1090-5138(99)00014-8

[12] Park JC. Effects of surgical factors on the outcomes of zygoma reduction malarplasty: A quantitative computed tomography study. Maxillofacial Plastic and Reconstructive Surgery. 2023;**45**:3. DOI: 10.1186/s40902-023-00371-z

Chapter 11

Osteotomy Challenges for Implant Placement in Posterior Mandible

Ibrahim H. Garoushi, Ramy R. Elbeialy, Amr Gibaly and Mohammed Atef

Abstract

The posterior mandibular region poses significant challenges for dental implantologists due to its unique anatomical constraints. This chapter delves into the complexities of inserting root-form dental implants in this region, focusing on the difficulties and complications that arise from anatomical considerations. A particular emphasis is placed on inferior alveolar nerve lateralization (IANL) surgical technique, which has expanded implant placement possibilities but is also linked with significant risks and drawbacks. The chapter provides an in-depth review of the history and progress of IANL methods, including their positive and negative aspects, as well as modifications made to reduce morbidity and neurosensory abnormalities. Additionally, the author presents their own integrated strategy for IANL, which combines bone graft compaction with collagen membrane nerve shielding to improve postoperative results. Beyond IANL, this chapter also explores alternative treatment options for the posterior mandibular region, including bone grafting and short implants. These techniques are crucial for overcoming the limitations imposed by atrophic ridges and promoting successful implant placement. The chapter concludes with practical advice on how to overcome these obstacles and achieve good results in this challenging region.

Keywords: posterior mandible, implant osteotomy, inferior alveolar nerve, short implants, bone augmentation

1. Introduction

Due to the inferior alveolar nerve's (IAN) near proximity to the alveolar ridge and the irreversible process of bone resorption that follows tooth loss, placing dental implants in the posterior mandibular region might be challenging. One of the main dental concerns that could have a detrimental effect on a patient's quality of life is the rehabilitation of patients who are either fully or partially edentulous [1].

A wide range of treatment options is available for patients with severely resorbed posterior edentulous mandibular ridge depending on the site and patient-related factors. Implant placement in particular is challenging and thus various treatment options exist such as the use of short implants or advanced surgical procedures (for instance, ridge augmentation or inferior alveolar nerve repositioning). Bone augmentation using blocks harvested from the patient is associated with increased cost, time, and the risk of morbidity for an implant-supported prosthesis [2, 3].

The height of bone superior to the mandibular canal in severely resorbed ridges and the poorer quality in comparison with its cortical counterpart is of insufficient length for the placement of ideal fixtures. The inferior alveolar nerve lateralization (IANL) procedure involves the exposure and deflection of the nerve laterally to allow the placement of longer implants engaging two cortices that provide good primary stability [4]. However, an attempt to place shorter dental implants will not provide a bi-cortical implant placement, and there is a high risk of injuring the nerve as a result of an effort by the operator to maximize the length of the implant [5–7].

Inferior alveolar nerve (IAN) repositioning to allow implant placement is an effective treatment option indicated in cases with severely atrophied posterior mandibular ridge. Transposition of the IAN includes the mental foramen in the procedure, while nerve lateralization is done through a window posterior to the mental foramen [1, 5].

Although the IAN lateralization procedure is an effective treatment option, it presents several drawbacks as the technique weakens the mandible temporarily and fracture could occur in association with implant placement. The risk of nerve damage and neurosensory disturbances is another disadvantage of the procedure. An additional concern about the use of barriers to isolate the implant from the nerve by resorbable membranes to be of benefit or not is a debate [8, 9].

2. Different treatment approaches

2.1 Posterior atrophic mandibular ridge treatment options

Although an extensively documented procedure, the outcomes of reconstructing vertically atrophic posterior mandibles using onlay bone grafts have not been encouraging. Several autogenous bone sources, including the iliac crest, calvaria, and symphysis menti, have been utilized as donor sites. In 1996, Vermeen et al. showed that the overall rate of bone resorption was about 50%, even with the use of autogenous onlay grafts. Consequently, it is crucial to avoid microrotation during the stiff fixation of the graft material since this may result in the nonunion or fibrous union of the graft material [10]. Dahlin and colleagues reported in 1991 that guided bone regeneration was proposed using expanded polytetrafluoroethylene (ePTFE) on exposed implant threads with a range of bone gain of 0.5 to 3.0 mm [11]. Expanded polytetrafluoroethylene membrane in conjunction with bone graft material is one therapeutic option for posterior mandibular reconstruction that has been used with varying degrees of effectiveness, as reported by Jovanovic et al. in 1992 [12].

Vertical augmentation is a very complex procedure; therefore, it is only predictable when the surgical protocol is followed accurately as Tinti et al. in 1998 concluded in their retrospective study [13]. Furthermore, ridge augmentation of the atrophied ridges vertically has been successful since they were introduced [14]. This is with the use of titanium mesh, which is fixed by titanium screws and autogenous bone grafts. It is said that, however, the fixing of titanium screws has a common complication that may result in the loss of grafted bone, resulting in failure of the procedure if infections occur [15].

Visor Osteotomy was believed to increase the entire height of the atrophic edentulous mandibular ridge using wires for fixation on the two bony parts. This is first defined by Harle in 1975 [16]. The implementation of this procedure for vertical ridge augmentation of the posterior mandible results in a reduction in the width of the ridge, attributable to the vertical splitting of the mandible. The technique where the bone block graft positioning is used between osteotomized bony segments is called the sandwich technique. This was established by Schettler [17] in 1974. In 2011, Scarano et al. reported in their case series study performed on nine patients using an inlay technique with xenograft for vertical ridge augmentation that the rigidity of blocks maintained the space and the technique eliminates the need of using screws [18].

2.2 Bone graft for posterior mandibular augmentation

Insufficient bone volume may result in implant placement being difficult or impossible if a significant vertical bone defect is present. The presence of the mandibular canal in the posterior mandible constitutes a further anatomic limitation that can be overcome with different surgical techniques. Such techniques include titanium mesh with autologous bone or biomaterials [19], alveolar osteodistraction [20], vertical guided bone regeneration (GBR) [21], block graft [22], and short implants [23].

The most scientifically supported methods for regenerating vertical lesions are block grafts, guided bone regeneration, and distraction osteogenesis [24]. Autogenous block grafts are shielded from surface resorption in horizontal augmentations by a collagen barrier made of bioabsorbable material and an organic bovine bone mineral, according to a 1999 clinical cohort research by Von Arx and Buser [25]. This has provided a clear illustration of how graft covering reduces resorption. Polytetrafluoroethylene membranes, which have been utilized to cover grafts, are another type of material that has been used with good clinical results but more problems than collagen membranes [26]. Furthermore, Aghaloo and Moy's 2007 analysis [27] made clear that implant survival might depend more on the remaining bone than on grafted bone to maintain the implant.

2.3 Inferior alveolar nerve transposition

Dental implants are commonly utilized in the posterior mandible to support fixed prostheses. After tooth extraction, this area typically has significant bone resorption, and the inferior alveolar nerve's vertical travel is limited (IAN). This constraint makes it challenging to insert implants at the proper sizes. In such circumstances, therapeutic approaches such as vertical bone grafting techniques to enhance crest height, prosthetic cantilever bridges, and short implants can be used. Shifting the IAN from the area via lateralization or transposition procedures is an additional strategy that has been documented in the literature [27].

Lateralization and transposition are the two distinct IAN repositioning methods. The process of implanting after exposure, laterally situating the IAN, and shifting it over implants is known as nerve lateralization. There is no interference with the mental foramen or incisive branch of the nerve during nerve lateralization. In contrast, nerve transposition involves cutting the incisive nerve branch and removing bone from the mental foramen region in order to realign the mental foramen posteriorly [28]. Alling transposed IAN for the first time in 1977 [29].

Jensen and Nock [30] reported the first instance of implant placement after IAN transposition in 1987. After making modifications to this procedure, the researchers assumed that implants may be placed in an atrophic crest using this technique. The change was to apply implants by opening a canal distal to the mental foramen, which made it possible for the IAN to move on the mandibular cortical layer with a large diameter round bur. When Rosenquist [31] used IAN transposition to put 26 implants in 10 patients in 1992, the results were positive after surgery. This lateralization of the IAN was then included as a substitute for the transposition method. Both of these approaches are in use today [2].

2.4 Lateralization and inferior alveolar nerve transposition

The inferior alveolar nerve (LIAN) lateralization procedure improves the possibility of direct view and enables implants to be installed in the ideal position or as near to it as possible [7]. The implant is enclosed in better-quality bone due to the mandibles' greater cortical and basal bodies than when it is placed in a repaired region using grafts [32]. When compared to reconstruction methods involving grafts, this lateralization procedure requires fewer donor areas, which reduces patient morbidity, lowers costs, allows for the prompt installation of long implants (since it utilizes all of the remaining jaw bone), and shortens the time patients must wait for treatment—up to 8 months in this case [33].

In comparison to the chin symphysis region, which is primarily composed of cortical bone, the posterior mandible has a larger proportion of marrow bone. The outcomes of the LIAN approach are biomechanically advantageous in the posterior region of the mandible. This method has been shown to provide an excellent match between the prosthesis and implant lengths [31]. On the other hand, the placement of short implants shows worse biomechanics and worse initial stability, which is linked to a unicortical anchor, even when the mandibular canal is preserved [34].

The use of dental implants in conjunction with inferior alveolar nerve transposition for the treatment of the atrophic posterior mandible was initially reported by Jensen and Nock in 1987 [30]. The approach was a modification of Alling's [29] lateralization operation on the inferior alveolar nerve, which was done to help denture patients with severely resorbed mandible feel less uncomfortable. These patients had severe discomfort and decreased patient satisfaction as a result of the prosthesis's pressure on their neurovascular bundle. Later in 1998, Dao and Mellor [35] found that all patients undergoing LIAN operations had temporary inferior alveolar nerve sensitivity abnormalities. As a result, they concluded that this treatment carries a substantial risk.

2.5 Short implant versus inferior alveolar nerve lateralization

Removable, complete, or partial dentures have historically been provided to individuals seeking dental care to restore both their functional and cosmetic appearance (referred to as Edentulous patients). However, wearing removable dentures causes those individuals to feel insecure, impair their ability to chew, and have low self-esteem [36]. The benefits of implant-supported prosthesis over traditional dentures, which have improved many patients' quality of life, give rise to implants as an alternative treatment option. The quantity and quality of bone appear to be closely correlated with the success rate [37].

Currently, there has been an increase in the use of short dental implants, which provide doctors with a systematic way to simplify prosthetic restorations when there is an anatomic limitation due to low alveolar bone height [38]. This is because the more aggressive methods frequently include bone augmentation, which entails bone grafting first and endosseous implant implantation second [39]. Since the discovery of the 10-mm implant length in 1971 [40], innumerable varieties of standard Branemark implants (3.75 mm) have been discovered and employed for the treatment of edentulous ridges.

In response to the increasing number of atrophic jaws requiring rehabilitation, the 7-mm standardized implant length was designed and released in 1979. In edentulous jaws, short implants were used either alone or in conjunction with lengthier implants [41]. The 1-, 3-, 5-, and 10-year findings demonstrated a prevalence of unsuccessful results among the short implants, given the role of these implants [42]. Wide-diameter implants were therefore developed in order to make it easier to replace a regular implant and to raise the success rate in situations when conditions are precarious [43]. Situations where there are insufficient or low-quality bones were the first to be addressed by Langer B et al.'s 1993 suggested wide-diameter implant [44]. According to certain research, wide-diameter implants worked well in situations where there was less residual alveolar height once the implant's length was compromised. Consequently, a correlation was observed between wider diameter and shorter implants.

Following augmentation surgeries without the use of short implants for the repair of the atrophic mandible, an increasing implant survival rate of 92.3% was seen after at least 10 years of follow-up. Short implants need to be thoroughly investigated before being used, as it is evident that their shortcoming—which is represented by the lack of data about the analysis of studies involving implants that are shorter than 7 mm—was discovered to be enhanced in certain ways. Thus, their review's objective was to provide a comprehensive overview of implant studies with a short length of ≤7 mm [45]. When there is an atrophied posterior mandible, there are two effective implant-based therapy options: short dental implants (SDI) and inferior alveolar nerve lateralization (IANL). Standard implants can be placed in IANL even with the hazards of malfunction, infection, and pathologic fractures [46].

A study in 2005 by Toledo Filho et al. [47] states that one option for prosthetic rehabilitation for patients with alveolar resorption (moderate to severe in the posterior mandible) or bone defects and intolerance to removable prosthesis is the lateralization of the inferior alveolar nerve. According to the research conducted by Garg et al. [48], bone resorption occurs after tooth extraction and is exacerbated by the use of removable prostheses. Bone pathogenesis is found to be fast and progressive. The degree and pattern of bone resorption seen in the alveolar process cause moderate to severe atrophy of the mandible. This moderate to severe mandibular atrophy can be attributed to both general systemic and local causes.

Silva et al.'s 1999 study [49] found that the alveolar ridge encounters an ongoing, permanent phase of bone resorption as a result of tooth loss. As a result, the posterior jaw resorption typically results in a depressed edge, making implant placement in these regions difficult. Since the posterior mandibular bone is of inferior quality to the anterior, short implants are placed to maintain the mandibular canal. Moreover, unicortical primary implant stability is seen [50]. The lateralization of the IAN is a modern procedure that has been shown to be a successful alternative treatment in cases of vertical atrophy [51]. To maximize the success of mandibular implant insertion, the inferior alveolar nerve lateralization procedure has been developed [52].

In 2004, Stellingsma et al. [53] reported that there are some forms of treatment for atrophic posterior mandibular short implants, termed tilted implants, as well as advanced surgeries such as distraction osteogenesis, interpositional graft, and lateralization of the inferior alveolar. Furthermore, Garcia Junior et al. [54] stated in 2006 that the technique of lateralization of IAN, without interference with the incisive nerve, consists of exposing the nerve and gently pulling it out of the mandibular canal laterally diverting its path and allowing implant placement. This practice has low morbidity and (if performed accurately) provides stable results and supports the fixation of implants in bi-cortical bone, hence increasing resistance to occlusal forces and guaranteeing a good proportion between the implant and the prosthesis.

Researchers have discovered through researches that the wider the implant's diameter, the greater the bone loss, and the higher the failure rate associated with shorter implants [55]. An implant's area of bone interaction is comparable to that of an implant with a diameter of 3.75 mm and a length of 10 mm for 5 mm and 6 mm, respectively [56]. Griffin et al. [57] suggested that implants shorter than 10 mm are associated with higher rates of dissatisfaction and that short implants ought to be paired together to improve outcomes [58].

Due to the possibility of numbness, paresthesia, or total loss of sensation in the affected area, IAN lateralization is a very risky surgical procedure [59]. The ability to perform this procedure successfully depends on the practitioners' proficiency in the field of operating technique, their knowledge of the local anatomy and the mandibular canal, and their physiological comprehension of the neurovascular bundle [60]. The patient must also receive complete explanations and consent to all possible dangers and problems, as noted by Kan et al. [61] and other authors in 1997. These consequences include temporary paresthesia that may become chronic as well as fractures to the jaw.

2.6 Surgical procedure for inferior alveolar lateralization

The surgical procedure for the inferior alveolar is performed using conscious sedation and local anesthesia. The anesthesia consists of a combination of epinephrine and a local anesthetic agent, which is administered through an epinephrine-containing anesthetic solution. Prior to the procedure, the oral cavity is rinsed with chlorhexidine mouthwash. A mid-crestal incision with both posterior and anterior oblique releasing incisions was used to expose the operative site, and full mucoperiosteal flap elevating was then performed (**Figure 1A**). The anterior vertical cut ought to be 5 mm posterior to the mental foramina, and the measurements for the lateral osteotomy should be made with the "Michigan-O" probe with Williams's markings [62].

A piezosurgery equipment is used to accomplish the rectangular osteotomy (**Figure 1B**). Using slow, careful tapping with chisels, the outside bony windows are removed, and the removed bone block is kept in a sterile solution of saline (**Figure 1C** and **D**). Using smooth blunt instruments, the inferior alveolar nerve (IAN) is gently excavated, its cortical sheath peeled off, and the nerve retracted and maintained in a deflected posture (**Figure 2A** and **B**) [62].

2.7 Osteotomy after inferior alveolar nerve lateralization

With the use of pilot-drilling guidance from radiography scan equipment, the sequential implant drilling process used sharp drills with stoppers to predefined lengths. In order to achieve bi-cortical engagement, implants with the appropriate diameters and lengths should be chosen. The implants were then implanted with a maximum torque of 25 N/cm to lower the chance of an unintentional mandibular fracture.

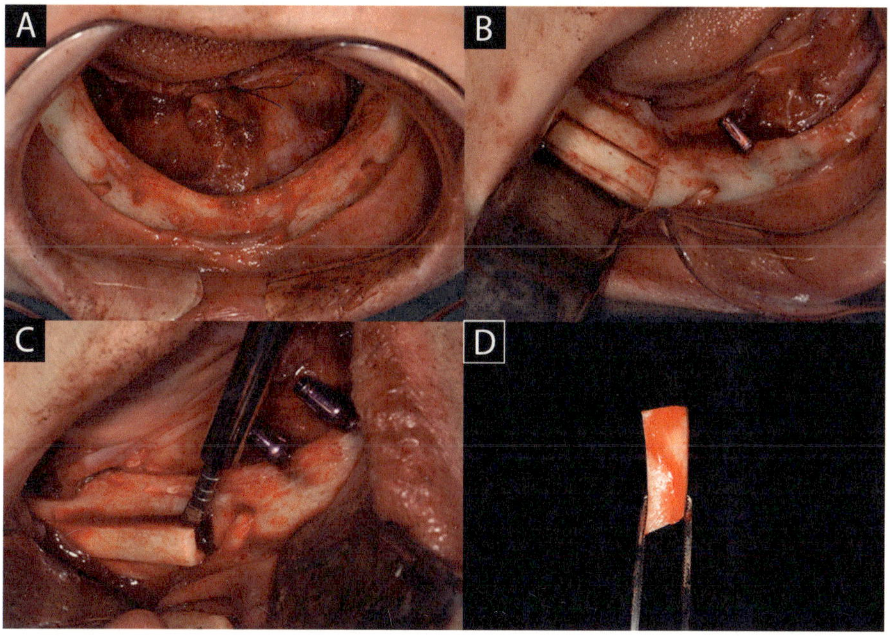

Figure 1.
(A) Mucoperiosteal flap elevation, (B) the osteotomy outline, (C) elevation of the bone window, and (D) the bone window retrieved.

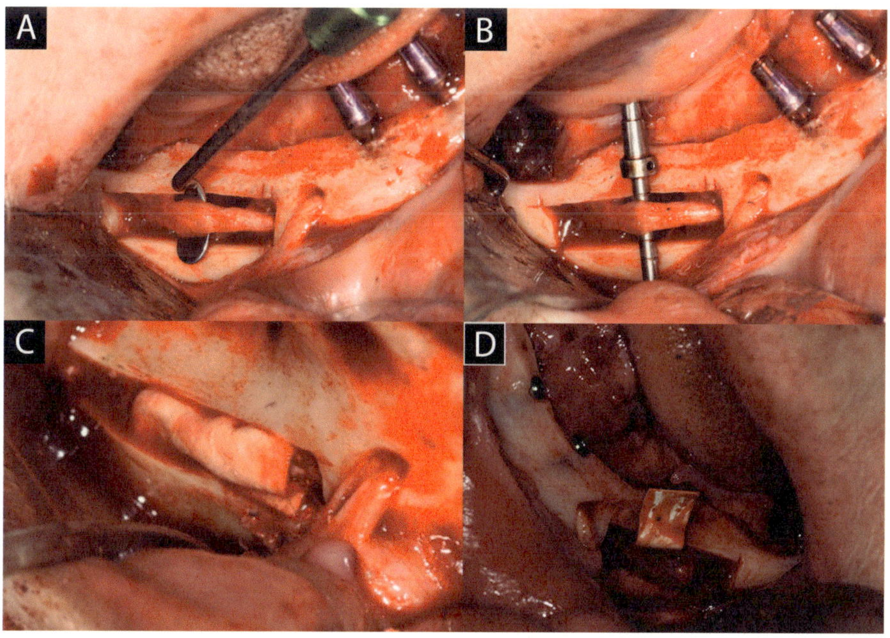

Figure 2.
(A) Retraction of the inferior alveolar nerve (IAN) by a blunt retractor, (B) the nerve retraction for implant placement, and (C and D) folding the membrane around the nerve.

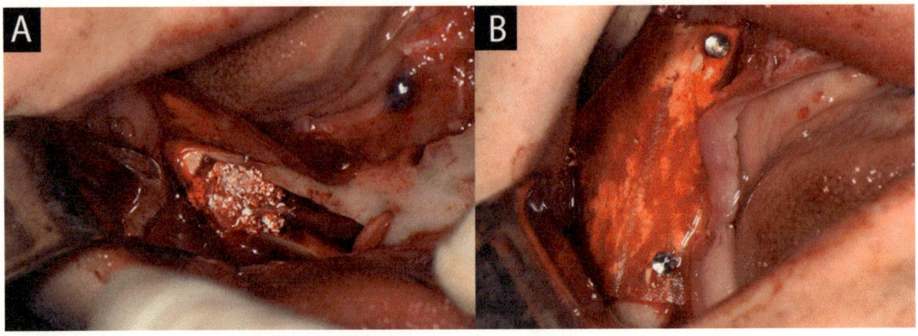

Figure 3.
(A and B) Bone particulate placement and collagen membrane fixation overlying the surgical site.

2.8 Inferior alveolar nerve after implant osteotomy

The outermost cortical bone layer is crushed into autogenous particles and combined 1:1 with anorganic bovine bone matrix (ABBM) after the IAN is pushed back to cover the implants underneath, either with or without collagen membrane isolation. Subsequently, the mixture is filled into the IAN site's rectangular osteotomy (**Figure 3**) [62].

Osteotomy and dental implant placement near sensitive anatomical structures such as nerves can be challenging. The IAN is a critical structure that supplies sensation to the lower teeth, and its damage can result in significant morbidity. Therefore, in order to minimize the potential of neural injury and enhance dental implant integration, innovative treatments are required. Dense cortical bone growth encircles the inferior alveolar canal, signifying the bone graft's effective integration. However, as compared to baseline readings, there was no discernible improvement in neurological complications, secondary implant stability, or marginal bone loss. Rehabilitation of severely resorbed posterior mandibular ridges requires careful consideration of anatomical, surgical, and biological factors. Treatment options include nerve lateralization, inferior alveolar nerve transposition, bone grafting, and implant placement. By understanding these treatment options and techniques, dentists can provide optimal care for patients with this condition.

Author details

Ibrahim H. Garoushi[1*], Ramy R. Elbeialy[2], Amr Gibaly[3] and Mohammed Atef[2]

1 Department of Oral and Maxillofacial Surgery, Faculty of Dentistry, Libyan International Medical University, Benghazi, Libya

2 Department of Oral and Maxillofacial Surgery, Faculty of Dentistry, Cairo University, Cairo, Egypt

3 Department of Oral and Maxillofacial Surgery, Faculty of Dentistry, Beni-Suef University, Beni-Suef, Egypt

*Address all correspondence to: ibrahim.garoushi@limu.edu

References

[1] Ramalho GC, Manzi MR, Pimentel AC, Sanches MA, Sendyk WR, Roman-Torres CV. Lateralization technique and inferior alveolar nerve transposition. Case Reports in Dentistry. 2016;**2016**:1-10. DOI: 10.1155/2016/4802637

[2] Lorean A, Kablan F, Mazor Z, et al. Inferior alveolar nerve transposition and reposition for dental implant placement in edentulous or partially edentulous mandibles: A multicenter retrospective study. International Journal of Oral and Maxillofacial Surgery. 2013;**42**(5):656-659. DOI: 10.1016/j.ijom.2013.01.020

[3] Anitua E, Murias-Freijo A, Alkhraisat MH, Orive G. Implant-guided vertical bone augmentation around extra-short implants for the Management of Severe Bone Atrophy. The Journal of Oral Implantology. 2013;**41**(5):563-569. DOI: 10.1563/aaid-joi-d-13-00131

[4] Castellano-Navarro JM, Castellano-Reyes JJ, Hirdina-Castilla M, Suárez-Soto A, Bocanegra-Pérez S, Vicente-Barrero M. Neurosensory issues after lateralisation of the inferior alveolar nerve and simultaneous placement of osseointegrated implants. The British Journal of Oral & Maxillofacial Surgery. 2019;**2018**:1-5. DOI: 10.1016/j.bjoms.2019.01.006

[5] Luna AHB, Passeri La, de Moraes M, Moreira RWF. Endosseous implant placement in conjunction with inferior alveolar nerve transposition: A report of an unusual complication and surgical management. The International Journal of Oral & Maxillofacial Implants. 2008;**23**(1):133-136. Available from: http://www.ncbi.nlm.nih.gov/pubmed/18416424

[6] Kan JY, Lozada JL, Goodacre CJ, Davis WH, Hanisch O. Endosseous implant placement in conjunction with inferior alveolar nerve transposition: An evaluation of neurosensory disturbance. The International Journal of Oral & Maxillofacial Implants. 1997;**12**(4):463-471

[7] Morrison A, Chiarot M, Kirby S. Mental nerve function after inferior alveolar nerve transposition for placement of dental implants. Journal of the Canadian Dental Association. 2002;**68**(1):46-50

[8] Khojasteh A, Hosseinpour S, Nazeman P, Dehghan MM. The effect of a platelet-rich fibrin conduit on neurosensory recovery following inferior alveolar nerve lateralization: A preliminary clinical study. International Journal of Oral and Maxillofacial Surgery. 2016;**45**(10):1303-1308. DOI: 10.1016/j.ijom.2016.06.003

[9] Vetromilla BM, Moura LB, Sonego CL, Torriani MA, Chagas OL. Complications associated with inferior alveolar nerve repositioning for dental implant placement: A systematic review. International Journal of Oral and Maxillofacial Surgery. 2014;**43**(11):1360-1366. DOI: 10.1016/j.ijom.2014.07.010

[10] Vermeeren JI, Wismeijer D, van Waas MA. One-step reconstruction of the severely resorbed mandible with onlay bone grafts and endosteal implants. A 5-year follow-up. International Journal of Oral and Maxillofacial Surgery. 1996;**25**:112-115

[11] Dahlin C, Lekholm U, Linde A. Membrane-induced bone augmentation at titanium implants. A report on ten fixtures followed from 1 to 3 years after loading. The International Journal of

Periodontics & Restorative Dentistry. 1991;**11**:273-281

[12] Jovanovic SA, Spiekermann H, Richter EJ. Bone regeneration around titanium dental implants in dehisced defect sites: A clinical study. The International Journal of Oral & Maxillofacial Implants. 1992;7:233-245

[13] Tinti C, Parma-Benfenati S. Vertical ridge augmentation: Surgical protocol and retrospective evaluation of 48 consecutively inserted implants. The International Journal of Periodontics & Restorative Dentistry. 1998;**5**:434-443

[14] Von Arx T, Hardt N, Wallkamm B. The TIME technique: A new method for localized alveolar ridge augmentation prior to placement of dental implants. The International Journal of Oral & Maxillofacial Implants. 1996;**11**:387-394

[15] Roccuzzo M, Ramieri G, Spada M, Bianchi S, Berrone S. Vertical alveolar ridge augmentation by means of a titanium mesh and autogenous bone grafts. Clinical Oral Implants Research. 2004;**15**:73-81

[16] Harle F. Visor osteotomy to increase the absolute height of the atrophic mandible. A preliminary report. Journal of Oral and Maxillofacial Surgery. 1975;**3**:257-260

[17] Schettler D. Sandwich technique with cartilage transplant for raising the alveolar process in the lower jaw. Fortschritte der Kiefer- und Gesichts-Chirurgie. 1976;**20**:61-63

[18] Scarano A, Carinci F, Assenza B, Piattelli M, Murmura G, Piattelli A. Vertical ridge augmentation of atrophic posterior mandible using an inlay technique with a xenograft without miniscrews and miniplates: Case series. Clinical Oral Implants Research. 2011;**22**:1125-1130

[19] Gupta A, Tiwari B, Goel H, Shekhawat H. Residual ridge resorption: A REVIEW. Indian Journal of Dental Sciences. 2010;**2**(2):7-11

[20] Kumar TA, Naeem A, Verma AK, Mariyam A, Krishna D, Kumar PK. Residual ridge resorption: The unstoppable. International Journal of Applied Research. 2016;**2**(2):169-171

[21] Tallgren A. The continuing reduction of the residual alveolar ridge in complete denture wearers; a mixed longitudinal study covering 25 years. The Journal of Prosthetic Dentistry. 1972;**27**:120-132. DOI: 10.1016/0022-3913(72)90188-6

[22] Jennings DE. Treatment of the mandibular compromised ridge: A literature review. The Journal of Prosthetic Dentistry. 1989;**61**:575-579

[23] Tideman H. Vestibulumplastiek met het vrije mucosa transplantaat. Acad. Thesis. University of Amsterdam; 1973. pp. 19-21

[24] Krenkel C, Grunert I. The Endo-distractor for preimplant mandibular regeneration. Revue de Stomatologie et de Chirurgie Maxillo-Faciale. 2009;**110**(1):17-26

[25] Von Arx T, Buser D. Horizontal ridge augmentation using autogenous block grafts and the guided bone regeneration technique with collagen membranes: A clinical study with 42 patients. Clinical Oral Implants Research. 2006;**17**:359-366

[26] Tonetti MS, Hämmerle CH. Advances in bone augmentation to enable dental implant placement: Consensus report of the sixth European workshop on periodontology. Journal of Clinical Periodontology. 2008;**35**(suppl):168-172

[27] Aghaloo TL, Moy PK. Which hard tissue augmentation techniques are the

most successful in furnishing bony support for implant placement? The International Journal of Oral & Maxillofacial Implants. 2007;**22**(suppl):49-70

[28] Rachmiel A, Emodi O, Aizenbud D. Reconstruction of the alveolar ridge by osteodistraction for implant placement. Refu'at ha-peh veha-shinayim. 2011;**28**:30-36

[29] Alling CC. Lateral repositioning of inferior alveolar neurovascular bundle. Journal of Oral Surgery. 1977;**35**:419

[30] Jensen O, Nock D. Inferior alveolar nerve repositioning in conjunction with placement of osseointegrated implants: A case report. Oral Surgery, Oral Medicine, and Oral Pathology. 1987;**63**:263-268

[31] Rosenquist B. Fixture placement posterior to the mental foramen with transpositioning of the inferior alveolar nerve. The International Journal of Oral & Maxillofacial Implants. 1992;**7**:45-50

[32] Schlee M et al. Piezosurgery: Basics and possibilities. Implant Dentistry. 2006;**15**(4):334-340

[33] Friberg B, Ivanoff CJ, Lekholm U. Inferior alveolar nerve transposition in combination with Brånemark replant treatment. International Journal of Periodontics & Restorative Dentistry. 1992;**12**:6

[34] Dario LJ, English R. Achieving implant reconstruction through bilateral mandibular nerve repositioning. Journal of the American Dental Association. 1939;**125**(3):305-309

[35] Dao TTT, Mellor A. Sensory disturbances associated with implant surgery. International Journal of Prosthodontics. 1998;**11**:5

[36] Jayme SJ, Ramalho PR, De Franco L, Jugdar RE, Shibli JA, Vasco MA. Comparative finite element analysis of short implants and lateralization of the inferior alveolar nerve with different Prosthesis Heights. Journal of Craniofacial Surgery. 2015;**26**(8):2342-2346

[37] Quirynen M, Naert I, Van Steenberghe D. Fixture design and overload influence marginal bone loss and fixture success in the Branemark system. Clinical Oral Implants Research. 1992;**3**:104-111

[38] Schliephake H, Neukam FW, Wichmann M. Survival analysis of endosseous implants in bone grafts used for the treatment of severe alveolar ridge atrophy. Journal of Oral and Maxillofacial Surgery. 1997;**55**:1227-1233

[39] Gentile MA, Chuang SK, Dodson TB. Survival estimates and risk factors for failure with 6 × 5.7 implants. The International Journal of Oral & Maxillofacial Implants. 2005;**20**:930-937

[40] Lekholm U. The Branemark implant technique. A standardized procedure under continuous development. In: Laney WR, Tolman DE, editors. Tissue Integration in Oral, Orthopedic and Maxillofacial Reconstruction. Chicago: Quintessence; 1992. pp. 194-199

[41] Adell R, Eriksson B, Lekholm U, Brånemark PI, Jemt T. A long-term follow up study of osseointegrated implants in the treatment of totally edentulous jaws. The International Journal of Oral & Maxillofacial Implants. 1990;**5**:347-359

[42] Jemt T. Failures and complications in 391 consecutively inserted fixed prostheses supported by Branemark implants in edentulous jaws: A study of

treatment from the time of prosthesis placement to the first annual checkup. The International Journal of Oral & Maxillofacial Implants. 1991;**6**:270-276

[43] Renouard F, Arnoux JP, Sarment DP. Five-mm-diameter implants without a smooth surface collar: Report on 98 consecutive placements. The International Journal of Oral & Maxillofacial Implants. 1999;**14**:101-107

[44] Langer B, Langer L, Hermann I, Erug M. The wide implant: A solution for special bone situations and rescue for the compromised implant. Part I. The International Journal of Oral & Maxillofacial Implants. 1993;**8**:400-408

[45] Davies JE. Mechanisms of endosseous integration. The International Journal of Prosthodontics. 1998;**13**:391-401

[46] Dursun E, Keceli HG, Uysal S, Güngör H, Muhtarogullari M, Tözüm TF. Management of limited vertical bone height in the posterior mandible: Short dental implants versus nerve lateralization with standard length implants. Journal of Craniofacial Surgery. 2016;**27**(3):578-585

[47] Toledo Filho J, Marzola C, Toro I, Toledo Neto JL. Transposição do plexo nervoso alveolar inferior para fixação de implantes. Revista de Odontologia da Academia Tiradentes de Odontologia. 2005;**5**(7):784-797

[48] Garg AK, Morales MJ. Lateralization of the inferior alveolar nerve with simultaneous implant placement: Surgical techniques. Practical Periodontics and Aesthetic Dentistry. 1998;**10**(9):1197-1204

[49] Silva AC et al. Osteotomia segmentar da mandíbula com lateralização do nervo alveolar inferior para restabelecer o adequado espaço entre os arcos dentários. Revista Odontológica do Brasil Central. 1999;**8**(26):39-42

[50] Rudolf MS et al. Quantification off bone resorption in the foramidal region off the atrophic mandible. The International Journal of Oral and Maxillofacial Implants. 2007;**22**(4):609-615

[51] Allhassani AA, Alghamdi AST. Inferior alveolar nerve injury in implant dentistry: Diagnosis, causes, prevention and management. Journal of Oral Implantology. 2010;**36**(5):401-407

[52] Di Pillo L, Rapoport A. Importância da lateralização donervo alveolar inferior para os implantes mandibulares. Revista Brasileira de Cirurgia da Cabeça e Pescoço(online). 2014

[53] Sttelingsma K et al. Implantology and the severly resorbed edentulous mandible. Critical Reviews in Oral Biology and Medicine, Alexandria. 2004;**15**(4):240-248

[54] Garcia Junior IR et al. Vestibularização da estrutura neurovascular para colocação de implantes dentais. Innovations Implant Journal. 2006;**01**(01):71-74

[55] Goodacre CJ, Kan JYK, Rungcharassaeng K. Clinical complications of osseointegrated implants. Journal of Prosthetic Dentistry. 1999;**81**:537-552

[56] Winkler S, Morris HF, Ochi S. Implant survival to 36 months as related to length and diameter. Annals of Periodontology. 2000;**5**:22-31

[57] Griffin TJ, Cheung WS. The use of short, wide implants in posterior areas with reduced bone height: A

retrospective investigation. The Journal of Prosthetic Dentistry. 2004;**92**:139-144

[58] Tawil G, Younan R. Clinical evaluation of short, machined-surface implants followed for 12 to 92 months. The International Journal of Oral & Maxillofacial Implants. 2003;**18**:894-901

[59] Hori M et al. Neurosensory function and implant survival rate following implant placement with nerve transpositioning: A case study. Journal of Oral Science, Tokyo. 2001;**43**(2):139-144

[60] Peleg M et al. Lateralization of the inferior alveolar nerve with simultaneous implant placement: A modified technique. International Journal of Oral & Maxillofacial Implants. 2002;**17**(101):101-106

[61] Kan JY, Lozada JL, Boyne PJ, Goodacre CJ, Rungcharassaeng K. Mandibular fracture after endosseous implant placement in conjunction with inferior nerve transposition: A patient treatment report. International Journal of Oral & Maxillofacial Implants. 1997;**12**(5):655-659

[62] Garoushi IH, Elbeialy RR, Gibaly A, Atef M. Evaluation of the effect of the lateralized inferior alveolar nerve isolation and bone grafting on the nerve function and implant stability. (randomized clinical trial). Clinical Implant Dentistry and Related Research. 2021;**23**(3):423-431. DOI: 10.1111/cid.13003

Chapter 12

Temporomandibular Disorders: Current Diagnosis and Treatment Methods

Seyide Tugce Gokdeniz, Zehra Irem Ozturk Barut, Arda Buyuksungur and Mehmet Eray Kolsuz

Abstract

The term temporomandibular disorders is used as a collective term for a group of musculoskeletal disorders that involve pain dysfunction in the masticatory muscles, temporomandibular joints, and related structures. Patients with temporomandibular disorders usually present to clinics with pain, limitation, and noise in jaw movement. While clinical examination is considered the most important process in the diagnosis of temporomandibular disorders, imaging methods selected according to the cases, are also considered important aids in diagnosis. The use of artificial intelligence in the diagnosis of temporomandibular disorders is also becoming increasingly common. Current studies on this subject recommend the use of deep learning models to facilitate diagnosis and increase diagnostic accuracy. The etiology of temporomandibular disorders is quite complex and multifactorial. Due to this complex etiology, current studies support conservative multidisciplinary treatment methods including behavioral therapy, physical therapy, and pharmacotherapy. The role of osteotomy in the treatment of temporomandibular joint disorders is also very important. It is also stated that temporomandibular joint dysfunctions decrease after osteotomies such as sagittal splint osteotomy, which corrects occlusion disorders. The purpose of this chapter is to provide an overview of the latest developments in the etiology, pathophysiology, diagnosis, and treatment of temporomandibular disorders.

Keywords: temporomandibular disorders, temporomandibular joint, diagnosis, treatment, osteotomy

1. Introduction

Temporomandibular disorders (TMD) is a common oral-maxillofacial disorder that causes pain and dysfunction in the masticatory muscles, temporomandibular joint (TMJ), and their associated structures [1]. Worldwide epidemiology studies indicate that approximately 33% of the world's population has a symptom of TMD [2]. Occlusal patterns, neuromuscular system disorders, social and emotional situations, etc. TMD is among the risk factors [3]. A localized pain in the preauricular region, acoustic changes, limitation in mouth opening, etc., symptoms may occur. In some patients, TMD remains asymptomatic without any symptoms, and pathologies can be detected during imaging studies [4]. Diagnostic and treatment approaches for TMD are quite complex. It is important to carry out clinical and radiological examinations together. In chronic TMD cases, it can cause significant effects on the patient's quality of life [5].

The purpose of this chapter is to provide an overview of the latest developments in the etiologies and classifications, imaging and other investigations, diagnosis of TMD, and treatment modalities.

2. Etiology and classifications

2.1 Etiology

The etiology of TMD is complex and multifactorial. Factors that increase the risk of TMD are called 'predisposing factors', factors that cause its onset are called 'initiating factors', and factors that accelerate the progression of TMD or prevent their recovery are called 'maintaining factors' [6]. Maintaining factors include behavioral, emotional, and psychosocial factors [7]. There is no single etiological factor or theoretical model that can interpret the onset of TMD [8]. TMD can occur or progress due to both physical and psychosocial factors. Therefore, diagnosis and classification are difficult when a patient presents with more than one TMD at the same time, which makes it impossible to attribute the condition to a single specific cause [9]. Although it cannot be reduced to a single cause, macrotrauma, occlusal factors, emotional factors, and parafunctional habits can be evaluated among the etiological factors.

2.1.1 Macrotrauma

Macrotraumas is one of the initiating factors for TMD. Blows to the head or neck play an important role in the development of TMJ pathologies [10]. TMD may occur in situations such as yawning or keeping the mouth open for a long time [11], as well as a result of traumatic extractions of third molar teeth [12]. In addition, endotracheal intubation is thought to be a risk factor for TMD [13].

2.1.2 Occlusal status

Occlusal relationships are risk factors for TMD [14]. Although different types of malocclusions cause signs and symptoms of TMD, some occlusal features reflect the result of TMD rather than the cause [15].

2.1.3 Emotional factors

It has long been known that there is a significant relationship between psychological and emotional factors and TMD [16]. Depression and anxiety are important factors affecting pain perception. These factors can also lead to the development of teeth clenching and grinding, muscle hypertrophy and TMD [17].

2.1.4 Parafunctional habits

All habits that are considered non-functional are parafunctional habits and may cause microtrauma to the TMJ [18]. Parafunctional habits such as clenching and grinding can create abnormal forces that cause degenerative changes [14]. Due to these forces, tissue damage, micro bleeding and pain occur in the TMJ area [19].

2.2 Classification

2.2.1 Disorders of the mastic muscles

The most common symptom of disorders of the masticatory muscles is pain during function. This pain increases with the use of the muscles [20]. Disorders of the masticatory muscles are divided into five.

2.2.1.1 Protective muscle contraction

It is the response to an injury that has occurred or will occur in the area where the muscles are located. The antagonist muscle group in the relevant area contracts to protect against pain [21]. It occurs in cases where the mouth remains open for a long time due to intraoral injections or high restorations. Pain and movement limitations are observed during function [22].

2.2.1.2 Local muscle pain

It develops when protective muscle contraction continues. It may develop due to trauma, muscle overwork or stress, and it is not inflammatory. In addition to pain during function, minimal pain is observed at rest. Muscle fatigue is observed [22].

2.2.1.3 Myofascial pain

Myofascial pain in the masticatory muscles is the muscles being affected, becoming tense, and eventually getting tired, causing pain [20]. Hypersensitive muscle bundles, called trigger points, cause local pain during palpation, and the patient experiences limitations in mouth opening [23]. Different factors such as stress, depression, anxiety, parafunctional habits, bruxism, autoimmune diseases, and systemic diseases can cause it and become chronic [24].

2.2.1.4 Myospasm

Myospasms are sudden and acute involuntary muscle contractions. Pain, limitation of movement, and muscle tension are observed during function and rest [22]. It is rare. Its etiology is multifactorial [21].

2.2.1.5 Myositis and others

Myositis is an acute or chronic inflammation of the muscles. Although it is mostly caused by infection, its etiology is multifactorial [24]. Long-term local muscle pain and myofascial pain can also cause myositis [21]. Pain and dysfunction are observed in the muscles around the joint [25].

2.2.2 TMJ disorders

2.2.2.1 Irregularity in condyle disc complex

It occurs due to the disruption of the normal position and function of the disc on the condyle. The most common etiological factor is trauma. It can occur due to microtraumas, such as bruxism, and macrotraumas, such as impacts [26].

2.2.2.1.1 Disc displacement

Disc displacement in TMJ is the displacement of the joint disc toward the front, back, inner, and outer sides in the closed position. It usually occurs toward the front and anteromedial sides. As a result, pain and limited movement may occur during mandibular movements [27]. It usually occurs due to forces of abnormal intensity and direction applied to TMJ area. The steepness of the articular tubercle, the morphological structure of the glenoid fossa and condyle, and the looseness of intra-articular structures may also affect the formation of disc displacement [21].

2.2.2.1.1.1 Reduced disc displacement

The articular disc, which is positioned in front of the condyle head when the mouth is closed, returns to its normal position at the condyle head when the mouth is opened (**Figure 1**) [28]. In reduced disc displacement, a first click occurs during mouth opening, and a second click occurs when the disc returns to its anterior displacement position during mouth closing. This sound is called a reciprocal click [21]. Pain, tenderness, limitation of mouth opening, and deviation to the displaced side may be observed [29]. The timing of the click sounds when the mouth is opened (early, middle, late) indicates the degree of disc displacement. If the click sound comes early, it indicates that the displacement is at an early level. If it comes late, it indicates that the displacement is at an advanced level [29].

2.2.2.1.1.2 Reductionless disc dislocation

Problems occur in disc positioning due to elasticity loss in the upper retrodiscal lamina. As the condyle slides forward, the articular disc is positioned in front of the condyle. The articular disc, which is displaced toward the front of the condyle head when the mouth is closed, cannot return to its normal position when the mouth is opened [28] (**Figure 1**). Pain, limitation of mouth opening, and deviation to the affected side are observed in acute nonreducible disc displacement cases. Deviation is not observed in cases where both joints are affected. In chronic cases, the pain disappears [29].

2.2.2.1.2 Disc perforation

TMJ disc perforation usually occurs due to prolonged anterior displacement and repetitive folding of the disc during the opening and closing of the jaw. Osteoarthrosis and trauma can also cause disc perforation [30].

2.2.2.2 Structural incompatibility of joint surfaces

It occurs due to changes in normal physiological joint functions and structures. The most common etiological factor is macrotrauma [21]. There are four types of structural incompatibilities of joint surfaces.

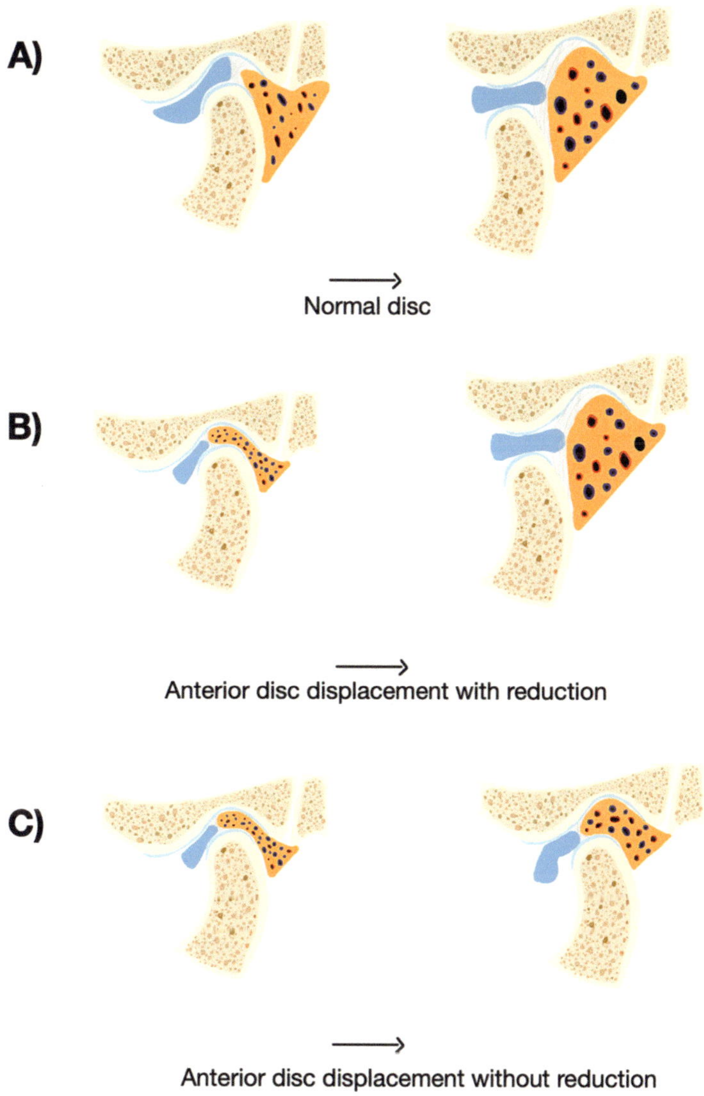

Figure 1.
Schematization of disc positions in the open and closed of the mouth (A) Normal disc (B) Anterior disc displacement with reduction (C) Anterior disk displacement without reduction.

2.2.2.2.1 Shape changes

Physiological aging or degeneration in the condyle, articular eminence, disc, or fossa causes the functions and structure of the joint to change. It can be seen as osteophytes, flattening, erosion, and subchondral cysts in the bone and as changes in thickness and perforation in the disc [31]. This situation causes dysfunction [20].

2.2.2.2.2 Adhesions

It is the long-term persistence of adhesions between the condyle and the disc or between the disc and the fossa. It may be due to fibrous connective tissue or decreased lubrication. It causes limitations in functional movements and mouth opening [20, 24].

2.2.2.2.3 Subluxation (hypermobility)

TMJ condyle passes anterior to the articular eminence during mouth opening. Causes include acute or chronic trauma, laxity of intra-articular ligaments, decreased height of the articular eminence, and abnormal position of the articular eminence. It is painless and spontaneous [21].

2.2.2.2.4 Spontaneous dislocation (open locking)

Dislocation of TMJ is the displacement of the mandibular condyle anterior to the decreased articular height and preventing it from returning to the fossa [32, 33]. Spasms of the masticatory muscles, laxity of the intra-articular ligaments, decreased height of the articular eminence, abnormal position of the articular eminence, arthritic changes in the condyle, or neurological problems may cause recurrent dislocations [34].

2.2.2.3 Inflammatory diseases

Diseases of inflammatory origin are usually characterized by severe and constant pain during function. Tactile sensitivity and protective contractions may also be observed [20]. These diseases are classified according to the structures involved in inflammation:

synovitis/capsulitis, retrodiscitis, arthritis, and others.

2.2.2.3.1 Synovitis/capsulitis

Synovitis is the inflammation of synovial tissues, and capsulitis is the inflammation of the capsular ligament [25]. Trauma may be the cause of synovitis and capsulitis. Limitation of jaw movements, pain, and tenderness on palpation may occur [20].

2.2.2.3.2 Retrodiscitis

It is an inflammation of the retrodiscal tissues. It occurs due to trauma or excessive pressure of the condylar head on the retrodiscal tissues. There is a limitation in jaw movements. Pain increases with clenching of teeth [20]. In cases where swelling occurs in the retrodiscal tissue, the condyle is pushed anteriorly, and acute malocclusion is observed on the same side [21].

2.2.2.3.3 Arthritis

Arthritis is inflammation of the articular surfaces of a joint. Signs of inflammation include pain, edema, warmth, redness, and loss of function. There are three types: osteoarthritis, osteoarthrosis and polyarthritis [20]. The most common type of TMJ is osteoarthritis, which is a destructive disease of the articular surfaces of the condyle and fossa. It may occur as a result of forces exerted on the joint exceeding the load-carrying capacity of the joint [35]. Polyarthritis develops due to rheumatic diseases. Among these, the ones that most affect TMJ are rheumatoid arthritis and ankylosing spondylitis [36].

2.2.2.3.4 Inflammative diseases of related structures

Inflammation of the tendon that attaches the temporal muscle to the coronoid process is called temporal tendonitis. It may occur as a result of bruxism and emotional stress. Pain and limitation of mouth opening are observed. Inflammation of the stylomandibular ligament is characterized by pain and limitation of mouth opening in the area where the ligament attaches to the mandible [21].

2.2.3 Chronic mandibular hypomobility

It is a long-term painless restriction of mouth opening. It is divided into three according to its etiology.

2.2.3.1 Ankylosis

Ankylosis is the development of adhesions on the articular surfaces of the joint, causing fusion between the mandible and the temporal bone [37]. It is divided into two: fibrous and osseous. If it develops as a result of fibrotic changes or fibrous adhesions in the capsular ligament, it is called fibrous ankylosis, and if it develops as a result of the union of bone structures due to the proliferation of bone cells, it is called osseous ankylosis [22]. In addition to limited movement, it causes difficulties in chewing and speaking, deterioration of oral health, facial asymmetry, and mandibular growth disorders [38, 39]. Depending on the type, degree, and age of onset of ankylosis, patients may present with various symptoms [40].

2.2.3.2 Muscle contractures

There are two types: myostatic contraction and myofibrotic contraction. Myostatic contraction occurs when the muscle remains tense for a long time. Myofibrotic contraction occurs due to myositis or trauma. Both result in painless restriction of mouth opening.In addition, lateral movements of the condyle were not affected by myofibrotic contraction [21].

2.2.3.3 Coronoid impedance (coronoid obstruction)

It occurs as a result of excessive elongation of the coronoideus process or the development of fibrosis in this area. It may occur due to surgical operation, trauma or infection. The deviation is observed on the affected side, but the deviation is not observed in cases where both joints are affected [21].

2.2.4 Developmental disorders

Developmental abnormalities of the bony components of TMJ include agenesis (absence of growth), hypoplasia (insufficient growth), hyperplasia (excessive growth), and neoplasia (uncontrolled destructive growth). Developmental disorders seen in the muscular components of the TMJ are hypotrophy (decrease in muscle size and strength), hyperplasia (increase in muscle size and strength) and neoplasia (uncontrolled destructive growth) [20].

3. Imaging and other investigations

TMJ region is a difficult area to image due to the complex structure of the hard and soft tissue components in this region, the overlapping of neighboring anatomical structures, changes in condyle morphology, limited mouth opening and lower jaw movements [41]. Different imaging methods are used to examine the functions and pathologies of TMJ. These vary in terms of usability, cost, bone and soft tissue imaging capabilities. Imaging methods used for the TMJ region are described below.

3.1 Conventional radiographies

Conventional radiographies are two-dimensional imaging methods used in TMJ imaging [42]. These methods are transcranio-oblique projection (schüller), transpharyngeal projection, transorbital projection, submentovertex projection, Reverse-Towne's projection, and posterioanterior radiography. The advantages of these methods are low radiation dose, easy accessibility and low costs [43]. The most important disadvantages of these methods are superposition, distortion, position errors, and inadequacy in soft tissue imaging. However, conventional radiography can be used for rapid and general assessment in emergency situations such as trauma [35, 43].

3.2 Panoramic radiography

Panoramic radiographs are two-dimensional imaging methods frequently used in dentistry and including ionizing radiation [42]. Teeth, jaw bones, temporomandibular joint, maxillary sinuses, and nasal cavity can be viewed simultaneously in a single image [44]. In this imaging technique, the central X-ray beam is oblique to the long axis of the condyle. Therefore, only the medial and lateral parts of the bony components of TMJ can be examined [45]. During imaging, because the mandible is positioned forward and partially open, information about condylar position and function cannot be provided. Due to superpositions, the relationship between the articular fossa and the condyle, the articular eminence, and slight bone changes cannot be determined. Significant bone changes, fractures, asymmetry, and pathological findings of TMJ can be evaluated [35, 41, 45, 46]. Other disadvantages of panoramic radiography include errors in patient positioning, the patient's inability to stand or maintain a straight neck position during the scan, the patient's inability to remain still during the scan, and artifacts that occur at any stage during the scan [47]. The advantages of panoramic radiography are relatively low radiation dose, easy accessibility, low costs, ability to combine with dental records, wide imaging field, condylar morphology, and ability to be evaluated in a short time [48]. New-generation panoramic radiography devices with special programs for imaging TMJ areas increase reliability by reducing superpositions [41, 44].

3.3 Arthrography

Arthrography is a technique in which radiopaque contrast material is injected to visualize soft tissues into both the upper and lower joint spaces to visualize the joint [42, 45]. While other imaging methods provide information on static images, arthrography can directly observe the joint condition through dynamic images and accurately determine the position, size and condition of the joint structure [49]. Disc perforations, disc position and morphology, adhesions, and internal irregularities can be detected by arthrography. Arthrography is the gold standard for diagnosing joint disc perforation [50]. The ability to perform arthrocentesis during arthrography is an important advantage. Disadvantages of arthroscopy include being an invasive technique, requiring experience, not providing detailed information about bone surfaces, high dose radiation, allergic reactions to iodinated contrast material, risk of disc perforation, risk of facial nerve injury due to the needle used, and risk of bleeding and infection [45, 46, 51].

3.4 Computed tomography (CT)

Computed tomography is a three-dimensional imaging technique that uses a fan-shaped X-ray beam [42]. Ct eliminates disadvantages such as superposition and distortion in two-dimensional imaging methods. Both the bone structures and soft tissues of TMJ can be evaluated [42]. Pathological changes in bone structure such as fractures, dislocations, ankylosis, osteophytes, condylar erosions, subchondral cysts, degenerative bone changes, arthritis, neoplasia, and developmental anomalies such as condylar hyperplasia can be detected by CT. Multidetector CT is more common today than conventional tomography [52]. Low-dose MDCT is useful in cases where MRI is contraindicated or not available. In addition, because of its superior soft tissue contrast, MDCT can detect pathologies that cannot be detected with CBCT [45, 46]. The most important disadvantages of CT are high radiation dose, longer scanning time, equipment accessibility, and cost compared to CBCT [45, 53]. CT is also weaker in imaging the joint disc than arthrography and MRI [45].

3.5 Cone-beam computed tomography (CBCT)

Cone-beam computed tomography is a three-dimensional imaging technique that uses a cone-shaped X-ray beam [42, 45]. It is used in the examination of the bone structures of TMJ, the evaluation of developmental anomalies, and the examination of pathologies such as osteophytes, erosions, flattening, ankylosis, fractures, subchondral sclerosis, and pseudocysts [54]. Without overlapping structures, the position and volume of the bony components of the joint can be determined and height, inclination measurements can also be made [48, 55]. In addition, it is also used to evaluate airway volume, sinuses, nasal cavity and congenital defects [53]. However, it is inadequate in the evaluation of soft tissues such as joint discs [56]. Additionally, CBCT allows the position of the condyle to be evaluated with minimal distortion, both in open and closed mouth positions [41]. CBCT is a reliable method for examining the bone components of TMJ in axial, sagittal, and coronal sections and is easy and reproducible [54]. In addition to having a lower radiation dose than CT, a shorter scanning time, and a smaller device, it also has a higher spatial resolution [41, 53]. Although it is a 3D imaging technique, 2D images can also be obtained [53]. Disadvantages of CBCT, very high density objects such as metal restorations, implants, root fillings or metal posts cause beam hardening artifacts. This negatively affects the diagnosis. The acquisition time is longer than that of conventional radiographs and panoramic radiography. This makes it difficult for patients to tolerate [57].

3.6 Ultrasonography (US)

Ultrasonography is a non-invasive imaging method that obtains real-time images using sound waves and does not contain ionizing radiation [42]. Fast and dynamic image acquisition, easy accessibility, and affordable cost are the advantages of US [58]. Pediatric patients can tolerate it more easily because it is not in a closed area and does not require sedation. And patients who cannot have an MRI scan due to claustrophobia can also tolerate it more easily [58, 59]. Soft tissues the position of the articular disc, type of intra-articular derangement, joint space, effusion, inflammation and ligament adhesion can be examined by US. In hard tissues, erosions and osteophytes occurring anterior and lateral to the condyle can be examined. However, the medial side of the condyle cannot be examined due to the superposition of the bony structures [45]. Because of the acquisition of dynamic images, disc mobility, condylar translation and anterior disc displacement can be evaluated [60]. However, changes in the medial part of the condyle and medial disc displacement cannot be examined with US. In addition, US imaging becomes difficult in cases of bone pathologies, preauricular swelling, and intra-articular effusion [51, 58]. Another disadvantage is that it depends on the operator's knowledge and experience [52]. US does not provide the same quality of detail as MRI, but it is suitable for TMJ evaluation due to its cost and ease of access [60]. US is not only used to detect the disease. It can also be used for disease tracking and the course of treatment [58, 59]. Because of the advances in technology, dynamic high-resolution US is more useful in evaluating TMD compared to static low-resolution US [58].

3.7 Magnetic resonance imaging (MRI)

Magnetic resonance imaging is a non-invasive three-dimensional imaging method that does not contain ionizing radiation, using magnetic fields and radiofrequency waves [42, 45]. Because it is non-invasive, it is safe for repeat shots [60]. MRI has high soft tissue imaging capability and provides important information about the soft tissue components of TMJ [48]. The disc's morphology and position, the retrodiscal tissues status, the associated muscles and the presence of inflammation can be evaluated with MRI in the open and closed mouth positions [50]. In addition to acute changes such as effusion, bone marrow edema, synovial thickening, chronic changes such as erosions, condylar changes, disc abnormalities, new bone tissue formation, soft tissue neoplasias, and neoplasia-like lesions can also be evaluated with MRI [58, 61, 62]. Although distortion in the articular disc can be visualized with MRI, disc perforation has still some limitations. A layer of synovial hyperplasia beneath the tortuous articular disc may lead to false-negative results. With new developments, it is also possible to visualize hard tissues in MRI, but these images are not yet detailed enough to be compared with CBCT or MDCT images [42, 50]. MRI with a contrast agent provides additional information about the soft tissues in TMJ area [61]. However, sedation or general anesthesia may be required due to the long imaging time and intravenous injection of contrast material,, especially in pediatric patients [58, 59]. Its disadvantages are its long imaging time, high cost, difficulty in transportation, equipment standards, the importance of parameter imaging, the need for the patient to be completely immobile during imaging, its dependence on the experience of the observer, its failure to be as successful as CBCT and CT in the evaluation of bone cortices, and its inability to be used in patients with claustrophobia, ferromagnetic intra-body implants, intracranial vascular clips, and pacemakers [45, 46, 51]. With dynamic MRI, joint mobility and disc function can be examined in detail during functional movements [60].

3.8 Nuclear medicine

It is the only imaging method that can detect the physiological effects of biochemical changes on functions [42]. Radionuclides used for imaging are injected into the patient intravenously and the reflected gamma rays are detected by a camera and transferred to the computer. In this way, the image is obtained [63]. The most commonly used radionuclide is technetium because it can be monitored at low radiation dose and has a short half-life (Tc-99 m) [42]. Nuclear imaging can be used to evaluate the skeletal development of TMJ and measure the degree of disease in patients with osteoarthritis. However, its most important disadvantages are its inadequacy in showing bone component morphology and disc displacements and the application of radioactive chemicals to the whole body by intravenous injection [63]. In addition to TMJ region, the entire maxillofacial region can be examined. It is divided into three types [45].

3.8.1 Scintigraphy

Images showing bone metabolic activity are obtained 2–3 hours after intravenous radionuclide injection [52]. Radioisotopes accumulate in areas with increased osteoblastic activity and are seen as 'hot' areas [45]. It is a non-specific examination but sensitive for detecting bone disorders such as growth, bone healing, active bone changes, trauma, infection, tumors and arthritic changes [52]. Scintigraphy can detect early changes related to the bone components of TMJ. In this way, malocclusion and facial asymmetry can be prevented early [64]. However, its routine use is limited due to high costs and radiation [65].

3.8.2 Spect (single proton emission computed tomography)

Images are obtained by recording radiation emissions using positron-emitting radionuclides with the help of a rotating gamma camera [45]. Although TMJ is a small joint in close proximity to the skull base and paranasal sinuses, it can be examined separately from other bones with SPECT. The morphological and functional status of hard tissues, degenerative bone changes and metabolic studies can be evaluated with SPECT [45, 66]. Condylar hyperplasia is the abnormal growth of the mandibular condyles. If this growth is excessive and unilateral, it causes facial asymmetry, malocclusions and related problems [67]. SPECT is superior to planar imaging methods for measuring differences in condylar growth in cases of condylar hyperplasia. In these cases, it is important to be able to detect growth activity, as facial asymmetry can only be treated when growth stops [46]. The most important disadvantage is that a non-anatomical examination. Although areas of improvement and high involvement can be quickly identified, their causes may not be determined [52].

3.8.3 Pet

A gamma camera and radiopharmaceuticals are used to detect metabolic processes, producing images that provide functional information. The most commonly used radiopharmaceutical is 2-fluoro-2-deoxyglucose labeled with fluoride-18 (18FDG) [52]. It is frequently used in the early diagnosis of neoplasms, staging of some tumors, radiotherapy planning, determining the location of the primary tumor and diagnosing response to treatment and recurrence [45]. The most important advantages are higher detection efficiency and spatial resolution than to scintigraphy [45]. PET can be used in combination with CT and MRI [52].

4. Diagnosis of TMD

Identifying the causes of TMD-related pain and dysfunction is very important as it affects the choice of treatment method. For example, different treatment options are often used to treat arthrogenous TMD and muscle-derived TMD. Patients with psychological comorbidities who exhibit TMD symptoms without an obvious physical cause may be best treated with psychological intervention [68]. Detection of more serious disorders that require urgent intervention is the most important part of TMD diagnosis [69]. For example, differential diagnosis is of great importance because some neoplasms, such as TMJ chondrosarcoma, may initially share the same signs and symptoms as some common diagnoses of TMD [70].

Although different diagnostic tools have been proposed for TMD, the most commonly used is the Diagnostic Criteria for Temporomandibular Disorders (DC/TMD) [71]. DC/TMD aims to provide a standardized and functional tool that combines physical examination (axis I) and screening for psychosocial-comorbid factors (axis II) for use in the diagnosis of TMD. This method of examination provides confirmation that any pain revealed during the examination is similar to or reproduces the same pain as a familiar pain that the patient has experienced in life [71]. This diagnostic tool recommends the use of a screening questionnaire called DC/TMD, TMD Pain Screen to simply and reliably assess the presence of painful TMD [71, 72]. This questionnaire cannot make specific TMD diagnoses but can provide rapid screening in busy clinical or research settings.

A further diagnostic axis (axis III) has been proposed to represent the underlying pathobiological processes of TMD, including diagnostic findings from genetics, epigenetics, and neuroscience [70]. This axis, which is not involved in DC/TMD, may have important implications for improving disease diagnosis and targeted management.

Artificial intelligence is rapidly taking its place among current diagnostic methods and helps physicians in diagnosis [73]. Since the ability of deep learning models to detect TMJ arthropathies with high sensitivity and specificity increases diagnostic accuracy, it is stated in current studies that this methodology can be used to evaluate TMD [74].

The use of biomarkers in saliva and serum for the diagnosis of TMD is another current study topic [75]. However, due to the lack of evidence on this subject, it is thought that more case-control studies are necessary [76].

5. Treatment modalities

Considering the complex biopsychosocial and multifactorial etiology of TMD, the use of multidisciplinary treatment methods may be required. In addition, the focus should be on pain management and psychosocial functionality. Since the majority of TMD cases undergo remission in the first 6–15 months, physicians recommend reversible conservative treatments.

However, each case should be evaluated on its own, and multimodal strategies should be included in the treatment plan, taking into account etiological factors. Therefore, it is important to know irreversible interventional treatments and to follow current treatment approaches. In this section, treatment methods are detailed under two main headings: 'Reversible and conservative treatments' and 'Irreversible and invasive treatments'.

5.1 Reversible and conservative treatments

5.1.1 Self-care techniques

An essential part of non-invasive conservative initial treatment is known as 'self-care' or 'self-management'. The components of a standard self-management program are education, self-exercise therapy, thermal modalities, self-massage therapy, diet and nutrition, parafunctional behavior [77]. It is important to detect, observe and prevent parafunctions such as gum chewing, nail biting, bruxism etc. Self-massage, therapeutic exercises, diet regulation and breathing exercises are also frequently used in treatments [77, 78].

5.1.2 Intraoral appliances

Occlusal splint is a widely accepted treatment for TMD worn over the upper and lower teeth, determining the occlusion and the condyle-mandibular fossa relationship [68]. Due to occlusal splints, occlusion is fixed and teeth are protected from excessive wear [79, 80]. There are also studies indicating that the use of occlusal splints is effective in relieving pain symptoms [81, 82].

5.1.3 Pharmacotherapy

A number of pharmacological treatments, such as analgesics, neuromodulatory agents, and intramuscular injections, are used for the treatment of TMD [78]. As with any drug treatment, all possible risks, side effects and interactions of the drug should be considered before prescribing [83]. Therefore, a comprehensive evaluation of medical history is very important in preventing allergic reactions and complications.

5.1.3.1 Nonsteroidal anti-inflammatory drugs (NSAID)

The use of NSAIDs is recommended in cases of acute temporomandibular arthritis caused by sudden disc displacement [68]. In acute temporomandibular arthritis, it is recommended to continue treatment for at least 2 weeks, and it is also recommended to use NSAIDs together with gastroprotective agents due to side effects on the gastrointestinal tract [84].

5.1.3.2 Corticosteroids

The use of corticosteroids is recommended for the treatment of moderate to severe TMD [68]. Corticosteroids have anti-inflammatory effects that help relieve pain. It is suitable for intra-articular injection or oral use. In intra-articular injection use, it can be combined with a local anesthetic (lidocaine, etc.) [85].

5.1.3.3 Myorelaxants

The use of muscle relaxants is important in the treatment of muscular TMD and chronic orofacial pain [68]. Muscle relaxants reduce skeletal muscle tone, thus helping to relieve muscle-related pain [86]. Cyclobenzaprine, metaxalone, methocarbamol are the most commonly used muscle relaxants [68]. Cyclobenzaprines are stated to relieve muscular pain and improve sleep quality [87].

Such medications can cause significant sedation. The use of muscle relaxants is contraindicated in patients with hyperthyroidism, heart failure, post-myocardial infarction, and heart rhythm disturbances [88]. A 10 mg dose at bedtime for 30 days followed by 2 weeks of medical follow-up is recommended [68].

5.1.3.4 Anticonvulsants

Gabapentin, a GABA analog anticonvulsant, can be used to reduce muscular pain, especially from the temporal and masseter muscles [68]. The pain-reducing effect of gabapentin is thought to occur through blocking neurotransmitter release and reducing postsynaptic excitability [89]. Gabapentins are generally well tolerated and are associated with temporary mild side effects (dizziness, drowsiness, dry mouth, weight gain and impaired concentration, etc.) [90].

5.1.4 Psychological and multimodal therapies

Behavioral approaches, which aim to reduce the frequency of behaviors that increase pain and increase the frequency of behaviors that increase health, are a multidimensional treatment method. Psychological and behavioral therapies are not only effective in alleviating the psychological crisis, but can also help the patient change his or her perception of pain. It also allows improving functionality in patients with chronic pain [91]. The duration of the program and the delivery of the treatment in an individual or group environment do not affect the therapeutic effect [68].

A study examining the effect of Cognitive Behavioral Therapy (CBT) shows that CBT provides long-term (>3 months) improvements in symptoms such as TMD pain and depression [92]. Patients with TMD and major psychological symptoms (anxiety, depression, etc.) have been shown to achieve greater improvement with multimodal treatment than TMD patients without major psychological symptoms [93]. It has been stated that biofeedback and relaxation training also have an important place in treatment [93].

5.1.5 Physical therapy

Physiotherapy is a health science discipline that aims to eliminate, alleviate, prevent and restore functional ability to dysfunctions involving the neuromuscular, musculoskeletal and other systems through movement and various physical factors [94]. Randomized clinical trials using postural exercises suggest relief of muscle pain and improvements in jaw mobility in TMD compared to education and cognitive behavioral therapy [95]. Combinations of jaw strengthening and coordination exercises and mobilization and posture exercises can also be applied together. Additionally, physical therapy techniques such as manual therapy, Kinesio Taping, Ultrasound and Transcutaneous Electrical Nerve Stimulation (TENS) are also frequently used in TMD [96].

5.1.6 Acupuncture, dry needling and substance injection for TMD myalgia

Acupuncture is frequently used in the treatment of chronic pain [97]. Acupuncture points generally correspond to points called trigger points and areas where the density of nerve endings transmitting the feeling of pain increases. The use of acupuncture has been shown to cause short-term improvement in TMD muscle pain compared to placebo acupuncture [97]. Dry needling has similarly been found to provide short-term improvements in TMD muscle pain [98]. Results are available on the effects of intramuscular botulinum toxin injections compared to placebo for TMD muscle pain [99].

5.2 Irreversible and invasive treatments

5.2.1 Surgical treatments and osteotomies for TMD

Interventions such as arthroscopy, arthrocentesis, arthroplasty, or joint replacement are irreversible invasive treatments used for patients with arthrogenic TMD [100]. These invasive procedures used in the treatment of TMD have been shown to be associated with significant morbidity [93].

It has been stated that surgical interventions (arthroscopy and arthroplasty) have no additional effect compared to medical treatment or non-surgical rehabilitation in patients with non-reducing disc displacement with limited mouth opening. It has also been reported that no difference was observed in pain intensity and frequency, mandibular range of motion, TMJ sounds or chewing disorder [101].

Open surgical treatment for TMD has become less common but is still used for certain indications and end-stage disease [102]. In fact, in cases such as ankylosis and neoplasms, relieving the ankylosis and removing the tumor may be the only viable option. With developing technologies, there is now an arthroscopic surgery option for procedures that were only performed with an open joint approach in the past. Disc repositioning, osteophyte removal, pathological tissue removal and TMJ biopsy can be performed with arthroscopic surgery [9].

Examining the effects of jaw osteotomies on TMJ is an important research area. Mandibular angle osteotomy with outer cortex grinding method is among the cosmetic procedures used to correct the square face form. To evaluate the safety of this procedure, analyzed the morphological stabilization of the TMJ and morphological changes in masseter muscle thickness after mandibular angle osteotomy [103]. It has been stated that mandibular angle osteotomy is safe and suitable for use in terms of occlusal function [104].

Sagittal split ramus osteotomy is a type of osteotomy commonly used to correct dentofacial deformities [105]. A study reported that 1 year after sagittal split ramus osteotomy, the tensile energy density in the articular disc was significantly reduced compared to before surgery [106]. In a study examining the effects of modified L-shaped intraoral vertico-sagittal ramus osteotomy and sagittal split ramus osteotomy on TMJ symptoms, it was found that modified L-shaped intraoral vertico-sagittal ramus osteotomy reduced TMJ symptoms more than sagittal split ramus osteotomy [107]. In the light of these information, it can be concluded that TMD symptoms can be alleviated by sagittal split ramus osteotomy and modified L-shaped intraoral vertico-sagittal ramus osteotomy, which correct the discrepancy in maxillofacial morphology.

6. Future predictions

Significant progress has been made in understanding the biological and psychological determinants of TMD but many factors remain missing and unexplained [108]. Future TMD etiological research will inevitably include a more detailed evaluation of life stressors, uncommon genetic variants, and genome associations [109, 110].

A study has investigated the effect of painless positioning of the head of the mandibular condyle in the joint fossa on postural and functional changes in the musculoskeletal system [111]. It can also be foreseen that in the future, dental diagnostic procedures for TMD may be combined with a posture examination.

Today, due to deep learning models, TMJ arthropathies can be detected with high sensitivity and specificity [73, 74]. The increased use of artificial intelligence will allow for increased diagnostic accuracy enabled by an evidence-based framework, objective measurements, and advanced analysis techniques.

There has been an observed improvement in the prognosis and longevity of alloplastic joint prostheses [112, 113]. Due to these successful results, it can be predicted that the popularity of alloplastic TMJ replacement will gradually increase in cases such as end-stage arthritic conditions, ankylosis, post-tumor resection and developmental anomalies of TMJ.

Examining the effects of jaw osteotomies on TMJ is among the current research topics [104]. There are studies examining sagittal split ramus osteotomy, modified L-shaped intraoral vertico-sagittal ramus osteotomy and mandibular angle osteotomies [104, 106, 107]. The number of studies examining the effects of other osteotomy methods involving the head and face region on the TMJ will continue to increase in the future.

In a study in which exosomes obtained from mesenchymal stem cells were used for the first time, successful results were obtained for the treatment of TMJ disc degeneration [114]. It is clinically promising that the use of bone marrow stem cells, a current treatment approach for TMJ disc degeneration, will continue to be investigated and that its use may increase in the future.

Author details

Seyide Tugce Gokdeniz[1*], Zehra Irem Ozturk Barut[1*], Arda Buyuksungur[2] and Mehmet Eray Kolsuz[1]

1 Dentomaxillofacial Radiology Department, Faculty of Dentistry, Ankara University, Ankara, Turkey

2 Basic Medical Sciences Department, Faculty of Dentistry, Ankara University, Ankara, Turkey

*Address all correspondence to: seyidetugce@gmail.com and z.iremozturk@hotmail.com

References

[1] Yap AU et al. Comparison of psychological states and oral health-related quality of life of patients with differing severity of temporomandibular disorders. Journal of Oral Rehabilitation. 2022;**49**(2):177-185

[2] Dworkin SF, LeResche L. Research diagnostic criteria for temporomandibular disorders: Review, criteria, examinations and specifications, critique. Journal of Craniomandibular Disorders. 1992;**6**(4):301-355

[3] De Boever JA, Carlsson GE, Klineberg IJ. Need for occlusal therapy and prosthodontic treatment in the management of temporomandibular disorders. Part I. Occlusal interferences and occlusal adjustment. Journal of Oral Rehabilitation. 2000;**27**(5):367-379

[4] Yadav S et al. Temporomandibular joint disorders in older adults. Journal of the American Geriatrics Society. 2018;**66**(6):1213-1217

[5] Abdel-Alim HM et al. Validity of cone-beam computed tomography in assessment of morphological bony changes of temporomandibular joints. The Journal of Contemporary Dental Practice. 2020;**21**(2):133-139

[6] Sharma S et al. Etiological factors of temporomandibular joint disorders. National Journal of Maxillofacial Surgery. 2011;**2**(2):116-119

[7] Chisnoiu AM et al. Factors involved in the etiology of temporomandibular disorders-a literature review. Clujul Medical Journal. 2015;**88**(4):473

[8] Chang CL et al. Functional disorders of the temporomandibular joints: Internal derangement of the temporomandibular joint. The Kaohsiung Journal of Medical Sciences. 2018;**34**(4):223-230

[9] Li DTS, Leung YY. Temporomandibular disorders: Current concepts and controversies in diagnosis and management. Diagnostics (Basel). 2021;**11**(3):165-179

[10] Fischer DJ et al. The association of temporomandibular disorder pain with history of head and neck injury in adolescents. Journal of Orofacial Pain. 2006;**20**(3):191-198

[11] Sahebi S et al. Effect of lengthy root canal therapy sessions on temporomandibular joint and masticatory muscles. Journal of Dental Research, Dental Clinics, Dental Prospects. 2010;**4**(3):95-97

[12] Huang GJ, Rue TC. Third-molar extraction as a risk factor for temporomandibular disorder. Journal of the American Dental Association (1939). 2006;**137**(11):1547-1554

[13] Dwivedi AN et al. Magnetic resonance imaging evaluation of temporomandibular joint and associated soft tissue changes following acute condylar injury. Journal of Oral and Maxillofacial Surgery. 2012;**70**(12):2829-2834

[14] Okeson JP. Temporomandibular disorders: Etiology and classification. In: Kandasamy S, Greene CS, Rinchuse DJ, Stockstill JW, editors. TMD and Orthodontics: A Clinical Guide for the Orthodontist. Cham: Springer International Publishing; 2015. pp. 19-36

[15] Pullinger AG, Seligman DA. Quantification and validation of predictive values of occlusal variables in temporomandibular disorders using

a multifactorial analysis. The Journal of Prosthetic Dentistry. 2000;**83**(1):66-75

[16] Ryalat S et al. Prevalence of temporomandibular joint disorders among students of the University of Jordan. Journal of Clinical Medicine Research. 2009;**1**(3):158

[17] Melo RA et al. Conservative therapies to treat pain and anxiety associated with temporomandibular disorders: A randomized clinical trial. International Dental Journal. 2020;**70**(4):245-253

[18] O'Connor RC, Shakib K, Brennan PA. Recent advances in the management of oral and maxillofacial trauma. British Journal of Oral and Maxillofacial Surgery. 2015;**53**(10):913-921

[19] Ingawale S, Goswami T. Temporomandibular joint: Disorders, treatments, and biomechanics. Annals of Biomedical Engineering. 2009;**37**:976-996

[20] Maini K, Dua A. Temporomandibular syndrome. In: StatPearls. Treasure Island (FL): StatPearls Publishing; 2024

[21] Okeson J. Management of Temporomandibular Disorders and Occlusion. Mosby: Elsevier; 2013. p. 129

[22] Yaltırık M et al. Temporomandibular joint disorders and diagnosis. Yeditepe Dental Journal. 2017;**13**:43-50

[23] García-de-la-Banda-García R, Cortés-Pérez I, Ibancos-Losada MdR, López-Ruiz MdC, Obrero-Gaitán E, Osuna-Pérez MC. Effectiveness of dry needling versus manual therapy in myofascial temporomandibular disorders: A single-blind randomized controlled trial. Journal of Personalized Medicine. 2023;**13**(9):1415

[24] Zlatanovska K et al. Classification of temporomandibular disorders. Knowledge-International Journal. 2021;**49**(4):693-698

[25] Zhang X et al. Low-intensity pulsed ultrasound in the treatment of masticatory myositis and temporomandibular joint synovitis: A clinical trial. Journal of Stomatology, Oral and Maxillofacial Surgery. 2024;**125**(1):101632

[26] Yun PY, Kim YK. The role of facial trauma as a possible etiologic factor in temporomandibular joint disorder. Journal of Oral and Maxillofacial Surgery. 2005;**63**(11):1576-1583

[27] Huang D et al. Association between chewing side preference and MRI characteristics in patients with anterior disc displacement of the temporomandibular joint. Journal of Stomatology, Oral and Maxillofacial Surgery. 2023;**124**(5):101484

[28] Young AL. Internal derangements of the temporomandibular joint: A review of the anatomy, diagnosis, and management. The Journal of Indian Prosthodontic Society. 2015;**15**(1):2-7

[29] Laskin DM, Greene CS, Hylander WL. TMDs, an Evidence-Based Approach to Diagnosis and Treatment. Chicago, IL: Quintessence Publishing; 2006

[30] Wang T et al. Application of modified articular disc anchorage in treating the perforation and rupture of temporomandibular joint disc. Hua Xi Kou Qiang Yi Xue Za Zhi. 2023;**41**(4):434-442

[31] Murakami S et al. Magnetic resonance evaluation of the temporomandibular joint disc position and configuration. Dento Maxillo Facial Radiology. 1993;**22**(4):205-207

[32] Chhapane A et al. Comparison of autologous blood injection and dextrose Prolotherapy in the treatment of chronic recurrent temporomandibular

dislocation: A randomized clinical trial. Journal of Oral and Maxillofacial Surgery. 2024;**23**(2):278-284

[33] Wroclawski C, Mediratta JK, Fillmore WJ. Recent advances in temporomandibular joint surgery. Medicina. 2023;**59**(8):1409

[34] Sharma NK et al. Temporomandibular joint dislocation. National Journal of Maxillofacial Surgery. 2015;**6**(1):16-20

[35] Harorlı A, Akgul M, Dagistan S. Diş Hekimliği Radyolojisi Kitabı. Erzurum: Eser Ofset Matbaacılık; 2012. pp. 80-150

[36] Yilmaz HH et al. Clinical and magnetic resonance imaging findings of the temporomandibular joint and masticatory muscles in patients with rheumatoid arthritis. Rheumatology International. 2012;**32**(5):1171-1178

[37] Bhalerao N et al. Temporomandibular joint ankylosis: Anesthetic challenge. Cureus. 2024;**16**(2):e54379

[38] Malik S, Haghighi P, Cunningham J, Stevens K. A systematic review of the clinical outcomes for various orthodontic and physiotherapy appliances used for the management of temporomandibular joint ankylosis. Journal of Cranio-Maxillo-Facial Surgery. Sep 2024;**52**(9):983-990

[39] Vagha K et al. Navigating complexity in mandibular condyle aplasia and temporomandibular joint Ankylosis in a five-year-old child: A case report. Cureus. 2024;**16**(5):e59615

[40] Mishra BP et al. Management of temporo-mandibular joint ankylosis using different surgical approaches. Bioinformation. 2023;**19**(13):1359-1364

[41] Başaran M, Yilmaztürk SS, Bozdemir E. Efficacy of panoramic radiography in determining bony changes in temporomandibular joint. Turkiye Klinikleri Journal of Dental Sciences. 2021;**27**(1):6-14

[42] White SC, Pharoah MJ. Oral Radiology: Principles and Interpretation. 7th ed. St. Louis, Missouri: Elsevier; 2014

[43] Tamimi D, Jalali E, Hatcher D. Temporomandibular joint imaging. Radiologic Clinics of North America. Jan 2018;**56**(1):157-175. DOI: 10.1016/j.rcl.2017.08.011. Epub 2017 Oct 6. PMID: 29157545

[44] Im Y-G et al. Diagnostic accuracy and reliability of panoramic temporomandibular joint (TMJ) radiography to detect bony lesions in patients with TMJ osteoarthritis. Journal of Dental Sciences. 2018;**13**(4):396-404

[45] Gupta A, Jain D, Sampath S. Conventional and contemporary diagnostic tools in temporomandibular disorders–an overview. International Journal. 2020;**3**(4):716

[46] Whyte A et al. Imaging of the temporomandibular joint. Clinical Radiology. 2021;**76**(1). p. 76. e21-76. e35

[47] Różyło-Kalinowska I. Panoramic radiography in dentistry. Clinical Dentistry Reviewed. 2021;**5**(1):26

[48] Schroder ÂGD et al. Diagnosis of TMJ degenerative diseases by panoramic radiography: Is it possible? A systematic review and meta-analysis. Clinical Oral Investigations. 2023;**27**(11):6395-6412

[49] Levring, Jäghagen E, Ahlqvist J. Arthrography of the temporomandibular joint and arthrography-guided steroid treatment. Imaging of the Temporomandibular Joint. 2019;(1):301-322

[50] Verhelst P-J et al. The agreement between magnetic resonance

imaging and arthroscopic findings in temporomandibular joint disorders. International Journal of Oral and Maxillofacial Surgery. 2021;**50**(5):657-664

[51] Azlağ Pekince K, Çağlayan F, Pekince A. The efficacy and limitations of USI for diagnosing TMJ internal derangements. Oral Radiology. 2020;**36**(1):32-39

[52] Nainoor N, Pani G. Imaging of Temporomandibular Joint. IntechOpen; 2024. DOI: 10.5772/intechopen.1004930

[53] Dhabale GS, Bhowate RR. Cone-beam computed tomography for temporomandibular joint imaging. Cureus. 2022;**14**(11):e31515

[54] Vasegh Z et al. Assessment of bony changes in temporomandibular joint in patients using cone beam computed tomography—A cross sectional study. Head and Face Medicine. 2023;**19**(1):47

[55] Dygas S, Szarmach I, Radej I. Assessment of the morphology and degenerative changes in the temporomandibular joint using CBCT according to the orthodontic approach: A scoping review. BioMed Research International. 2022;**2022**(1):6863014

[56] Sezgin ÖS. Temporomandibuler Bozukluklarda Konik Işınlı Bilgisayarlı Tomografi Bulguları. Turkiye Klinikleri Oral and Maxillofacial Radiology-Special Topics. 2015;**1**(1):96-100

[57] Boquete-Castro A et al. Applications and advantages of the use of cone-beam computed tomography in endodontics: An updated literature review. Saudi Endodontic Journal. 2022;**12**(2):168-174

[58] Rotolo RP et al. Comparison between ultrasound and magnetic resonance imaging of the temporomandibular joint in juvenile idiopathic arthritis: A systematic review. Journal of Oral Rehabilitation. 2023;**50**(10):1082-1092

[59] Tonni I et al. Temporomandibular joint involvement in patients with juvenile idiopathic arthritis: Comparison of ultrasonography and magnetic resonance imaging in assessing the periarticular space width. Oral Radiology. 2023;**39**(4):750-758

[60] Zaman MU, Alam MK, Alqhtani NR, et al. Effectiveness of ultrasonography in the diagnosis of temporomandibular joint disorders: A systematic review and meta-analysis. Journal of Oral Rehabilitation. 2024:1-11

[61] Suenaga S, Nagayama K, Nagasawa T, Indo H, Majima HJ. The usefulness of diagnostic imaging for the assessment of pain symptoms in temporomandibular disorders. Japanese Dental Science Review. Nov 2016;**52**(4):93-106

[62] Tamimi D, Kocasarac HD, Mardini S. Imaging of the temporomandibular joint. In: Seminars in Roentgenology. Elsevier; 2019

[63] Ozcan I. Diş Hekimliğinde Radyolojinin Esasları: Konvansiyonelden Dijitale. İstanbul: İstanbul Tıp Kitapevi; 2017

[64] Jo JH et al. Limited implication of initial bone scintigraphy on long-term condylar bone change in temporomandibular disorders—Comparison with cone beam computed tomography at 1 year. Journal of Oral Rehabilitation. 2021;**48**(8):880-890

[65] Shim JS et al. Correlation between TM joint disease and rheumatic diseases detected on bone scintigraphy and clinical factors. Scientific Reports. 2020;**10**(1):4547

[66] Naaz S et al. Diagnostic imaging of temporomandibular joint-a review.

Saudi Journal of Oral and Dental Research. 2024;**9**(7):151-159

[67] Haider SMM et al. Comparison of bone scan and SPECT/CT in detection of condylar hyperplasia. Pakistan Journal of Medical & Health Sciences. Jan 2022;**16**(1):189-191

[68] Garstka AA et al. Accurate diagnosis and treatment of painful temporomandibular disorders: A literature review supplemented by own clinical experience. Pain Research and Management. 2023;**2023**:1002235

[69] Kumar A, Brennan MT. Differential diagnosis of orofacial pain and temporomandibular disorder. Dental Clinics of North America. 2013;**57**(3):419-428

[70] Ohrbach R, Dworkin SF. The evolution of TMD diagnosis: Past, present. Journal of Dental Research. 2016;**95**(10):1093-1101

[71] Schiffman E et al. Diagnostic criteria for temporomandibular disorders (DC/TMD) for clinical and research applications: Recommendations of the international RDC/TMD consortium network* and orofacial pain special interest group†. Journal of Oral and Facial Pain and Headache. 2014;**28**(1):6-27

[72] Gonzalez YM et al. Development of a brief and effective temporomandibular disorder pain screening questionnaire: Reliability and validity. Journal of the American Dental Association (1939). 2011;**142**(10):1183-1191

[73] Iwase Y et al. Deep learning classification performance for diagnosing condylar osteoarthritis in patients with dentofacial deformities using panoramic temporomandibular joint projection images. Oral Radiology. 2024;**40**(4):538-545

[74] Rokhshad R et al. Deep learning for temporomandibular joint arthropathies: A systematic review and meta-analysis. Journal of Oral Rehabilitation. 2024;**51**(8):1632-1644

[75] Eslami H, Azizi B, Katebi K, Hoseini Z. Association between temporomandibular joint disorders and salivary cortisol levels: A systematic review and meta-analysis. Shiraz E-Medical Journal. 2023;**24**:e137608

[76] Eslami H et al. The relationship between oxidative stress markers and temporomandibular disorders: A systematic review and meta-analysis. Journal of Research in Medical Sciences : The Official Journal of Isfahan University of Medical Sciences. 2024;**29**:33

[77] Durham J et al. Self-management programmes in temporomandibular disorders: Results from an international Delphi process. Journal of Oral Rehabilitation. 2016;**43**(12):929-936

[78] Palmer J, Durham J. Temporomandibular disorders. BJA Education. 2021;**21**(2):44-50

[79] Hamata MM, Zuim PR, Garcia AR. Comparative evaluation of the efficacy of occlusal splints fabricated in centric relation or maximum intercuspation in temporomandibular disorders patients. Journal of Applied Oral Science. 2009;**17**(1):32-38

[80] Sabhlok A et al. Practice of occlusal splint therapy for treating temporomandibular disorders by general dentists of Jabalpur—A cross-sectional survey. Journal of Pharmacy and Bioallied Sciences. 2021;**13**(Suppl. 2):S1079-s1083

[81] Kuzmanovic Pficer J et al. Occlusal stabilization splint for patients with temporomandibular disorders:

Meta-analysis of short and long term effects. PLoS One. 2017;**12**(2):e0171296

[82] Al-Ani MZ et al. WITHDRAWN: Stabilisation splint therapy for temporomandibular pain dysfunction syndrome. Cochrane Database of Systematic Reviews. 2016;**2016**(1):Cd002778

[83] Durham J, Aggarwal V, Davies SJ, Harrison SD, Jagger RG, Leeson R, et al. Temporomandibular Disorders (TMDs): An Update and Management Guidance for Primary Care from the UK Specialist Interest Group in Orofacial Pain and TMDs (USOT). London, UK: Royal College of Surgeons; 2013

[84] Hijos-Mallada G, Sostres C, Gomollón F. NSAIDs, gastrointestinal toxicity and inflammatory bowel disease. Gastroenterología y Hepatología. 2022;**45**(3):215-222

[85] Kim SB et al. Anatomical consideration of ultrasonography-guided intraoral injection for temporal tendinitis. Clinical Anatomy. 2024;**37**(6):628-634

[86] Borenstein DG, Korn S. Efficacy of a low-dose regimen of cyclobenzaprine hydrochloride in acute skeletal muscle spasm: Results of two placebo-controlled trials. Clinical Therapeutics. 2003;**25**(4):1056-1073

[87] Moldofsky H et al. Effects of bedtime very low dose cyclobenzaprine on symptoms and sleep physiology in patients with fibromyalgia syndrome: A double-blind randomized placebo-controlled study. The Journal of Rheumatology. 2011;**38**(12):2653-2663

[88] Boulesteix G et al. Intratracheal intubation without muscle relaxant with the use of remifentanil-propofol. Annales Françaises d'Anesthèsie et de Rèanimation. 1999;**18**(4):393-397

[89] Sills GJ. The mechanisms of action of gabapentin and pregabalin. Current Opinion in Pharmacology. 2006;**6**(1):108-113

[90] Haviv Y et al. Myofascial pain: An open study on the pharmacotherapeutic response to stepped treatment with tricyclic antidepressants and gabapentin. Journal of Oral and Facial Pain and Headache. 2015;**29**(2):144-151

[91] Syrop SB. Initial management of temporomandibular disorders. Dentistry Today. 2002;**21**(8):52-57

[92] Aggarwal VR et al. The effectiveness of self-management interventions in adults with chronic orofacial pain: A systematic review, meta-analysis and meta-regression. European Journal of Pain. 2019;**23**(5):849-865

[93] List T, Axelsson S. Management of TMD: Evidence from systematic reviews and meta-analyses. Journal of Oral Rehabilitation. 2010;**37**(6):430-451

[94] Medlicott MS, Harris SR. A systematic review of the effectiveness of exercise, manual therapy, electrotherapy, relaxation training, and biofeedback in the management of temporomandibular disorder. Physical Therapy. 2006;**86**(7):955-973

[95] Shimada A et al. Effects of exercise therapy on painful temporomandibular disorders. Journal of Oral Rehabilitation. 2019;**46**(5):475-481

[96] Kasat V et al. Transcutaneous electric nerve stimulation (TENS) in dentistry—A review. Journal of Clinical and Experimental Dentistry. 2014;**6**(5):e562-e568

[97] Fernandes AC et al. Acupuncture in temporomandibular disorder myofascial pain treatment: A systematic review.

Journal of Oral and Facial Pain and Headache. 2017;**31**(3):225-232

[98] Machado E et al. A systematic review of different substance injection and dry needling for treatment of temporomandibular myofascial pain. International Journal of Oral and Maxillofacial Surgery. 2018;**47**(11):1420-1432

[99] Häggman-Henrikson B et al. Pharmacological treatment of oro-facial pain—Health technology assessment including a systematic review with network meta-analysis. Journal of Oral Rehabilitation. 2017;**44**(10):800-826

[100] Durham J, Newton-John TR, Zakrzewska JM. Temporomandibular disorders. BMJ. 2015;**350**:h1154

[101] Schiffman EL et al. Effects of four treatment strategies for temporomandibular joint closed lock. International Journal of Oral and Maxillofacial Surgery. 2014;**43**(2):217-226

[102] Chowdhury SKR et al. Evaluation of total alloplastic temporomandibular joint replacement in TMJ ankylosis. Journal of Oral and Maxillofacial Surgery. 2019;**18**(2):293-298

[103] Dvoranova B et al. Does orthognathic surgery affect mandibular condyle position? A retrospective study. Oral and Maxillofacial Surgery. 2024;**28**(2):639-643

[104] Huang Y, Liu F, Lu J, Teng L. Morphological changes of the temporomandibular joint and masseter muscle after mandibular angle osteotomy. The Journal of Craniofacial Surgery. Oct 2024;**35**(7):2059-2062

[105] Nishimura M et al. Transitional joint effusion in the mandibular prognathic surgery patient: Intraoral vertical ramus osteotomy versus sagittal split ramus osteotomy. Journal of Oral and Maxillofacial Surgery. 2004;**62**(5):545-548

[106] Murakami K et al. Changes in strain energy density in the temporomandibular joint disk after sagittal split ramus osteotomy using a computed tomography-based finite element model. Journal of Orofacial Orthopedics. 2024;**85**(4):289-305

[107] Kikuta S et al. Improvement of the temporomandibular joint symptoms due to the condylar position change following modified L-shaped intraoral vertico-sagittal ramus osteotomy: A single-center, retrospective study. Oral and Maxillofacial Surgery. 2024;**28**(3):1365-1374

[108] Bair E et al. Multivariable modeling of phenotypic risk factors for first-onset TMD: The OPPERA prospective cohort study. The Journal of Pain. 2013;**14**(12 Suppl):T102-T115

[109] Alshahrani AA et al. The association between genetic factors and temporomandibular disorders: A systematic literature review. Archives of Oral Biology. 2024;**166**:106032

[110] Slade GD et al. Summary of findings from the OPPERA prospective cohort study of incidence of first-onset temporomandibular disorder: Implications and future directions. The Journal of Pain. 2013;**14**(Suppl. 12): T116-T124

[111] Garstka AA et al. Cause-effect relationships between painful TMD and postural and functional changes in the musculoskeletal system: A preliminary report. Pain Research and Management. 2022;**2022**:1429932

[112] Sultan D, Pellecchia R, Mercuri LG. Alloplastic TMJ replacement in the skeletally immature patient—A systematic review. Journal of Cranio-Maxillo-Facial Surgery. 2024;**52**(7):821-828

[113] Dang RR, Mehra P. Alloplastic reconstruction of the temporomandibular joint. Journal Istanbul University Faculty of Dentistry. 2017;**51**(3 Suppl. 1):S31-s40

[114] Yang Y et al. Mesenchymal stem cells-derived exosomes alleviate temporomandibular joint disc degeneration in temporomandibular joint disorder. Biochemical and Biophysical Research Communications. 2024;**726**:150278

Chapter 13

Use of Statins after Bone Osteotomy and Augmentation and their Antibacterial Effect: Narrative Review of Literature

Tomislav Katanec, Tihomir Kuna and Dragan Gabrić

Abstract

Statins, a class of cholesterol-loweringdrugs, have been investigated for their potential benefits in oral surgery, particularly in bone osteotomy and augmentation procedures. Recent studies suggest that statins may stimulate bone formation and enhance the osseointegration of dental implants. This review examines the current evidence on the effects of statins on bone osteotomy and augmentation in oral surgery. The available data indicates that while patients with a history of bisphosphonate use may not face a higher risk of dental implant failure or marginal bone loss, they may be more susceptible to bisphosphonate-related osteonecrosis of the jaw. Further research is needed to fully elucidate the impact of antiresorptive drugs, including statins, on dental implant outcomes and to identify optimal strategies for managing patients undergoing oral surgical procedures. The practice of fixed bridges and partial prosthesis can be and are iatrogenic to the existing teeth and bone. Dental implants have become a viable treatment option when there is sufficient quantity and quality of bone to achieve the desired functional and esthetic results. Horizontal ridge augmentation and contextual implant placement with a resorbable membrane and particulate grafting material can be used to reconstruct three-dimensional atrophic edentulous areas of the jaws, allowing for correct implant positioning and avoiding mechanical and prosthetic failures. The reduction in bone volume has many etiologies, including periodontal disease, pneumatization of the maxillary sinus, long-term ill-fitting dentures, and the general progression of osteoporosis with aging. Interestingly, recent studies suggest that statins, a class of cholesterol-lowering drugs, may have a positive effect on bone osteotomy and augmentation in oral surgery. Statins have been found to stimulate bone formation and enhance the osseointegration of dental implants.

Keywords: statins, bone osteotomy, bone augmentation, dental implants, oral surgery

1. Introduction

Dental implantology is a rapidly evolving field that aims to improve dental implant systems by integrating materials science and surface technology [1]. Statins, a class of drugs primarily used to lower cholesterol levels, have also been studied for their potential role in enhancing osseointegration, the process by which dental implants bond with the surrounding bone [2]. Studies have shown that statins can promote bone regeneration and enhance osseointegration in animal models. One study conducted on rabbits found that local application of simvastatin (SIM), a commonly used statin, significantly increased bone-to-implant contact and implant stability compared to control groups. Another study on rats showed that systemic administration of atorvastatin, another type of statin, improved implant stability and enhanced bone formation around the implant [1, 2].

These findings suggest that statins may have potential as an adjunct therapy in dental implantology to improve osseointegration and long-term implant success. Overall, the use of statins in dental implantology holds promise for improving osseointegration and long-term implant success [2].

Therefore, more research is needed to determine the optimal dosage, duration, and administration method of statins in dental implantology, as well as to evaluate their potential adverse effects and interactions with other medications. In summary, the use of statins in dental implantology shows promise for improving osseointegration and long-term implant success.

2. Review of literature on statins' role in dental treatment

Periodontal and peri-implant diseases are complex conditions that can have a significant impact on oral health and overall well-being. In recent years, there has been growing interest in the potential relationship between these diseases and the use of statins, a class of drugs commonly prescribed to lower cholesterol levels.

Research suggests that statins may have anti-inflammatory and immunomodulatory effects that could potentially benefit individuals with periodontal and peri-implant diseases. Additionally, some studies have shown that statins may have a positive impact on bone metabolism, which is particularly relevant in the context of peri-implant diseases where the stability of the bone surrounding dental implants is crucial [3].

Ting et al. showed literature review of the effect of SIM on different oral pathogens and microorganisms. The best effect of SIM was on Aggregatibacter actinomycetemcomitans and Porphyromonas gingivalis and against most dental plaque bacteria, including Streptococcus mutans. Also there was some antifungal impact on Candida albicans, Aspergillus fumigatus, and Zygomycetes spp. The most important antibacterial effects show that statins may have antibacterial properties by inhibiting the growth of certain bacteria, including Staphylococcus aureus and Escherichia coli. This suggests a potential role for statins in combating bacterial infections and potentially reducing the risk of certain complications. Atorvastatin showed better antibacterial effect than rosuvastatin.

In addition to their antibacterial properties, statins have also been investigated for their antiviral effects. Research indicates that statins may exert antiviral activity against a range of viruses, including influenza virus, hepatitis C virus, and human immunodeficiency virus. These findings have sparked interest in exploring the potential use of statins in the treatment or prevention of viral infections. Atorvastatin, fluvastatin, and SIM exhibit comparable anti-HCMV effects. SIM has the highest inhibitory potency (50% antiviral effective concentration [EC50] = 3 nM) compared with atorvastatin and fluvastatin (EC50 = 30 nm). Furthermore, there is emerging evidence suggesting that statins may possess antifungal properties, contributing to the management of fungal infections. By targeting key pathways in fungal cells, statins have shown promise in inhibiting the growth and proliferation of certain fungi, highlighting their potential as adjunctive or alternative antifungal agents [4].

Moraschini et al. in systematic review aimed to assess the scientific evidence on the effect of statins on the osseointegration of titanium dental implants. All included studies showed a positive effect of statins on increasing osteogenesis around dental implants in animals. In this review, they used review literature on studies based on 478 rats and dogs. The positive effect of statins on osteogenesis around implants is likely due to the increased expression of BMP-2 and stimulation of osteoblasts. Statins also demonstrated a decrease in osteoclast activity, as evidenced by a reduction in the histological marker tartrate-resistant acid phosphatase in blood serum. The studies included in the review were assessed for quality according to ARRIVE guidelines. Delivery methods of statins for efficient treatment are currently not optimal, but efforts are being made to develop more effective methods such as hydrogels and nanoparticles. The positive effects of statins on osteogenesis around dental implants, as highlighted in the review, shed light on the potential for improving the success rate of dental implant procedures. The increased expression of BMP-2 and stimulation of osteoblasts indicate promising avenues for enhancing the integration of titanium dental implants in clinical practice. Furthermore, the observed decrease in osteoclast activity due to statin administration suggests a multifaceted approach to promoting implant stability and longevity [5].

In the field of osteoporosis research, studies conducted on animal models play a crucial role in evaluating the efficacy and safety of potential treatment options. One study conducted by Ayukawa et al. aimed to investigate the effects of SIM, a commonly used statin medication, on bone parameters in rats. Ayukawa et al. conducted a study involving 10 female rats. These rats were injected daily with 10 mg/kg of SIM for a period of 20 days. The researchers used rough Kyocera material as the implant and measured various parameters to assess the impact of SIM on bone. The results showed that all parameters measured, including bone-implant contact (BIC) and bone volume (BV), significantly increased, indicating a positive effect of SIM on bone parameters in rats [6]. Another study conducted by Moriyama et al. explored the effects of fluvastatin, another statin medication, on bone parameters in rats. For their study, Moriyama et al. used a larger sample size of 60 female rats. These rats were not given any specific treatment prior to the study. The researchers topically applied three different concentrations (3, 15, and 75 mg) of fluvastatin to the rat bone-implant interface. They used rough Kyocera material as the implant and assessed BIC and BV and performed a mechanical push-out test to evaluate the effects of fluvastatin on bone parameters. The results of Moriyama et al.'s study showed that all parameters measured, including BIC, BV, and mechanical push-out test results, significantly increased with the application of fluvastatin, indicating a positive effect on bone parameters in rats [7]. In a study conducted by Du et al., 54 osteoporotic female rats were used to evaluate the effects of SIM on bone parameters. In this study, the rats were not given any specific treatment prior to the experiment. They treated the rats with SIM and assessed various bone parameters. The authors used an animal level analysis and found that all parameters increased; however, specific details regarding which parameters were measured were not provided [8]. Furthermore, it is important to note that the delivery method of SIM in these studies was different. Ayukawa et al. injected SIM daily, while Moriyama et al. topically applied fluvastatin. The delivery method of SIM in Du et al.'s study was not specified [7, 8]. In a study conducted by

Moriyama et al., the researchers used 60 female rats at the animal level to investigate the effects of topical application of fluvastatin. The rats were divided into different groups and subjected to topical application of fluvastatin at three different dosages: 3, 15, and 75 mg. After a period of 4 weeks, the researchers performed a BIC test, BV analysis, and a mechanical push-out test to evaluate the impact of fluvastatin on bone density. The results showed that all parameters significantly increased in the first two weeks of the study, indicating an improvement in bone density. However, at the 4-week mark, there was no significant difference observed between the rats treated with fluvastatin and those in the placebo group [9]. In the study conducted by Masuzaki et al., the researchers aimed to investigate the effects of fluvastatin, a statin medication commonly used to reduce cholesterol levels, on bone metabolism and biomechanical testing in rats. The study used 40 female rats and divided them into two groups: a treatment group receiving fluvastatin and a control group receiving a placebo. The rats in the treatment group were given percutaneous injections of fluvastatin after the completion of implant surgery. The researchers administered a dosage of 0.5 mg/kg and 1 mg/kg of fluvastatin to the rats in the treatment group. The effects of fluvastatin on bone metabolism and biomechanical testing were evaluated through various measurements including bone mineral density, BV fraction, serum biochemistry, bone metabolism markers, and biomechanical testing. The results of the study showed that the rats in the treatment group exhibited increased bone mineral density, BV fraction, and improved biomechanical properties compared to the rats in the control group. The serum biochemistry test, however, did not show any significant difference between the rats in the treatment group and the control group. These findings suggest that fluvastatin has a positive effect on bone metabolism and biomechanical properties in rats [10]. Nyan et al. conducted a study in which 36 male rats were divided into different groups and treated with SIM through topical application at dose levels of 25 mg and 50 mg. The researchers evaluated BIC, bone mineral density, and performed micro-CT scans. They found that only BIC showed a statistically significant increase. Tan et al. conducted a study with 48 female rats, in which SIM was applied topically at doses of 5 mg and 10 mg. They assessed BIC, mineral apposition rate, micro-CT scans, immunohistochemistry, and mechanical push-in tests. They reported that all parameters showed an increase, indicating a positive effect of SIM on BIC and bone parameters. In another study conducted by Fang et al., 36 female rats were treated with SIM for a duration of 72 hours. Fang et al. observed the effects of SIM treatment on implant surface in these rats. They found that SIM treatment had a positive effect on BIC and bone parameters. In vitro studies have also shown promising results regarding the effects of SIM on bone cell mineralization. According to the studies conducted by Nyan et al., Tan et al., and Fang et al., it can be concluded that SIM has a positive effect on BIC and bone parameters in rats [11–13]. Karanicola et al. conducted a study about effects of diclofenac and SIM on bone healing. The study used male Wistar rats and divided them into groups based on the route of drug administration and type of defect healing. Diclofenac was administered intramuscularly, while SIM was administered both systemically and locally. A total of 144 male Wistar rats were used in the study. The study also included subgroups based on the duration of the study (2, 4, or 8 weeks). The histomorphometric data provided valuable information on the percentage of new bone formation, shedding light on the potential impact of these medications on bone healing [14]. Littuma et al. analyzed biofunctionalized prosthetic abutment different properties and characteristics of a titanium disc coated with polylactic-co-glycolic acid (PLGA) incorporating SIM. The study employed different methods to achieve its objective. The methods involved distributing titanium discs into four groups, including pure titanium, titanium coated with PLGA, titanium coated with PLGA incorporating 6% SIM, and titanium coated with PLGA incorporating 0.6% SIM. The use of PLGA as a coating material for titanium discs was prepared through the chloroform evaporation technique. After the complete dissolution of PLGA, SIM was diluted in the solution. The study then proceeded to dipcoat the titanium discs with PLGA and different concentrations of SIM. The sources provided were relevant and supported the study's objective. In vitro bone formation was evaluated using alkaline phosphatase and von Kossa assays over a period of 16 days. The results showed that saponified SIM and OG-PLG significantly increased alkaline phosphatase expression, while all three, SIM, saponified SIM, and OG-PLG, enhanced mineralization. In conclusion, the biofunctionalized prosthetic abutment proposed in this study shows promising potential for enhancing bone formation. The incorporation of SIM into the titanium disc coated with PLGA demonstrated increased alkaline phosphatase expression and enhanced mineralization. Additionally, the evaluation of SIM release from the PLGA coatings and its effect on bone cell mineralization provides valuable insights into potential biomedical applications. Further research and development in this area could lead to significant advancements in prosthetic abutment technology, ultimately benefiting patients in need of dental implants [15]. There is also similar study from Sordi et al. who concluded that the addition of SIM to the PLGA + HA/βTCP scaffold positively impacts the osteoinductive capacity of stem cells from human exfoliated deciduous teeth (SHED). This is an important discovery as it demonstrates the potential for SIM to enhance the performance of tissue engineering scaffolds in promoting bone formation. Further research in this area could lead to the development of improved scaffolds for bone regeneration, with potential applications in the treatment of bone defects and injuries. They evaluated the effect of embedding simvastatin on the osteoinductive capacity of PLGA + HA/βTCP scaffolds in SHED [16]. However, new study from Ozturk et al. [17] showed 16 male New Zealand rabbits which were on high-cholesterol diet for 8 weeks, and hyperlipidemia was created. A critical-sized defect was created in the mandible. The defect was closed with xenograft and membrane. Oral 10 mg/kg atorvastatin was started in the experimental group, and no drug was administered in the control group. At the 16th week, animals were sacrificed. In conclusion, the study provides valuable insights into the potential impact of atorvastatin on bone regeneration in dental implantology in individuals with hyperlipidemia. New bone area (45,924 μm^2, $p < 0.001$) and AP intensities (105.645 ± 16.727, $p = 0.006$) were higher in the atorvastatin group than in the control group, and TRAP intensities in the control group (82.192 ± 5.346, $p = 0.021$) were higher than those in the atorvastatin group [17]. Yamashita et al. investigate the effects of SIM on tumor necrosis factor alpha (TNF-α) suppression of bone morphogenetic protein-induced Runx2 expression and alkaline phosphatase activity. SIM is tested in combination with BMP-2 and TNF-α to determine its impact on the regulation of Runx2 expression and ALP activity. SIM (3–30 μM) is used in combination with BMP-2 (100 ng/ml) and TNF-α (10 and 30 ng/ml) for 48 hours. In conclusion, the results of the study suggest that SIM has a potential role in mitigating the suppression of bone morphogenetic protein-induced Runx2 expression and alkaline phosphatase activity by TNF-α. The combination of SIM with BMP-2 and TNF-α demonstrated a significant impact on the regulation of Runx2 expression and ALP activity. These findings hold promise for potential therapeutic interventions in conditions where TNF-α negatively affects bone formation [18].

However, the existing literature and animal studies suggest that statins have the potential to enhance osseointegration and improve long-term implant success in dental implantology. The mechanisms underlying the effects of statins on osseointegration are not fully understood, and more research is needed to evaluate their clinical efficacy and safety in human patients. Additionally, studies have shown that statins can promote bone formation, inhibit bone resorption, and have anti-inflammatory effects, which are all beneficial for osseointegration in dental implants. Animal studies have shown that statins can increase bone formation around dental implants, improve implant stability, and reduce complications such as peri-implantitis. These findings suggest that statins could be a promising adjunctive therapy in dental implantology. Furthermore, some authors have suggested that statins may have a potential role in reducing the risk of implant failure in patients with systemic conditions such as osteoporosis or diabetes. Overall, the available literature and animal studies indicate that statins have potential benefits in dental implantology by improving osseointegration and long-term implant success. However, it is important to note that more research is needed to fully understand the optimal dosage, duration, and administration method of statins in dental implantology, as well as to evaluate their potential adverse effects and interactions with other medications [17, 18].

3. The effect of statins on bone metabolism and bone formation

Statins, a widely prescribed class of medications primarily used for the management of hyperlipidemia, have garnered significant attention in recent years for their potential to influence bone metabolism and promote new bone formation. This paper aims to review the current scientific understanding of the mechanisms by which statins exert their effects on bone homeostasis and their potential therapeutic implications.

Bone is a dynamic tissue that undergoes continuous remodeling, a process regulated by the delicate balance between bone formation by osteoblasts and bone resorption by osteoclasts [19]. Interestingly, numerous studies have demonstrated that statins, in addition to their well-established lipid-lowering properties, can also significantly modulate bone metabolism through complex mechanisms. Statins have been found to influence the differentiation and activity of both osteoblasts, the cells responsible for bone formation, and osteoclasts, the cells that mediate bone resorption. By regulating the balance between these two cell types, statins can promote the overall process of bone remodeling and potentially enhance new bone formation. This multifaceted effect of statins on bone metabolism has garnered significant interest in the field of bone health and osteoporosis management [19, 20]. One of the proposed mechanisms by which statins exert their osteogenic activity is through the inhibition of the mevalonate pathway, a key metabolic pathway involved in the synthesis of cholesterol and other important lipid molecules. By inhibiting this pathway, statins can modulate the production of intermediates such as farnesyl pyrophosphate and geranylgeranyl pyrophosphate, which play crucial roles in the regulation of osteoblast and osteoclast function. This inhibition leads to increased osteoblast differentiation and activity, as well as reduced osteoclast formation and bone resorption, ultimately promoting new bone formation and maintaining bone homeostasis.

Furthermore, statins have also been found to exhibit anti-inflammatory and antioxidant properties, which can contribute to their beneficial effects on bone health. Chronic inflammation and oxidative stress are known to be key contributors to the development and progression of various metabolic bone diseases, including osteoporosis. By counteracting these detrimental factors, statins may help to create a more favorable microenvironment for bone regeneration and maintenance.

In addition to these direct effects on bone cells, statins have also been reported to influence bone metabolism through indirect mechanisms. For instance, some studies have suggested that statins can stimulate the production of bone morphogenetic proteins, a family of growth factors that play a crucial role in the differentiation and activity of osteoblasts [21]. This indirect pathway may further enhance the osteogenic potential of statins and contribute to their bone-protective effects.

While the beneficial effects of statins on bone metabolism have been widely documented, it is important to note that the magnitude and clinical significance of these effects may vary depending on factors such as the type of statin, the dosage, and the individual patient's response.

Ongoing research and clinical trials are aimed at further elucidating the precise mechanisms by which statins influence bone metabolism and evaluating their potential therapeutic applications in the management of metabolic bone diseases, such as osteoporosis. These investigations seek to optimize the use of statins as a treatment option for improving bone health and reducing the risk of fractures, particularly in high-risk populations.

In conclusion, the available evidence suggests that statins, in addition to their well-established cardiovascular benefits, possess the potential to positively impact bone metabolism and promote new bone formation [22, 23]. The understanding of the underlying mechanisms and the development of targeted therapeutic strategies incorporating statins may contribute to the improvement of bone health and the management of metabolic bone diseases in the future. Further research is needed to fully elucidate the complex interactions between statins and bone metabolism, as well as to determine the optimal dosing and treatment regimens for maximizing their bone-protective effects. By leveraging the versatile properties of statins, clinicians may be able to develop more effective interventions for preserving skeletal integrity and reducing the burden of debilitating conditions like osteoporosis [24].

4. The molecular mechanism of statins in promoting newly formed bone

Statins, a class of medications primarily used to lower cholesterol levels, have garnered significant attention in the field of bone biology due to their potential role in promoting the formation of new bone. The discovery of statins' bone anabolic properties has led to numerous investigations into their use for the treatment of bone catabolic diseases, such as osteoporosis.

The molecular mechanism by which statins influence bone metabolism is multifaceted and involves several key pathways. Statins act by inhibiting the enzyme 3-hydroxy-3-methylglutaryl coenzyme A reductase, the rate-limiting step in hepatic cholesterol biosynthesis [25]. This inhibition results in a reduction of serum cholesterol levels, which has been linked to increased bone mineral density and a decreased risk of osteoporosis-related fractures [26].

One of the primary mechanisms by which statins promote bone formation is through the upregulation of the bone morphogenetic protein-2 gene. This gene is a potent inducer of osteoblast differentiation, leading to enhanced mineralization and the formation of new bone.

Additionally, recent studies have uncovered a link between cholesterol metabolism and bone homeostasis, mediated by the oxysterol 27-hydroxycholesterol.

This cholesterol metabolite has been shown to decrease osteoblast differentiation and enhance osteoclastogenesis, resulting in increased bone resorption. Statins, by modulating cholesterol metabolism, can counteract the negative effects of 27-hydroxycholesterol on bone, thereby promoting a more favorable bone remodeling balance [25, 26].

Statins have also been found to have anti-inflammatory properties, which can contribute to their bone-promoting effects. Inflammation is a known risk factor for osteoporosis, and by reducing inflammatory cytokines and mediators, statins can create an environment more conducive to bone formation and repair.

Despite the promising results from in vitro and animal studies, the efficacy of systemic statin administration in the treatment of osteoporosis in humans has been somewhat limited. However, alternative dosing strategies, such as local applications of statins or the development of bone-targeting systemic preparations, may prove to be more effective in the future.

In conclusion, the molecular mechanism by which statins promote the formation of new bone involves a complex interplay between their effects on cholesterol metabolism, bone morphogenetic signaling, and anti-inflammatory properties. Statins inhibit the enzyme 3-hydroxy-3-methylglutaryl coenzyme A reductase, which reduces cholesterol levels and leads to increased bone mineral density. They also upregulate the bone morphogenetic protein-2 gene, enhancing osteoblast differentiation and bone mineralization. Furthermore, statins can counteract the negative effects of the cholesterol metabolite 27-hydroxycholesterol on bone homeostasis, and their anti-inflammatory properties create a more favorable environment for bone formation and repair [27].

5. The effect of statins on soft tissue healing in the oral cavity

The cardioprotective effects of statins are well-established, with numerous studies demonstrating their ability to enhance endothelial function, exert anti-inflammatory and anti-atherothrombotic properties, and modulate the immune system [28, 29]. However, recent investigations have uncovered the potential benefits of statins in promoting soft tissue healing within the oral cavity.

One of the key mechanisms by which statins may contribute to improved soft tissue healing in the oral cavity is through their influence on the body's inflammatory response. Statins have been shown to possess anti-inflammatory properties, reducing the production of pro-inflammatory cytokines and mediators, which can impede the natural healing process. By mitigating inflammation, statins may create an environment more conducive to the repair and regeneration of soft tissues, such as the gingiva, oral mucosa, and periodontal tissues.

Moreover, statins have been observed to enhance the proliferation and migration of cells involved in tissue repair, such as fibroblasts and endothelial cells. This increased cellular activity can accelerate the deposition of extracellular matrix components, promote angiogenesis, and facilitate the overall healing of soft tissues within the oral cavity.

Interestingly, the potential benefits of statins on soft tissue healing in the oral cavity may extend beyond their direct effects on the tissues themselves. Statins have been found to exert positive impacts on bone metabolism, potentially improving the integration and stability of dental implants or promoting the healing of periodontal defects [21, 30].

While the research in this area is still ongoing, the existing evidence suggests that the use of statins may hold promise in the management of various oral soft tissue conditions, such as gingivitis, periodontitis, and postsurgical healing. In particular, the anti-inflammatory and cell-proliferative effects of statins have been shown to potentially enhance the healing and regeneration of gingival, mucosal, and periodontal tissues, which could lead to improved outcomes in the treatment of common oral health issues. Furthermore, the potential benefits of statins on bone metabolism may also contribute to better integration and stability of dental implants, as well as the healing of periodontal defects. Overall, the promising findings warrant further investigation to fully elucidate the role of statins in promoting soft tissue healing within the oral cavity [31].

Author details

Tomislav Katanec[1,2]*, Tihomir Kuna[1,2] and Dragan Gabrić[1,2]

1 Department of Oral Surgery, School of Dental Medicine, Zagreb, Croatia

2 Department of Oral Surgery, University Hospital Centre, Zagreb, Croatia

*Address all correspondence to: tkatanec@sfzg.hr

References

[1] Taylor TD, Agar JR. Twenty years of progress in implant prosthodontics. The Journal of Prosthetic Dentistry. 2002;**88**(1):89-95

[2] Khan SN, Ramachandran M, Senthil Kumar S, Krishnan V, Sundaram R. Osseointegration and more–a review of literature. Indian Journal of Dentistry. 2012;**3**(2):72-76

[3] Di Spirito F, Schiavo L, Pilone V, Lanza A, Sbordone L, D'Ambrosio F. Periodontal and Peri-implant diseases and systemically administered statins: A systematic review. Dental Journal. **2021**;*9*:100

[4] Ting M, Whitaker EJ, Albandar JM. Systematic review of the in vitro effects of statins on oral and perioral microorganisms. European Journal of Oral Sciences. 2016;**124**(1):4-10

[5] Moraschini V, Almeida DCF, Calasans-Maia JA, Diuana C-MM. The ability of topical and systemic statins to increase osteogenesis around dental implants: A systematic review of histomorphometric outcomes in animal studies. International Journal of Oral and Maxillofacial Surgery. 2018;**47**(8):1070-1078

[6] Ayukawa Y, Okamura A, Koyano K. Simvastatin promotes osteogenesis around titanium implants. A histological and histometrical study in rats. Clinical Oral Implants Research. 2004;**15**:346-350

[7] Moriyama Y, Ayukawa Y, Ogino Y, Atsuta I, Koyano K. Topical application of statin affects bone healing around implants. Clinical Oral Implants Research. 2008;**19**:600-605

[8] Du Z, Chen J, Yan F, Xiao Y. Effects of simvastatin on bone healing around titanium implants in osteoporotic rats. Clinical Oral Implants Research. 2009;**20**:145-150

[9] Moriyama Y, Ayukawa Y, Ogino Y, Atsuta I, Todo M, Takao Y, et al. Local application of fluvastatin improves peri-implant bone quantity and mechanical properties: A rodent study. Acta Biomaterialia. 2010;**6**:1610-1618

[10] Masuzaki T, Ayukawa Y, Moriyama Y, Jinno Y, Atsuta I, Ogino Y, et al. The effect of a single remote injection of statin-impregnated poly (lactic-co-glycolic acid) microspheres on osteogenesis around titanium implants in rat tibia. Biomaterials. 2010;**31**:3327-3334

[11] Nyan M, Hao J, Miyahara T, Noritake K, Rodriguez R, Kasugai S. Accelerated and enhanced bone formation on novel simvastatin-loaded poroustitanium oxide surfaces. Clinical Implant Dentistry and Related Research. 2014;**16**:675-683

[12] Tan J, Yang N, Fu X, Cui Y, Guo Q, Ma T, et al. Single-dose local simvastatin injection improves implant fixation via increased angiogenesis and bone formation in an ovariectomized rat model. Medical Science Monitor. 2015;**21**:1428-1439

[13] Fang W, Zhao S, He F, Liu L, Yang G. Influence of simvastatin-loaded implants on osseointegration in an ovariectomized animal model. BioMed Research International. 2015;**2015**:831504

[14] Karanikola T, Cheva A, Sarafidou K, Myronidou-Tzouveleki M, Tsavdaridis I, Kontonasaki E, et al. Effect of diclofenac and simvastatin on bone defect healing-an in vivo animal study. Biomimetics (Basel). 2022;**7**(4):143

[15] Littuma GJS, Sordi MB, Borges Curtarelli R, Aragonês Á, da Cruz ACC, Magini RS. Titanium coated with poly(lactic-co-glycolic) acid incorporating simvastatin: Biofunctionalization of dental prosthetic abutments. Journal of Periodontal Research. 2020;**55**(1):116-124

[16] Sordi MB, Curtarelli RB, Mantovani IF, Moreira AC, Fernandes CP, Cruz ACC, et al. Enhanced osteoinductive capacity of poly(lactic-co-glycolic) acid and biphasic ceramic scaffolds by embedding simvastatin. Clinical Oral Investigations. 2022;**26**(3):2693-2701

[17] Öztürk K, Kuzu TE, Ayrıkçil S, Gürgan CA, Önder GÖ, Yay A. Effect of systemic atorvastatin on bone regeneration in critical-sized defects in hyperlipidemia: An experimental study. The International Journal of Implant Dentistry. 2023;**9**(1):50

[18] Yamashita M, Otsuka F, Mukai T, Otani H, Inagaki K, Miyoshi T, et al. Simvastatin antagonizes tumor necrosis factor-α inhibition of bone morphogenetic proteins-2-induced osteoblast differentiation by regulating Smad signaling and Ras/rho-mitogen-activated protein kinase pathway. Journal of Endocrinology. 2008;**196**(3):601-613

[19] Breathwaite E, Weaver J, Odanga J, dela Pena-Ponce M, Lee JB. 3D bioprinted osteogenic tissue models for *in vitro* drug screening. Molecules. 2020;**25**(15):3442

[20] Cottrell JA, Vales FM, Schachter D, Wadsworth S, Gundlapalli R, Kapadia R, et al. Osteogenic activity of locally applied small molecule drugs in a rat femur defect model. Journal of Biomedicine and Biotechnology. 2010 Jan;**1**(2010):1-11

[21] Liao JK, Laufs U. Pleiotropic effects of statins. Annual Review of Pharmacology and Toxicology. 2005;**45**(1):89-118

[22] Almuti K, Rimawi R, Spevack D, Ostfeld RJ. Effects of statins beyond lipid lowering: Potential for clinical benefits. International Journal of Cardiology. 2006;**109**(1):7-15

[23] Sassano A, Platanias LC. Statins in tumor suppression. Cancer Letters. 2008;**260**(1-2):119

[24] Svec A, Adameova A. Facts and ideas on statins with respect to their lipophilicity: A focus on skeletal muscle cells and bone besides known cardioprotection. Molecular and Cellular Biochemistry. 2022;**478**(8):1661-1667

[25] Mundy G, Garrett R, Harris S, Chan J, Chen D, Rossini G, et al. Stimulation of bone formation *in vitro* and in rodents by statins. Science. 1999;**286**(5446):1946-1949

[26] Nelson ER, DuSell CD, Wang X, Howe MK, Evans GL, Michalek RD, et al. The oxysterol, 27-hydroxycholesterol, links cholesterol metabolism to bone homeostasis through its actions on the estrogen and liver X receptors. Endocrinology. 2011;**152**(12):4691-4705

[27] Toledano JE, Partridge NC. Statins: Not just for cholesterol? Trends in Endocrinology and Metabolism. 2000;**11**(7):255-256

[28] Chen PY, Sun JS, Tsuang YH, Chen MH, Weng PW, Lin FH. Simvastatin promotes osteoblast viability and differentiation via Ras/Smad/Erk/BMP-2 signaling pathway. Nutrition Research. 2010;**30**(3):191-199

[29] Mihos CG, Pineda AM, Santana O. Cardiovascular effects of statins,

beyond lipid-lowering properties. Pharmacological Research. 2014;**88**:12-19

[30] Zhang Y, Bradley AD, Wang D, Reinhardt RA. Statins, bone metabolism and treatment of bone catabolic diseases. Pharmacological Research. 2014 Oct;**88**:53-61

[31] Degala S, Bathija NA. Evaluation of the efficacy of simvastatin in bone regeneration after surgical removal of bilaterally impacted third molars-a Split-mouth randomized clinical trial. Journal of Oral and Maxillofacial Surgery. 2018 Sep;**76**(9):1847-1858

Chapter 14

The Effect of Different Osteotomy Techniques on Implant Stability in Implant Socket Design

Levent Ciğerim and Zeynep Dilan Orhan

Abstract

Dental implant surgery is one of the most common oral and maxillofacial surgical procedures performed today. While standard drilling protocols recommended by implant manufacturers can be used for routine cases, routine osteotomies may not be sufficient for implant stability in different bone types or in cases where the bone structure differs due to local or systemic reasons. The use of various modified osteotomy (drilling) protocols to solve such cases contributes positively to primary implant stability.

Keywords: dental implant, osteotomy, drilling, primary stability, socket design

1. Introduction

Extensive knowledge of physics and mechanics, along with a strong emphasis on the soft and hard tissues around dental implants, is necessary for oral and maxillofacial surgery. The introduction of different osteotomy techniques has greatly impacted the field of implant stability in implant socket design. These techniques have been developed to improve the initial stability of dental implants and to enhance the long-term success of osseointegration [1, 2].

The current osteotomy technique is classified based on the tip of the osteotomy, the major osteotomy, and the manipulation. The severity of the effects of implant therapy, the final stability of the implant removal technique, and the mechanical and anatomical movements in the positioning direction of the implant are the determinants of implant-to-bone stability.

Implant stability for implantology can be defined as the remaining mechanical implant system and good quality bone at the end of the recipient bed. Bone quality can be seen in terms of the quantity and quality of the operating receiver bones. The mechanical properties of the implant operating receiver are closely related to the type of office implant to be used, the volume of bone in the width of the implant operating receiver, and the operating volume of the bone receiver in the length of the implant [3, 4].

The effect of different osteotomy techniques on implant stability in implant socket design is a critical aspect of implant surgery. Its resistance after being placed, leading to a decrease in the required number of turns for placement and ultimately ensuring stability of the implant influences the mechanical properties of the implant receiver.

The main objective of this chapter is to explore the correlation between different osteotomy methods and the stability of dental implants. The goal is to offer important perspectives for dental practitioners [5].

2. Anatomy and physiology of the alveolar bone

The maxillofacial skeleton is formed by the cranial bone in the axial region. The dental alveolus forms a complex anatomically formed by the bone, cementum, periodontal ligament, and gingival lining the individual teeth. The alveolar bone can be classified into cortical (compact) bone, supporting bone (cancellous), and buccal or palatal flanges (**Figure 1**). The alveolar bone is attached to the base of the maxilla or the mandible and supports and protects the roots of the teeth.

The proteins produced by the overall molecular biology processes reach every part of a dental implant; the term for immobilization of implant body and surface is osseointegration (**Figure 2**). An adequate bone volume or the use of bone grafts significantly influences the success of osseointegration in a dental implant. The major determinant in the mechanical biologic performance of bone instability is due to strength (content of mineralized collagen), remodeling, and turnover (established by estrogen, management, etc.). The alterations in bone affect the implant's initial stability in addition to the implant's physical properties (length, width, surface area) in creating primary stability by the depth of osteotomy site. Wireless length and stability of phonetic are high for the posterior region than the anterior region and the portal area in the maxilla. The process of placing a metal implant or device within the mandible or maxilla is called osteotomy or bone cutting. There are, however, various types and methods of surgical options [6–9].

2.1 Structure of the alveolar bone

The typical configuration of the alveolar bone consists of denser, cortical external tables surrounding medullary bone. The external tables are composed primarily of compact bone, which provides strength and support to the surrounding structures. The internal tables, on the other hand, are made up of cancellous bone, which is more porous and provides a greater surface area for blood supply and bone remodeling. In addition, the alveolar bone is composed of both cortical and cancellous bone, which contribute to its overall strength and density. This structural composition plays a crucial role in determining the success of different osteotomy techniques in implant socket design.

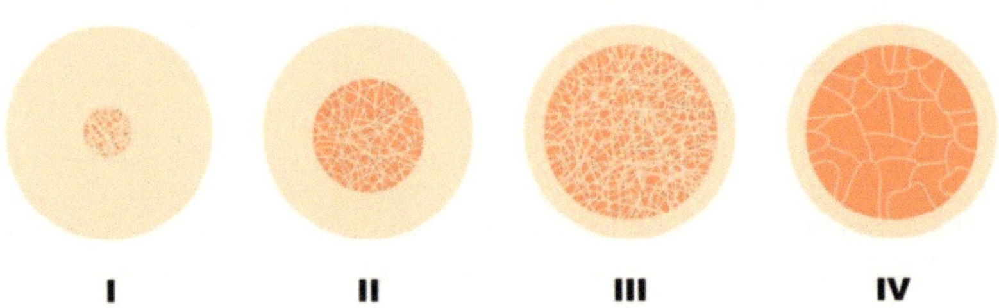

Figure 1.
Bone quality classification; Type I: Dense, uniform cortical bone with minimal marrow space. Type II: Thick cortical bone with a noticeable marrow cavity. Type III: Thin cortical bone with dense trabecular bone, suitable for implants despite the thinner cortex. Type IV: Thin cortical bone with low-density trabecular bone. Source: Ref. [6].

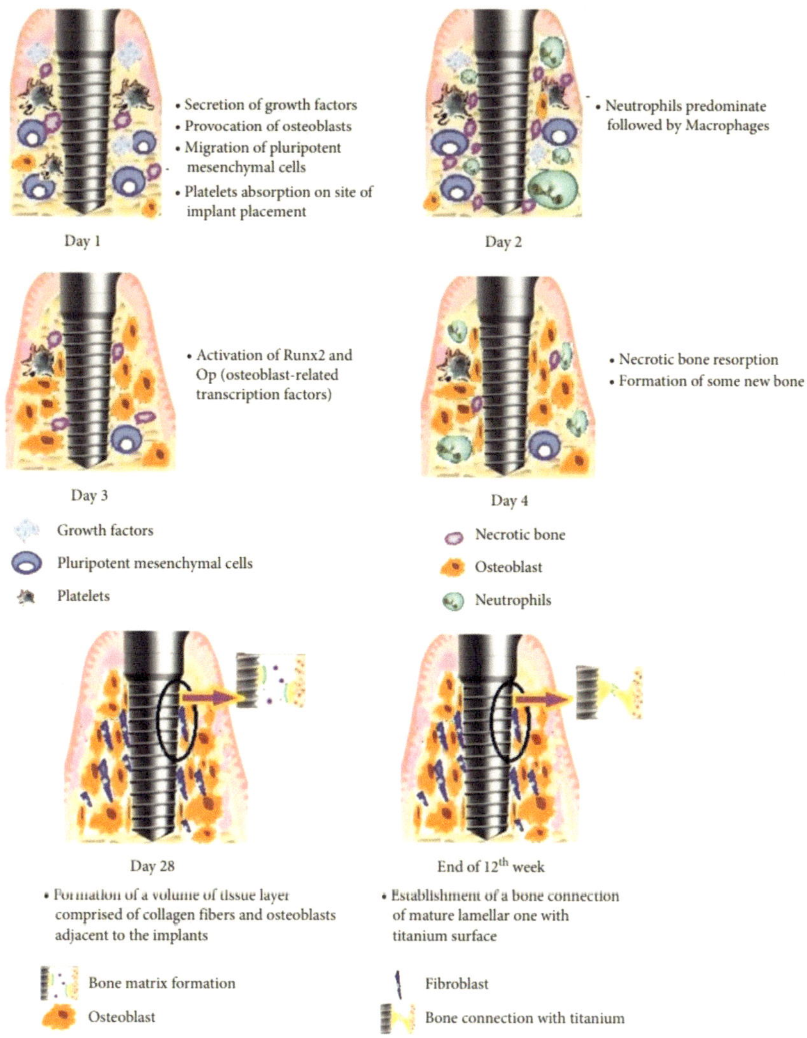

Figure 2.
Osseointegration after implant placement Ref. [7].

The density and quality of the alveolar bone are important factors that contribute to implant stability and successful osseointegration. Nonetheless, a certain variability in the microarchitecture could be found. The medullary bone may have intertrabecular porosities containing bone marrow tissues. In contrast, the cortical bone contains abundant osteocytes distributed among its lateral and terminal channels. These osteocytes have the potential to play an essential role when deciding the surgical protocol in dental implantology, which involves bone drilling or osteotomy procedures. Specifically, the drilling techniques commonly employed, include the steel bur drills and the piezosurgical tips. For the osteotomy, both hard tissue and soft tissue cutting techniques could be applied. Bone cutting may include chiseling, the ultrasonic and piezoelectric osteotome, and bur osteotomy. The cutting of the soft tissue may include filtration and fibrotomy [10–12].

3. Implant stability

Osseointegration is very important for the success of implant application. The achievement of direct contact between the bone and implant is most important for achieving osseointegration. The implant stability is the initial key for the early osseointegration. The implant stability is affected by the surgical procedure. In particular, mini implants are easily influenced by the surgical procedure. Everything can be counted as a factor of the implant stability in compliance with the definition in the relevant literature. For this purpose, the primary stability was defined, particularly in implantology, and a rigid connection was created by adding a part onto the implants, in order to eliminate the screw connection and negatively affect the initial stability in the first stage. This process has provided better prosthetic treatments without problems. The diameter changes of the implant and the bone-implant contact surface are very important for osseointegration [11, 13–16].

In the case of making implant applications to the edentulous areas, the lateral bony wall thickness and height are important for obtaining the primary mechanical stability. In conditions where tooth loss is out of control, width and height changes occur in the bone, which causes the oral tissues to be deformed in a structural manner. It is important to know the alveolar bone structure in pre-implant planning. At this stage, it is important to evaluate the socket before placing the implant and to make the necessary modifications in the bone [17–19].

Implant stability relies on micromotion. Motion restriction threshold and decreased primary stability are critical for cell development and osseointegration. Rapid insertion, stability repetition, and bone condensation aid bone adaptation. Biological and mechanical factors affect primary implant stability, evaluated through insertion torque and resonance frequency analysis. Torque provides initial stability while resonance frequency analysis measures the stability over time [20].

3.1 Factors affecting implant stability

Macro-design factors are important to achieve primary stability in the implants. To achieve this, a few variables should be selected and standardized from the design features among theoretically proposed variables such as thread geometry, pitch, shoulder form, surface characteristics, and the implant design factors. In addition, the structure of the implant bed, bone type, direction of torque application, and the presence of micro-threads are among the main factors affecting the primary stability of the implant [21–23].

Additionally, considering age, sex, smoking, bone properties, implant type, intraoperative surgical parameters such as surgical experience, the osteotomy technique, implant design, and dental care can increase the implant stability and have a positive influence on the structural connection interface between bone and implant. Since optimum implant stability results in a faster operation process, the first practice is the acquisition of primary implant stability and successful osseointegration. Increasing and accelerating the healing response after implant installation can be done by enhancing the bone-implant contact (BIC) ratio and increasing the mechanical bonding of the implant to the surgical bed. Factors affecting the reaching of a balance between these two processes are surgical-dental factors such as implant diameter, implant shape and length, bone quality, quantity, and contact with the neighboring anatomical structures as well as biological factors [1, 24–26].

3.2 Methods for assessing implant stability

Implant stability can be assessed by measuring the stability or placement amount of an implant at a certain time, and it changes with the osseointegration process. The implant stability can be measured directly and indirectly by various tests (**Figure 3**). The most commonly used methods for measuring implant stability are resonance frequency analysis (RFA), insertion torque (IT), and removal torque (RT) [1, 2, 27].

RFA, the method of percussion sounds is a qualitative method to assess implant primary stability. This is a palpation with a small bone tap with a length of about 3 cm that has a round or flat end and an edge diameter of about 3 mm. This percussion is performed successively over the dominal and apical endings of the implant, the stability of which is determined. The lower the sounds, the more stable the implant is. At the moment of implant placement, a surgical kit's gauge is used to measure the insertion torque of the implant. The insertion torque applied to the implant's surroundings produces densification of the bone and, therefore, an increase in primary stability. It is important to use a torque wrench with the handle parallel to the vertical axis to avoid false measurements. To achieve adequate primary stability, the average insertion torque values are between 20 and 30 N/cm, depending on the quantity and quality characteristics of the bone. The condition is that the insertion torque should not be less than 10–15 N/cm to avoid overloads on the implant, which can decrease the success and osseointegration of the implant. Another traditional method for evaluating the strength of implant-to-bone contact is removal torque test. This test is performed using a torque wrench. The torque wrench measures the rotational force required to remove the implant from the bone [28–32].

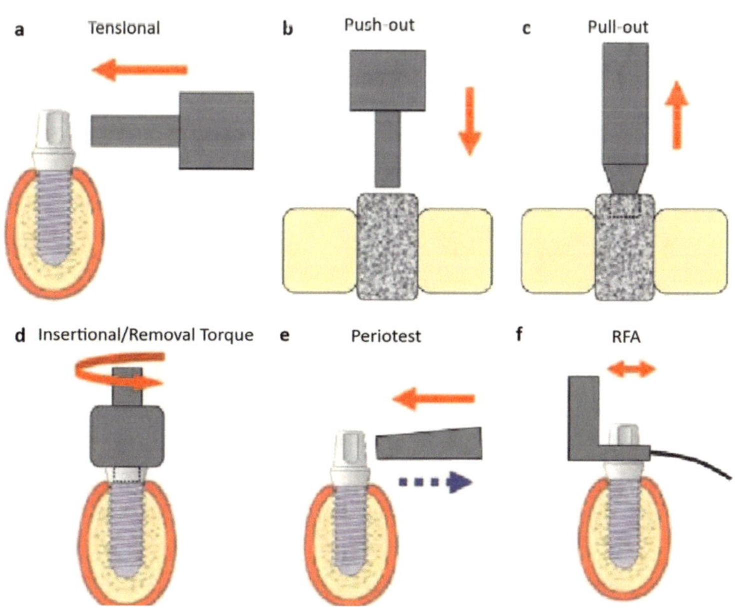

Figure 3.
Methods for measuring implant stability. Source: Ref. [8].

4. Osteotomy techniques

There are several different osteotomy techniques that can be used to prepare the implant site, and the choice of technique can have a significant impact on the stability of the implant. For example, the use of conventional drilling techniques may result in greater implant stability initially, but the bone may undergo more remodeling over time. On the other hand, the use of piezoelectric or osseodensification techniques may lead to reduced initial stability but less bone remodeling in the long term. These techniques have been found to be beneficial in certain clinical scenarios [25, 26].

4.1 Conventional osteotomy technique

The conventional osteotomy technique is the classic therapy for bone drilling, and this method is the reference standard for all drilling instruments. A medical drill that includes a rotating bur used for drilling through bones or teeth is hand-held mechanical but is often driven by a motor or a rotary drill. A modern surgical drill is a drill used by surgeons and dentists to perform a bone removal procedure, by segmental en bloc resection or by transplant resection, to excise various portions of the bone including tumors, cysts, and foreign materials. The surgical technique presented here, which employs the conventional method of implant site preparation, is founded on conventional rotary cutting systems and involves the use of drills with different diameters and lengths to create an osteotomy site that is suitable for implant placement (**Figure 4**).

In comparison to all other current techniques, this device creates wider or narrower bony fractures with less force, less microfracture, and less trauma. This helps to increase the peri-implant bone vascularization and the new bone formation, which aids in the overall healing process. The goal is to create minimal bone loss and decrease surgical duration. The conventional osteotomy technique plays a crucial role in the stability of implants within the implant socket design. It is widely used in dental implant surgeries and has been extensively studied for its impact on implant stability. This time-honored approach has been extensively utilized due to its remarkable effectiveness and success rate in achieving optimal results [1, 34, 35].

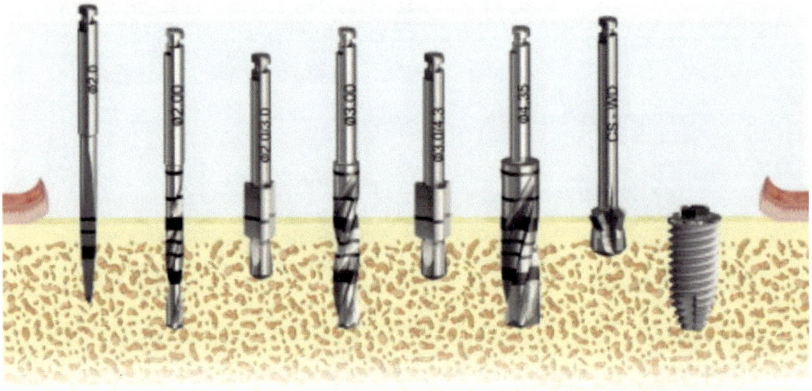

Figure 4.
Conventional osteotomy drills in an ascending order. Source: Ref. [33].

The goal of drilling techniques is to produce an ideal cavity smooth wall profile with the desired undercuts. Three essentially different methods accomplish this task: Sequential drilling, step-drilling, and bone compression drilling.

4.1.1 Sequential drilling technique

Sequential drilling is an approach of implant site preparation done through a series of increasing diameter drills. This method produces the deepest undercut on the topmost layer of the cavity wall, and since the mechanical profile of the drilling tool is wider than that of the pre-drill, osteotomy would not progress beyond the depth of the pre-drill. When the larger drill is activated, milled layers of bone are generated until the completion of the widener drill. Once implant pre-drilling is completed, the wedging action induced by the implant would start pushing bone toward the adjacent regions of the implant and this would create secondary undercuts on the cavity side walls [36, 37].

4.1.2 Step-drilling technique

In this technique, the pilot is drilled either to the depth of the pre-prepared treatment plan or drilled slightly into the bone at superficial levels. Initially, a pilot hole with a small diameter is drilled and then the hole is gradually enlarged with larger diameter drills. This method helps to prevent overstretching of the bone with slow and controlled expansion and prevent possible fractures.

While, by using step-drilling one can be more systematic in the enlargement of the area for the hole, in using the sequential drilling one will be in a better position to control the size of the hole together with its depth. Step-drilling is mainly concerned with the increase in the diameter of the bone while sequential drilling controls both, the diameter and the depth. With regard to the extent of enlargement, sequential drilling provides a much safer and more manageable process of enlargement in comparison with step-drilling while, regarding the accuracy of preparation of the hole, the second type provides better results than the first one [1, 2, 38].

4.1.3 Bone compression drilling technique

Bone compression drilling is an autoimpaction osteotomy technique that relies on the compacting intrinsic device curvature rotational motion. This motion produces continuous compressing, plasticizing, and displacing forces that work against the bone tissue. These bone expansion and compaction effects occur without burr cutting and the generation of voided osteotomy, but, instead, the creation of bone-imbedded osteotomy. Since implant insertion is equal to the osteotomy expansion and avoids cutting action, the compression drilling device diameter would be larger than the implant body.

This technique is different from the conventional and under-preparation techniques and creates inherently different surgical and biomechanical scenarios. On the one hand, the bone-compressing dental implant approach positively affects bone biomechanical support and immediate primary stability. On the other hand, bone-imbedding osteotomy negatively affects the dental implant rotation during placement, thus, deriving higher bone-imbedded forces and nonyielding torque [36, 39].

4.2 Piezoelectric osteotomy technique

Piezoelectric ultrasonic osteotomy is a method wherein mechanical oscillations or vibrations of very high frequency are imposed on an oscillating tip and the sine wave

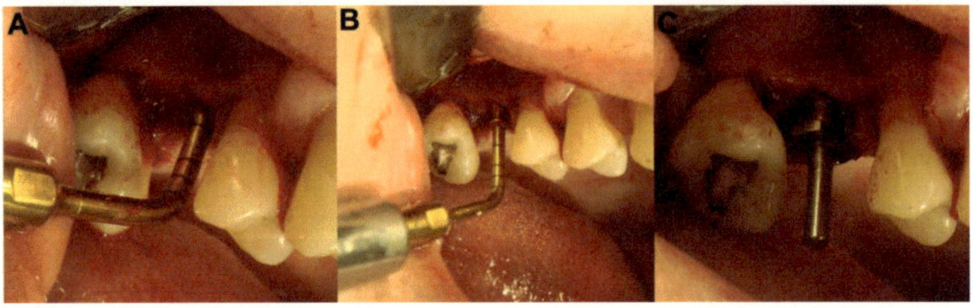

Figure 5.
Piezoelectric osteotomy technique, using different tips in an ascending order A-C. Source: Ref. [40].

energy applied is processed into a well-defined oscillation pattern that can be exclusively selected. Application of the tip to mineralized tissues leads to piezoelectricity allowing for almost perfect cutting precision without affecting surrounding soft tissues by the selective cutting of bone during dental implant surgeries (**Figure 5**).

Ultrasonic osteotomy systems comprise two key parts: an ultrasonic stimulator or generator, usually mounted in a box, and a handpiece with an oscillating metal tip. The vibrations generated by the ceramic pellets contained in the handle of the instruments induce a high-frequency almost linear reciprocal motion of the metallic tip of the instrument. In a piezoelectric bone surgery unit, the handpiece vibrates at a similar frequency to the ultrasonic piezoelectric dental scaler, however, it is three to six times more powerful. At frequencies of 25–35 kHz, the instrument is only cutting mineralized tissue leaving the soft tissue virtually untouched. Soft tissue, such as periosteum, vibrates without rupture at the same frequency as the tip of the instrument, this also favors the preservation of the surrounding vascularized pericranium and better healing.

Although implantation may be successful using conventional procedures, there remains a considerable risk of adjacent bone or tooth tissue damage because of the difficulty in managing the drilling force, leading to an increase in temperature at the osteotomy sites. The piezoelectric osteotomy technique has some advantages over traditional rotary and oscillating techniques. It is a non-invasive device and patient safety is practiced in all procedures, in addition to the greatest comfort and safety in all bone-cutting procedures. It also produces clean cuts and can be placed very close to soft tissues and tooth structures without the risk of damaging these structures, which are cut selectively, does not produce thermal damage, and allows for better healing rates as compared to the others. Additionally, it is possible to not create a pressure image, minimizing surgical risks and even the incorporation of the patient's medical history (congenital or acquired bone osseous tissues of the systemic disease-description layer) before the surgery, with the ability to section the high volume tissue. Furthermore, the gradual use of new ultrasonic tips with different geometries has broadened the use of this modality in the field of implantology, tools that are quite easy to handle and highly flexible in terms of clinical application, since they can be used to expand all types of the implant bed in both the horizontal and axial positions. In summary, piezoelectric techniques in dental implant surgery might very well develop into an ideal method for cutting hard tissues and drilling implants [40–45].

4.3 Recent advances and innovations in osteotomy techniques

Recent advances in osteotomy techniques are exciting for dental implant surgery. Computer-Aided Design and Manufacturing (CAD/CAM) is being used more frequently in surgery and dentistry. A new approach of CAD/CAM was developed with a titanium mesh for a pre-planned osteotomy and implant placement. This technique is easier and provides accurate results compared to conventional methods. Metal 3D printing complements CAD/CAM and allows for precise placement of implants. Research is being conducted to optimize implant position and improve bone formation. Robot-assisted osteotomy is also being developed for accurate cutting. CAD/CAM in osteotomy allows for total control during surgery. Robotic technology has been integrated into surgical procedures, including dental implants. While there are challenges, a dual-robot system has been developed to increase flexibility in the implant process [46–48].

5. Implant socket design

Socket design is the understood shape/geometry of the dental implant after it is placed in the body, which directly affects the success of the dental implant by either improving or impairing osseointegration. Hence, socket design needs to be scrutinized for its different advantages and disadvantages over the others. Generally, sockets can be classified on the basis of the timing of placement and hence two main sockets comprise either immediate implant placed sockets or delayed implant placement sockets. Socket designs are generally cylindrical, tapered, wide/narrow grooves, serrated designs, self-tapping, and thread designs.

Designs of the implant also include screw implants, cylinder implants, and blade implants. Modern designs comprise of screws only. Further detailing in screw designs comprises a smooth neck, grooves turned on the body of screws, serrated designs, undercut designs, and self-threading screw designs. These modern designs of implants supposedly grip the bone tightly imparting mechanical stability. It has been found that more than 70% of bone to implant contact occurs within 3 weeks of initial placement [49, 50].

Osteotomy is a significant procedure during the placement of dental implants. Effectiveness and bone injury in osteotomy are necessary for the long-term success of an implant. Implant sockets have various types, and their designs influence implant primary stability. Implant sockets include conventionally expanded, self-drilling, and self-tapping. The implant is advanced within the bone, twisting and compressing the surrounding immediate bone. All implant sockets have features both in drilling protocols and their self-tapping components, but their osteotomy techniques are different from each other. Drill entry, drilling sequence, and design of each implant socket can also be factors affecting the clinical and radiographic outcomes of an implant. In this issue, implant socket design can respond to the question of different osteotomy techniques and their effect on implant stability in the particular buccal region of the anterior mandible. However, this issue cannot be predicted exactly [1, 2].

Bone quality and quantity are crucially important factors for long-term implant success. A flat rationale should not be employed in socket design for all tooth-type models. Poor bone quality (D3-D4) would demand a larger platform implant with a wider (4.3 mm) diameter so that more bone surface area is acted upon, leading to superior mechanical fixture stability. The amount of resorbed bone height following extraction is found to be better preserved in molars compared to incisors, premolars, and canines. Therefore, it is reasonable to design a socket for posterior teeth that compensates for normal resorption animations. Maxillary tuberosity area is often proposed as a location for additional bone, since under normal situation-wide horseshoe-shaped septum bone is left following extraction. Of the common placing sites of implants, the posterior mandible having innervated sub-mental vessels would demand particular socket design consideration to accommodate for the possibility of accidental vessel perforation. Another site, in less flexibility ridge, would be the canine [51, 52].

There are several types of implant sockets that can be used in different osteotomy techniques to enhance implant stability. The most common types include tapered and cylindrical implant sockets. Each type of implant socket has its own advantages and disadvantages. For example, when comparing different types of implant sockets, it is important to consider their impact on both initial stability and stress on the surrounding bone. A tapered implant socket may offer superior initial stability, ensuring a secure fit from the start. However, this increased stability can also result in heightened stress on the surrounding bone tissue. On the contrary, a cylindrical implant socket may distribute stress more evenly, reducing the strain on the surrounding bone. Nevertheless, this can also lead to reduced initial stability [53].

6. Conclusion

In conclusion, the osteotomy technique used to place the implant significantly affects implant stability. It is important to know the interplay between different osteotomy techniques and implant socket design. Implant primary stability directly relates to surgical cell loads and, together with the ability to disperse forces with a high friction coefficient, is determinant in deciding the proper osteotomy technique. Therefore, it is a mandatory requirement to reduce trauma. Although bone quality predicts primary stability, there are alternatives designed for low-quality bone in cases where no adequate bone is present. Furthermore, it is important to evaluate the effect of the engagement of threads on implant stability during the osteotomy process.

Conflict of interest

The authors declare no conflict of interest.

Author details

Levent Ciğerim* and Zeynep Dilan Orhan
Department of Oral and Maxillofacial Surgery, Faculty of Dentistry, Van YuzuncuYil University, Van, Turkey

*Address all correspondence to: levent139@hotmail.com

References

[1] Palaskar JN, Joshi N, Shah PM, Gullapalli P, Vinay V. Influence of different implant placement techniques to improve primary implant stability in low-density bone: A systematic review. The Journal of Indian Prosthodontic Society. 2020;**20**(1):11-16

[2] Ikar M, Grobecker-Karl T, Karl M, Steiner C. Mechanical stress during implant surgery and its effects on marginal bone: A literature review. Quintessence International. 2020;**51**(2):142-150

[3] Foster AL, Moriarty TF, Zalavras C, Morgenstern M, Jaiprakash A, Crawford R, et al. The influence of biomechanical stability on bone healing and fracture-related infection: The legacy of Stephan Perren. Injury. 2021;**52**(1):43-52

[4] Olmedo-Gaya MV, Romero-Olid MN, Ocaña-Peinado FM, Vallecillo-Rivas M, Vallecillo C, Reyes-Botella C. Influence of different surgical techniques on primary implant stability in the posterior maxilla: A randomized controlled clinical trial. Clinical Oral Investigations. 2023;**27**(7):3499-3508

[5] Comuzzi L, Tumedei M, De Angelis F, Lorusso F, Piattelli A, Iezzi G. Influence of the dental implant macrogeometry and threads design on primary stability: An in vitro simulation on artificial bone blocks. Computer Methods in Biomechanics and Biomedical Engineering. 2021;**24**(11):1242-1250

[6] Li J, Jansen JA, Walboomers XF, van den Beucken JJ. Mechanical aspects of dental implants and osseointegration: A narrative review. Journal of the Mechanical Behavior of Biomedical Materials. 1 Mar 2020;**103**:103574

[7] Pandey C, Rokaya D, Bhattarai BP. Contemporary concepts in osseointegration of dental implants: A review. BioMed Research International. 2022;**2022**(1):6170452

[8] Kittur N, Oak R, Dekate D, Jadhav S, Dhatrak P. Dental implant stability and its measurements to improve osseointegration at the bone-implant interface: A review. Materials Today: Proceedings. 2021;**43**:1064-1070

[9] Gil J, Sandino C, Cerrolaza M, Pérez R, Herrero-Climent M, Rios-Carrasco B, et al. Influence of bone-level dental implants placement and of cortical thickness on osseointegration: in silico and in vivo analyses. Journal of Clinical Medicine. 2022;**11**(4):995

[10] de Elío OJ, del Canto DA, del Canto DM, Orea CJ, del Canto PM, Calvo JS. Alveolar bone density and width affect primary implant stability. Journal of Oral Implantology. 2020;**46**(4):389-395

[11] Noaman AT, Bede SY. The effect of bone density measured by cone beam computed tomography and implant dimensions on the stability of dental implants. Journal of Craniofacial Surgery. 2022;**33**(3):e241-e247

[12] Ivanova V, Chenchev I, Zlatev S, Mijiritsky E. Correlation between primary, secondary stability, bone density, percentage of vital bone formation and implant size. International Journal of Environmental Research and Public Health. 2021;**18**(13):6994

[13] Rues S, Schmitter M, Kappel S, Sonntag R, Kretzer JP, Nadorf J. Effect of bone quality and quantity on the primary stability of dental implants in a simulated bicortical placement. Clinical Oral Investigations. 2021;**25**:1265-1272

[14] Do TA, Le HS, Shen YW, Huang HL, Fuh LJ. Risk factors related to late failure of dental implant—A systematic review of recent studies. International Journal of Environmental Research and Public Health. 2020;**17**(11):3931

[15] Huang H, Wu G, Hunziker E. The clinical significance of implant stability quotient (ISQ) measurements: A literature review. Journal of Oral Biology and Craniofacial Research. 2020;**10**(4):629-638

[16] Rameh S, Menhall A, Younes R. Key factors influencing short implant success. Oral and Maxillofacial Surgery. 2020;**24**(3):345-350

[17] Ibrahim A, Heitzer M, Bock A, Peters F, Möhlhenrich SC, Hölzle F, et al. Relationship between implant geometry and primary stability in different bony defects and variant bone densities: An in vitro study. Materials. 2020;**13**(19):4349

[18] Monje A, Roccuzzo A, Buser D, Wang HL. Influence of buccal bone wall thickness on the peri-implant hard and soft tissue dimensional changes: A systematic review. Clinical Oral Implants Research. 2023;**34**(9):999-1013

[19] Farronato D, Pasini PM, Orsina AA, Manfredini M, Azzi L, Farronato M. Correlation between buccal bone thickness at implant placement in healed sites and buccal soft tissue maturation pattern: A prospective three-year study. Materials. 2020;**13**(3):511

[20] Farronato D, Manfredini M, Stocchero M, et al. Influence of bone quality, drilling protocol, implant diameter/length on primary stability: An in vitro comparative study on insertion torque and resonance frequency analysis. Journal of Oral Implantology. 2020;**46**(2):191-199

[21] Jeong KW, Kim JC, Yeo IS. Clinical significance of internal friction connection and micro-threads in implant-supported prostheses: A literature review. Recent Progress in Materials. 2020;**3**(12):1227-1238

[22] Heimes D, Becker P, Pabst A, Smeets R, Kraus A, Hartmann A, et al. How does dental implant macrogeometry affect primary implant stability? A narrative review. International Journal of Implant Dentistry. 2023;**9**(1):20

[23] Kreve S, Ferreira I, da Costa Valente ML, Dos Reis AC. Relationship between dental implant macro-design and osseointegration: A systematic review. Oral and Maxillofacial Surgery. 2024;**28**(1):1-4

[24] Abrahamsson I, Carcuac O, Berglundh T. Influence of implant geometry and osteotomy design on early bone healing: A pre-clinical in vivo study. Clinical Oral Implants Research. 2021;**32**(10):1190-1199

[25] Yeh YT, Chu TM, Blanchard SB, Hamada Y. Effects on ridge dimensions, bone density, and implant primary stability with osseodensification approach in implant osteotomy preparation. International Journal of Oral & Maxillofacial Implants. 2021;**36**(3):533-540

[26] Attanasio F, Antonelli A, Brancaccio Y, Averta F, Figliuzzi MM, Fortunato L, et al. Primary stability of three different osteotomy techniques in medullary bone: An in vitro study. Dentistry Journal. 2020;**8**(1):21

[27] Huang YC, Huang YC, Ding SJ. Primary stability of implant placement and loading related to dental implant materials and designs: A literature review. Journal of Dental Sciences. 2023;**18**(4):1121-1134

[28] Poudrel AS. Vibro-acoustic characterization of implant biomechanical stability. In: HAL Archives ouvertes. Lyon, France: HAL Open Science; 2022 [Internet]. Available from: https://hal.archives-ouvertes.fr/hal-02982972

[29] Sharma N, Nagpal A, Kundal A, Singla A, Jindal V. Axis of success: Primary and secondary stability of implant. Indian Journal of Dental Sciences. 2021;**13**(2):141-145

[30] Joshi S, Dhatrak P, Nimbalkar S, Gherde C. An effect of various parameters on insertion torque to improve the success rate of dental implantation: A review. Materials Today: Proceedings. 2021;**46**:163-169

[31] Dahdal S, Alkhori I, Shihabi S. Evaluation of the effectiveness of high insertion torques on implant stability quotient (ISQ) and marginal bone loss of implants in posterior mandible. International Journal of Dentistry and Oral Science. 2021;**8**(4):1241-1249

[32] Romeo D, Chochlidakis K, Barmak AB, Agliardi E, Lo Russo L, Ercoli C. Insertion and removal torque of dental implants placed using different drilling protocols: An experimental study on artificial bone substitutes. Journal of Prosthodontics. 2023;**32**(7):633-638

[33] Elias CN, Meyers MA, Valiev RZ, Monteiro SN. Ultrafine grained titanium for biomedical applications: An overview of performance. Journal of Materials Research and Technology. 2013;**2**(4):340-350

[34] Yu X, Chang C, Guo W, Wu Y. Primary implant stability based on alternative site preparation techniques: A systematic review and meta-analysis. Clinical Implant Dentistry and Related Research. 2022;**24**(4):453-467

[35] Ibrahim AM, Ayad SS, ElAshwah A. The effect of osseodensification technique on implant stability (clinical trial). Alexandria Dental Journal. 2020;**45**(2):1-7

[36] Al-Almaie S. Immediate dental implant placements using osteotome technique: A case report and literature review. Journal of Oral Implantology. 2016;**42**(6):551-560

[37] Andrés Bastidas D, Roldan L, Ramirez P, Munera A. A segmental osteotomy with 3D virtual planning to move a malpositioned dental implant. Journal of Prosthodontics. 2021;**30**(7):698-704

[38] Misch CE. Dental Implant Prosthetics. Amsterdam, Netherlands: Elsevier; 2005

[39] Adriano Costa J, Manuel Mendes J, Salazar F, Júlio Pacheco J, et al. Osseodensification vs. conventional osteotomy: A case series with cone beam computed tomography. Implant Dentistry. 2024;**33**(1):45-53

[40] Stübinger S, Stricker A, Berg BI. Piezosurgery in implant dentistry. Clinical Cosmetic and Investigative Dentistry. 2015;**7**:115-124. DOI: 10.2147/CCIDE.S63466

[41] Thomas M, Akula U, Ealla KKR, Gajjada N. Piezosurgery: A boon for modern periodontics. Journal of Clinical Periodontology. 2017;**44**(3):265-273

[42] Shubhangini C, Arvina R. Piezo-surgery in periodontics. Journal of Periodontology and Implant Dentistry. 2022;**13**(4):289-295

[43] Hennet P. Piezoelectric bone surgery: A review of the literature and potential applications in veterinary

Oromaxillofacial surgery. Veterinary Surgery. 2015;**44**(8):1043-1052

[44] Almawla SAF. The initial primary stability of dental implants via various osteotomy preparation techniques: An ex vivo comparative study utilizing two distinct non-invasive techniques. Journal of Dental Research. 2023;**102**(10):1408-1415

[45] Singla A. Post insertion stability of dental implants following osteotomy site preparation with conventional versus piezoelectric drilling protocol—A comparative study. Implant Dentistry. 2020;**29**(6):600-608

[46] Pellegrino G, Pavanelli F, Ferri A, Lizio G, et al. Ultrasonic navigation for the treatment of medication-related jaw osteonecrosis involving the inferior alveolar nerve: A case report and protocol review. Journal of Oral and Maxillofacial Surgery. 2020;**78**(11):1853-1860

[47] Altieri F, Iezzi G, Luzzi V, Di Giorgio G, et al. Computer-guided bone biopsy: A technical note with the description of a clinical case. Journal of Clinical and Diagnostic Research. 2021;**15**(12):ZC65-ZC70

[48] Unsal GS, Turkyilmaz I, Lakhia S. Advantages and limitations of implant surgery with CAD/CAM surgical guides: A literature review. Journal of Prosthetic Dentistry. 2020;**124**(1):70-76

[49] Pal U, Kumar Dhiman N, Singh G, Singh RK, et al. Evaluation of implants placed immediately or delayed into extraction sites. Journal of Oral Implantology. 2011;**37**(5):547-554

[50] Kim JJ, Ben Amara H, Chung I, Koo KT. Compromised extraction sockets: A new classification and prevalence involving both soft and hard tissue loss. Journal of Clinical Periodontology. 2021;**48**(5):685-694

[51] Vairo G, Sannino G. Comparative evaluation of Osseointegrated dental implants based on platform-switching concept: Influence of diameter, length, thread shape, and In-bone positioning depth on stress-based performance. Journal of Oral Rehabilitation. 2013;**40**(9):699-709

[52] Khaohoen A, Sornsuwan T, Chaijareenont P, Poovarodom P, Rungsiyakull C, Rungsiyakull P. Biomaterials and clinical application of dental implants in relation to bone density—A narrative review. Journal of Clinical Medicine. 2023;**12**(21):6924. DOI: 10.3390/jcm12216924

[53] Kamal MN. Implant stability and Peri-implant marginal bone loss around two different threads design implants. Egyptian Dental Journal. 2020;**66**(4):2759-2770